# WHAT TO EAT FOR WHAT AILS YOU

## How to Treat Illnesses by Changing the Food and Vitamins in Your Diet

## WINNIE YU

**FAIR WINDS**
PRESS

Copyright © 2007 Fair Winds Press

First published in the USA in 2007 by
Fair Winds Press, a member of
Quayside Publishing Group
33 Commercial Street
Gloucester, MA 01930

11 10 09 08 07    1 2 3 4 5

ISBN-13: 978-1-59233-236-6
ISBN-10: 1-59233-236-6

Library of Congress Cataloging-in-Publication Data available

Cover design by Howard Grossman/12E Design
Book design by Yee Design
Photography by Steve Galvin

Printed and bound in Canada

*This book is not intended to replace the services of a physician. Any application of the recommendations set forth in the following pages is at the reader's discretion. The reader should consult with his or her own physician or specialist concerning the recommendations in this book.*

# WHAT TO EAT FOR
# WHAT AILS YOU

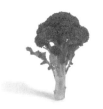

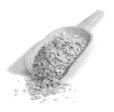

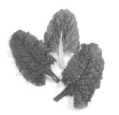

*To Margie, Randy, and Alison.*

# CONTENTS

# FOREWORD

FOOD IS A TREMENDOUSLY IMPORTANT part of our daily lives; yet, many of us don't ever stop to think that what we put in our mouths may actually play a role in how we feel.

As a physician who practices nutritional medicine, it has been eye-opening to me to watch people take control of their eating habits and start to feel better in the process. When this happens, patients are able to reduce their reliance on prescription medications. The overuse of prescription drugs is the sixth-leading cause of death in this country, so being able to replace drugs with food is critical for long-term health.

Our ancestors knew that food was a powerful healer, but that simple concept has gotten lost through the years, as the food delivery system in this country has become more consolidated and industrialized. Cheap food and cheap ingredients have changed and reshaped the American palate during the past four decades at an unprecedented rate. Prior to the 1970s, Americans consumed the same amount of fat, protein, and carbohydrates as they had at the turn of the century; obesity rates were constant; and disease rates were falling.

Since the 1970s, obesity rates have skyrocketed—two-thirds of all Americans now have a weight problem. The amount of sugar and carbohydrates consumed has gone from less than 10 percent of the average diet to greater than 60 percent, and rates have climbed for diseases that we bring upon ourselves—heart disease, diabetes, and osteoarthritis, to name a few. It is estimated that if we don't do something drastic to stem this tide, our youngest generation will have a lower life expectancy than the one before it for the first time in history.

These are the reasons why *What to Eat for What Ails You* is such an important book. It gets to the root of many common maladies that do not have to be treated with medications. This book shows that the food you eat is an important part of how you feel—not a novel concept, but certainly provocative in our modern society.

Winnie Yu has done an amazing job of putting so much information together in one book. She has managed to take complicated information and format it in a simple and easy-to-use manner. It is possible to use this resource and decrease the number of visits to your family physician by at least half—the information is that powerful.

Learning about proper nutrition has changed my life and my career. The information in Winnie Yu's book can have that same effect on you and your family. This book makes nutritional supplement recommendations for the ailments, but, unlike other books of this nature, it emphasizes the foods that heal, not the pills. This is not another book pushing nutritional supplements.

I prescribe many nutritional supplements for my patients, but I always tell them that there are not enough pills in the world to help you unless you start with eating correctly, eating the foods that have evolved through the millennia to help heal you. I see eating properly as the foundation for good health—without it, nothing else you do will have any value in the long run.

*What to Eat for What Ails You* can teach you exactly what you need to know in order to take charge of your health. It can be used as a powerful reference guide for when you have a particular ailment. But most important, it is a book that contains timeless and near-forgotten informa-

tion. Use it, read it, follow its advice, and, most of all, remember to pass this information to your children and grandchildren.

Fred Pescatore, M.D., M.P.H., C.C.N.
Author of *The Hamptons Diet* and
*Thin for Good*

# INTRODUCTION

THE LINK BETWEEN FOOD AND HEALTH is nothing new, but the connection these days is often a negative one. Eat too many high-fat foods, and you'll clog your arteries. Drink too much coffee, and you'll lose sleep. Don't get enough fiber, and you'll be bogged down by constipation. Even important macronutrients—namely fats and carbs— have been demonized for their role in America's rapidly expanding waistline, when in reality, they're essential to your health.

Lost in those messages is the power of food to heal, nourish, and sustain. That's where this book comes in. In *What to Eat for What Ails You*, you'll find a wealth of information that links specific foods to common conditions that affect so many of us today. The information is arranged in short, easy-to-read chapters, all of which have been reviewed by health care professionals who use nutrition to help heal their patients and clients. The information is by no means a substitute for a doctor's care or meant to replace any medications that are necessary for your treatment. But it is intended to help you lessen your symptoms and to improve your quality of life.

Even before you start reading, it's a safe bet that you probably know more about food's healing properties than you realize. You're using food as medicine every time you eat chicken soup for a cold, relieve a urinary tract infection with cranberry juice, or eat yogurt to wipe out a yeast infection. You're also making the most of food's healing potential when you nibble on crackers to quell your nausea, sip ginger ale after you vomit, and drink milk to strengthen your bones.

But those are only the obvious ones. As it turns out, there are so many other ways in which our diets influence our health and specific foods can affect specific conditions. The oils in cold-water fish have the potential to alleviate arthritis pain, dry eyes, and the chill in the fingers of a Raynaud's sufferer. Soy in tempeh can help tame hot flashes in menopausal women. The fiber in whole grains, fruits, and vegetables can relieve the symptoms of irritable bowel syndrome. Even drinking water can play a major role in alleviating many symptoms.

What you don't eat is just as important as what you do. Too many saturated fats, refined carbohydrates, and sugar can wreak havoc on your health. These foods can aggravate the inflammation of autoimmune illnesses, worsen your heart condition, and put you in a bigger slump if you have depression or another mood disorder.

For many people, good nutrition also means taking supplements. Health supplements have become a staple in the American medicine cabinet. We take zinc for colds, melatonin for sleep, and glucosamine to tame our arthritis. And while some health supplements really do seem to work, remember that the science for many supplements is weak and inconclusive.

Before you take any supplement, even the ones that you know are good for you, it's absolutely essential that you talk to your doctor first. At high levels, even the most essential vitamins can become toxic and cause unpleasant symptoms. For example, too much vitamin A, which is vital for healthy eyes, can cause liver damage and bone and joint pain. Certain supplements can also interact with other medications. Some may cause allergies. Others may cause bothersome side effects. Your doctor can help you decide what's best for you. And notice that no dosages are mentioned in this book—you'll need to get those from your doctor or another qualified health care professional.

Keep in mind too, that supplements aren't as tightly regulated as medications. Health supplements are classified as food, not drugs. The U.S. Food and Drug Administration regulates dietary supplements under the Dietary Supplement Health and Education Act of 1994 (DSHEA), which says the manufacturer is responsible for ensuring that a supplement is safe before it is marketed. FDA approval is not required before selling dietary supplements. But if a product is deemed unsafe, the FDA can prohibit its sale.

Just because something is natural does not mean it's safe. Choose products made by well-established manufacturers and those that are "standardized," which means that the manufac-

turer has measured and guarantees the amount of active ingredient in the pill, not just the amount of the herb. Beware of supplements that claim to diagnose, treat, cure, or prevent disease—they're typically lacking in scientific proof. Without scientific evidence, such claims violate federal regulations, and the product is considered an unapproved drug.

A healthy diet, although important, is never a substitute for the care of a good doctor. Many conditions in this book warrant medical attention, and you should never attempt to self-diagnose or self-treat with food, or anything else for that matter.

It's also important to realize that no single diet will work for every individual or even a group of people suffering from the same ailment. The best foods for your particular condition depend on many factors, including the medications you take, your age, your allergies, your lifestyle, and other health concerns. Your best bet is to work closely with a registered dietitian to figure out the eating plan that is right for you.

The bottom line is this: No matter what anyone tells you or what you read in this book or elsewhere, the final decision on what to eat is up to you. But one thing is for sure—choosing your foods wisely can make a world of difference in how you feel.

# ACNE

ZITS. PIMPLES. ACNE. By the time you're 16, you're probably familiar with the unsightly bumps that crop up on your skin at the most inopportune times. Many people are lucky enough to get by with just an occasional pimple on an otherwise clear complexion. Others, who are less fortunate, may be plagued with acne on their face, chest, neck, back, arms, and shoulders. It can even continue well into adulthood. The condition can be emotionally upsetting and potentially disfiguring. Left untreated, acne can lead to permanent scarring.

Acne is caused by the overproduction of sebum, an oily substance manufactured in the sebaceous glands of the skin. Under normal conditions, the sebum seeps into the hair follicles, then flows into the skin, acting as a natural lubricant. During puberty, the body secretes androgens, a hormone in both girls and boys that stimulates the sebaceous glands, causing them to become larger and produce more sebum. When the sebaceous glands produce too much sebum, the follicles get clogged. Some people may be especially sensitive to androgens.

Acne can occur in any one of several forms. Whiteheads and blackheads are both comedones, a plug made up of sebum and dead skin in a hair follicle. Whiteheads are closed comedones that are sealed up and not exposed to air. Blackheads are open comedones, which have darkened as the result of exposure to the air, causing the melanin in the skin to become oxidized. Pimples are red, oil-filled pustules. And if you have deep pus-filled lumps, you are said to have cystic acne.

The severity of acne varies a great deal from one person to the next, but most people outgrow acne in their late teens. Others, however, may continue to have acne well into their adult years. Although the onset of puberty is the most common trigger of acne, it can also occur during times of stress or with certain illnesses such as Cushing's syndrome, in which there is excess corticosteroid hormones. Women may develop acne or experience a reprieve from acne during times of hormonal upheaval such as pregnancy and menopause.

Although there is no cure for acne, the condition can be controlled and managed to prevent breakouts. Topical creams, gels, or lotions with benzoyl peroxide or retinoid cream are sometimes prescribed. Injections of corticosteroids may be used on large red bumps that don't go away. Sometimes patients are prescribed antibiotics, and women may be prescribed birth control pills.

## ¶¶ What to Eat

The link between diet and acne is uncertain, but according to Ray Sahelian, M.D., a family practice physician who hosts a Web site on dietary supplements at www.raysahelian.com, eating fish can help tame the inflammation at the root of acne. Fish contains omega-3 fatty acids such as eicosapentaenoic acid (EPA) and docosahexaenoic acid (DHA). More specifically, he recommends halibut, salmon, tuna, and sardines, which are rich in omega-3s.

He also suggests increasing your intake of water, particularly by drinking a glass or two upon waking in the morning, which will help move the bowels and flush the body of toxins.

Beyond that, acne sufferers should try to eat a lot of fresh vegetables, such as broccoli, spinach, carrots, red peppers, and sweet potatoes, which are high in vitamin A, an antioxidant that can protect body cells from disease and free radical damage. According to Sahelian, the combination of fish and vegetables is most likely the healthiest diet.

Some experts also tout zinc as a good nutrient for acne control. Zinc is used in cell reproduction and tissue growth and repair and is involved in the healthy functioning of the sebaceous glands. Zinc is found in meat, seafood, and liver.

## ⊘ What Not to Eat

In general, there is no scientific data that shows any food makes acne worse. Instead, if you have acne, you should strive to eliminate foods that seem to aggravate your acne. Common culprits include peanuts, almonds and other nuts, and peanut butter. Some experts recommend that you should also steer clear of processed foods, refined foods, and any foods high in sugar, including soda and fruit juices. In addition, they might recommend that you limit your intake of fried foods and greasy food, which may also perpetuate your condition.

Anyone who has been on antibiotics for prolonged periods may benefit from a diet free of yeast products. The chronic use of antibiotics can destroy healthy bacteria and allow the yeast *Candida albicans* to thrive, setting the stage for acne breakouts. If you suspect an underlying problem with *Candida*, try eliminating any foods that contain yeast, mold, and starches for three months.

### Does Chocolate Cause Acne?

Good news for chocolate lovers: The connection between acne and chocolate has never been scientifically proven. Anecdotally, however, some people say that their acne is aggravated when they eat chocolate.

Finally, some research has suggested avoiding milk and dairy products. A study published in *The Journal of the American Academy of Dermatology* in 2005 found a link between acne and the intake of milk and skim milk. The reason for the link is uncertain, but some experts believe it may be due to the high iodine content of milk or the presence of hormones and bioactive molecules in milk.

But because the link to milk is so uncertain, some experts are hesitant to discourage milk consumption. "As a registered dietitian, I recommend three servings of skim milk or its equivalent daily, whether a person has acne or not," says Christine Gerbstadt, M.D., R.D., a spokesperson for the American Dietetic Association. "I always recommend organic milk without hormones, as hormones have been the probable culprit in the acne and milk link. I don't think you can tell anyone to avoid or limit an excellent source of protein, calcium, and vitamin D if there is no strong evidence."

## 🗒 Stay-Healthy Strategies

- **WASH YOUR FACE DAILY** with a mild cleanser and water. Although acne isn't caused by a lack of good hygiene, keeping the skin clean can help. But don't wash too often or too vigorously, which can make acne worse.

- **AVOID USING TOO MUCH MAKEUP.** Look for makeup that is labeled noncomedogenic, which means it should not cause whiteheads or blackheads. Products labeled non-acnegenic should not cause acne.

- **HIDE ACNE WITH A FLESH-TINTED ACNE LOTION.** You can also try applying a loose powder over an oil-free foundation to help cover up your blemishes.

- **TRY TO MINIMIZE STRESS.** Although stress is a part of life, taking steps to avoid stressful situations, altering your perception of bothersome events, and incorporating relaxation into your daily routine can help reduce its effects.

- **DO NOT PICK, POP, OR SQUEEZE PIMPLES.**

- **SLEEP ON YOUR BACK,** so that your skin isn't aggravated by friction against your pillow.

# ADVANCING AGE

GETTING OLDER ISN'T EXACTLY A DISEASE, though some people may view it that way. In reality, it's simply a passage of life, one that more and more people are enjoying, but one that poses its own unique set of health challenges.

But aging is not something that happens in a single defining moment. It is a gradual process that occurs over time. Along with aging comes physiological changes in body cells and body function. Metabolism slows. Vital organs no longer function at top capacity. Cholesterol levels and blood sugar levels naturally rise. No one knows exactly why the aging process occurs, but along with these physiologic changes come changes in nutritional needs.

## What It Looks Like

To some extent, everyone is familiar with the process of aging, but it becomes more apparent when people reach their 60s and 70s. We see it in graying hair, wrinkled skin that bruises more easily, and the slower, more cautious movements of an elderly person. We hear it in their softening voices. We recognize it in their hesitancy as they tally up numbers or read a manual.

Specific changes in the aging process can affect your nutritional status. For starters, your sense of taste and smell diminishes with age, making it harder for you to appreciate the appeal of food and to enjoy it. You may also have trouble with vision, which can make it hard to shop for food and prepare a meal. In addition, you may have gum disease, which can make it difficult for you to chew food. Older adults also experience a reduction in—or cessation of—the skin's ability to manufacture vitamin D. In some cases, they don't get enough sunshine, while in other cases their cells no longer make it.

Social factors can also influence nutritional status. Seniors are more likely to live alone and less likely to take time to prepare a balanced meal. They also may not shop often and may be living on limited budgets—factors that can restrict their access to fresh fruits and vegetables.

Many older adults also take medications that can affect their nutritional status. Certain drugs such as digitalis (Digoxin), prescribed for heart failure, can cause you to lose your appetite, which puts you at risk for malnutrition and weight loss. Other drugs, such as cholestyramine (Questran), a cholesterol-lowering agent, may inhibit the absorption of vital nutrients such as vitamins A, D, E, and K. Diuretics for high blood pressure, heart failure, or edema can cause the loss of important electrolytes in the urine, including potassium.

While it's impossible to prevent most changes that occur with aging, a healthy diet can definitely make an impact by helping to minimize the aforementioned effects, keep you active, and slow the onset of disease. For these and many other reasons, a healthy diet continues to remain essential in elderly adults. At the same time, the elderly do have some specific nutrient needs that warrant attention.

## ¶¶¶ What to Eat

Older adults need about 25 percent fewer calories than younger people. For most people, that means eating a 1,600-calorie diet. The reduction in caloric needs is the result of a slowdown in metabolic rate and a decrease in your muscle, or lean body, mass.

Beyond a healthy, well-balanced diet, older adults need to make sure they get certain nutrients. In particular, elderly people are at risk for deficiencies of B vitamins. A deficiency of B12 is especially common, since the ability to absorb it frequently diminishes with age. Sometimes the lack of B12 can cause symptoms that resemble dementia, including tingling, numbness, weakness, and a lack of coordination. Good sources of B12 include meat, poultry, eggs, and dairy foods.

It's also important to get enough B6 in your diet. B6 is essential for the production of important body chemicals including insulin, hemoglo-

bin, and antibodies. It can be found in chicken, liver, fish, and pork as well as whole grains, legumes, and nuts. In addition, pay attention to your folic acid intake. Folic acid is essential to the production of red blood cells and helps lower levels of homocysteine, an amino acid that, in excess, can increase risk of heart disease. Without enough, you may be at risk for anemia and age-related hearing loss. Good sources of folic acid include leafy greens, fortified breads and cereals, legumes, and wheat germ.

Another essential nutrient is vitamin C, an antioxidant that can help stave off disease and illness. You also need to make sure you get enough fiber, which can help you avoid constipation (a common problem in older adults), slow the absorption of sugars, and lower insulin levels. Many foods that are rich in vitamin C are also high in fiber. These foods include citrus fruits, berries, baked potatoes, spinach, legumes, and beans.

### Long Life Ahead

Most people today can expect to live well into their 70s. According to the National Center for Health Statistics, life expectancy for men in 2002 was 74.5 years, while that for women was 79.9. By 2030, the number of older Americans is expected to more than double to seventy million, or one in every five Americans, according to the Centers for Disease Control and Prevention.

It's also important to eat foods high in calcium and vitamin D, such as low-fat milk, yogurt, and fortified orange juice. Both calcium and vitamin D can help strengthen bones and reduce risk of falling, which is more common in seniors.

Finally, make sure to drink plenty of water. The ability to sense thirst diminishes with age, and elderly people are at risk for dehydration. Water also helps to soften the stool and prevent constipation. So make an effort to get plenty of fluids.

## What Not to Eat

Steer clear of foods that contain too much saturated fat and that are high in calories, including red meat, processed foods, and rich desserts. Because your energy needs are less in your senior years, excess calories will be stored as the more dangerous fat around your abdomen, which can exacerbate health problems.

Seniors should also avoid foods high in sodium, a mineral that contributes to heart failure, poor blood pressure control, and fluid retention. Foods high in sodium are often not obvious, but many canned foods, tomato sauces, and processed meals contain large amounts of sodium. Pre-packaged frozen dinners are also high in sodium, so use moderation.

Be wary of alcohol, too, especially if you take medication. Certain drugs, taken with alcohol, can cause health problems. In addition, alcohol suppresses appetite and can decrease the absorption of many vitamins.

## Supplements for Advancing Age

All elderly adults should take a multivitamin, according to Marie Savard, M.D., author of *The Body Shape Solution for Weight Loss and Wellness*. Look for a multivitamin with 100 percent of the recommended daily allowance of most vital nutrients. "But get the 'silver' variety, which doesn't contain iron," Savard says. "Extra iron can mask an underlying bleeding problem, contribute to constipation, and may even play a role in heart disease."

Seniors who take the blood thinner warfarin (Coumadin) should avoid multivitamins with vitamin K in them, Savard adds. If you decide to take any other supplements, consult your physician or a registered dietitian to make sure you are taking the proper amount and that the supplements don't interact with any of your medications.

### CALCIUM AND VITAMIN D

Older people should get 1,200 mg of calcium a day, but often they don't get enough in their diets. To make matters worse, postmenopausal women lack the bone-protecting effects of estrogen. Elderly people are also at risk for having a vitamin D deficiency for many reasons, including less exposure to sunlight, lessened ability to make vitamin D in their skin and kidneys, and low vitamin D intake.

Consider adding a calcium supplement to your diet, especially one that contains vitamin D.

A study in the *Archives of Internal Medicine* found that long-term supplementation with vitamin D and calcium could reduce the risk of falls in ambulatory women by 46 percent. In less-active older women, the effects were even more pronounced—those who received the supplement lowered their odds of falling by 65 percent.

## MAGNESIUM

Magnesium deficiency is common among the elderly and can cause fatigue, low appetite, confusion, weakness, and insomnia. Supplementation can help relieve these symptoms and enhance energy levels.

## Stay-Healthy Strategies

- **MAKE AN EFFORT TO EXERCISE.** Even small amounts of movement can boost energy levels, improve mobility, and lessen arthritis pain.

- **SOFTEN UP YOUR FOODS** if you have dental problems. Good choices include ripe bananas, baked sweet potatoes, and steamed vegetables.

- **TRY TO STAY MENTALLY ACTIVE.** Do a crossword puzzle. Read books and magazines. Participate in volunteer activities.

- **STAY SOCIALLY ENGAGED.** Get together with friends regularly. Social involvement nourishes the soul and helps keep depression at bay.

## The Raw Foods Diet

Some people believe that the aging process may be slowed by following what is known as the raw foods diet.

Proponents believe that raw foods contain enzymes that are destroyed in the heating process and so advocate eating foods in their raw form or with minimal cooking (foods are not supposed to be cooked at temperatures above 160°F).

Raw foods are considered easier to digest and contain helpful microorganisms that stimulate immunity and minimize illness. The diet is composed of raw fruits, vegetables, nuts, seeds, sprouts, grains, beans, and seaweed.

Not everyone, however, believes the raw foods diet is a healthy option. The American Dietetic Association says that while the raw foods diet encourages eating more fruits and vegetables, which increases fiber intake, it may put people at risk of foodborne illness if foods are not adequately cooked. The diet also encourages eating sprouts, which may contain unhealthy bacteria. A raw foods diet may also be harmful to people at risk for osteoporosis, those who are underweight, and those with dental problems.

# AIDS/HIV INFECTION

BACK IN THE LATE 1970s, doctors noticed a surge in rare types of pneumonia, cancer, and other diseases. These conditions were especially prevalent among gay men in metropolitan areas. By 1982, scientists coined the phrase "acquired immunodeficiency syndrome," or AIDS, to describe these infections. A year later, experts had traced these infections to the human immunodeficiency virus (HIV). Now, almost three decades later, there are approximately one million people in the United States who are living with AIDS and/or HIV infection, and not all of them are gay or living in cities.

HIV is transmitted through bodily fluids. Most people become infected when they have sexual contact with an infected person. But it can also be acquired through the use of shared needles among drug users, or acquired by children before or during birth or while breastfeeding. Once inside the body, HIV replicates and progressively destroys immune cells essential to preventing infections and certain types of cancer. Left unchecked, HIV will progress to AIDS, the most serious stage of HIV infection.

Diagnosing AIDS requires several blood tests that look for HIV infection as well as significant reductions in levels of CD4+, a type of immune cell that is attacked by HIV. You must also have one or more AIDS-defining diseases, such as tuberculosis, pneumocystis carinii pneumonia, and Kaposi's sarcoma, a type of cancer. These types of illnesses are extremely uncommon in people who have healthy immune systems and so are used to help diagnose AIDS.

In 1996, the introduction of anti-retroviral drugs dramatically slowed the progression of HIV infection to full-blown AIDS. Other advances helped treat some of the illnesses caused by HIV infection. But HIV infection and AIDS still pose a serious health problem in modern society, and the incidence of infection is even growing in some populations, such as women. Strategies to prevent AIDS, such as the use of condoms and not sharing needles, are still promoted to help prevent the spread of HIV infection and AIDS.

These days, high-risk populations are encouraged to get tested. Like most illnesses, the earlier the infection is detected, the more likely AIDS can be prevented. Part of any treatment plan for AIDS or HIV infection is healthy eating.

## 🔍 What It Looks Like

At first, many people infected with HIV look perfectly healthy and feel well too. Some people may remain free of symptoms for as long as eight or nine years. It's only with the use of a blood test for HIV antibodies that you can know for sure if you're infected.

But after a while, as the infection lingers, you may notice flu-like symptoms such as swollen lymph nodes, fever, chills, fatigue, coughing, and shortness of breath. You may also develop blurred vision, weight loss, and frequent diarrhea.

Eventually, the disease may progress to AIDS, and you'll have one or more of the rare diseases that defines AIDS, such as cervical cancer, lymphoma, or Kaposi's sarcoma. Other diseases include mycobacterium avium complex, cytomegalovirus, and tuberculosis. Symptoms at this point may include soaking night sweats, chronic diarrhea, oral thrush, changes in taste, rashes, persistent fatigue and headaches, high fever for extended periods, and prolonged swelling of the lymph nodes that lasts more than three months.

## 🍴 What to Eat

A healthy diet is essential for proper immune function. So when it's compromised by HIV, it's important to eat well in order to boost immunity, says Milton Stokes, M.P.H., R.D., a spokesperson for the American Dietetic Association. A diet filled with whole grains, fruits, vegetables, nuts, seeds, and lean proteins such as fish and poultry can help ensure that. Many experts also recommend whey protein as a way to prevent weight loss and strengthen immunity.

### Fermented Foods Helped Him Heal

Can pickled cabbage, kimchi, and miso soup help you live more healthfully with AIDS? Sandor Katz thinks so. Katz, affectionately known as Sandorkraut, is the author of *Wild Fermentation: the Flavor, Nutrition, and Craft of Live-Culture Food* and host of the www.wildfermentation.com Web site. He credits fermented foods with helping him live better with HIV/AIDS.

The process of fermentation involves converting carbohydrates into alcohols or acids and is used in the production of wine and beer as well as sauerkraut, pickles, yogurt, tempeh, and cheese. Wild fermentation, Katz says, involves creating conditions in which naturally occurring organisms thrive and proliferate. Eating a variety of live fermented foods promotes the growth of many diverse microbial cultures in your body, which may in turn help boost immunity.

Other aspects of your diet will depend in large part on the symptoms you're experiencing. Many people with more advanced HIV infection or AIDS have diarrhea. These people should avoid high-fiber diets and focus on bland foods such as bananas, applesauce, rice, and plain poultry, fish, and lean meat. Plain pasta, breads, and crackers are also good choices. In addition, still eat some vegetables, but stick with certain cooked or canned varieties, such as carrots, green beans, spinach, and zucchini. And to help maintain adequate fluid levels, consider drinking broth soups.

Some people will experience strange tastes in their mouth that can interfere with proper nutrition. To make food taste better, the Association of Nutrition Services Agencies offers these tips:

- Marinate foods in soy sauce, fruit juice, wine, Italian dressing, marinade, or sweet and sour sauce.

- Use bacon, ham, garlic, or onion to add flavor to foods.

- Try stronger seasonings, such as basil, oregano, rosemary, tarragon, lemon or lime juice, garlic, or mint.

- Give tart foods a try. Orange, cranberry, or pineapple juice are good options. Try eating pickles, lemons, and tart lemon yogurt, which can help eliminate a metallic taste.

Some people may experience weight loss, especially if they lose their appetite. On those days, try to make your meals more enjoyable with music, friends, and candles. Also, make up for low-appetite days by eating more on days when you do feel hungry and have more energy. On days when you're feeling tired, opt for convenience foods such as cut up fruits and veggies, boneless chicken breast, and frozen pizza topped with your own veggies and lean meats. Finally, be creative with meals. If you'd rather have an omelet at dinner or a peanut butter sandwich at breakfast, then go for it.

## What Not to Eat

Any food that taxes the immune system should be omitted from your eating plan. Limit your intake of refined sugars, processed foods, fried foods, and high-fat fast foods, which stress the immune system. Eliminate alcohol, which can also strain immunity.

If you have AIDS or HIV, pay attention to how food is prepared and handled. Foodborne pathogens (disease-causing microorganisms) can be devastating for someone with HIV and can grow when food is not properly handled or cooked thoroughly. For that reason, be wary of raw or undercooked poultry, and make sure all eggs are thoroughly cooked and fresh. Both are sources of *Salmonella*.

Improperly handled or cooked poultry is also at risk for contamination with *Campylobacter jejuni* bacteria. In addition, people with AIDS or HIV should be wary of unpasteurized cheeses and ready-made foods such as hot dogs or deli meats, which may be contaminated with *Listeria*.

To make food preparation safe, be vigilant about frequent hand washing while cooking and before eating. And watch for cross contamination. For instance, make sure to wash your hands after handling raw meats and before preparing vegetables. Don't prepare meat and vegetables on the same cutting board. Check out the U.S. Department of Agriculture's Food Safety and Inspection Service Web site at www.fsis.usda.gov for specific tips on food safety.

## 💊 Supplements for AIDS

People with HIV infection or AIDS should take a multivitamin/mineral supplement for overall health. But beyond that, you should approach the use of any supplement or herbal remedy with caution. Some supplements may interact with medications and may not be suitable to your particular condition. Always ask your doctor or a registered dietitian about any supplement you're considering. Supplements you may hear about include the following:

### ANTIOXIDANT VITAMINS

The antioxidant vitamins A, C, and E support immune function and may be beneficial in people who have AIDS. But consult a registered dietitian before taking any, because high levels may be harmful.

### B VITAMIN COMPLEX

Some people with AIDS or HIV are lacking in B vitamins. A quality B vitamin complex would replenish levels of biotin, choline, folic acid, inositol, para-aminobenzoic acid (PABA), and the six "numbered" B vitamins: vitamin B1 (thiamin), B2 (riboflavin), B3 (niacin), B5 (pantothenic acid), B6 (pyridoxine), and B12 (cobalamin).

### SELENIUM

Some doctors may suggest selenium supplements to help strengthen the immune system. Selenium is an antioxidant that may help slow the progression of AIDS.

### SPIRULINA

Spirulina is a blue-green algae, rich in amino acids and many other nutrients, such as B vitamins, carotenoids, and antioxidant vitamins. Some experts recommend it as a supplement for AIDS, but there is no firm scientific evidence yet to back up its effectiveness.

## 📋 Stay-Healthy Strategies

- **FIND A DOCTOR WHO SPECIALIZES IN AIDS TREATMENT.**

- **FOLLOW YOUR DOCTOR'S ORDERS.** Keep all appointments, and take any and all medications appropriately.

- **PROTECT YOURSELF AGAINST INFECTIONS** with routine immunizations for diseases such as influenza and pneumonia.

- **STOP SMOKING, AND QUIT ANY ILLICIT DRUGS.** These substances compromise your immune system even further.

- **KEEP OTHERS SAFE.** Practice safe sex and do not share needles, toothbrushes, or razors. Alert partners to your infection.

---

### Garlic: Not So Helpful for AIDS

Some people with HIV/AIDS used to take garlic to boost their immune system. But a study in 2001 by the National Institutes of Health found that garlic disrupted blood levels of an antiretroviral drug called saquinavir. So ignore the advice of anyone who recommends taking garlic if you're taking this medication.

---

# ALCOHOLISM

FOR MOST PEOPLE, A GLASS OF WINE or a bottle of a beer is an innocent accompaniment to dinner or a sporting event. But for approximately eighteen million Americans, indulging in these drinks is part of a disease known as alcoholism.

Alcoholism is a serious health condition that can raise your risk for deadly illnesses such as cancer, cirrhosis of the liver, and brain damage. Alcoholics are also more likely to be killed in car accidents and occupational injuries and to be involved in suicides or homicides. And as the alcoholism worsens, many people experience devastating life-changing consequences.

According to the National Institute on Alcohol Abuse and Alcoholism, 17.6 million adults in the United States abuse alcohol or are alcoholics. While some people used to believe that alcoholism was a weakness, experts now know that it is a chronic disease with a strong genetic component. Having family members who are alcoholics raises your risk, but the development of alcoholism may also be influenced by lifestyle. Your friends, your access to alcohol, and the amount of stress you have can all play a role in whether you become an alcoholic.

But alcoholism is just one problem associated with alcohol. Some people may abuse alcohol by drinking too much too often. These people may encounter some of the same health and lifestyle problems that alcoholics do. The difference is that they do not become dependent on alcohol.

Treating alcoholism requires a combination of medications and therapy. Many alcoholics also join support groups such as Alcoholics Anonymous in their quest for recovery.

## What It Looks Like

Not everyone who drinks a lot of alcohol is an alcoholic, though they may certainly be abusing alcohol. Alcoholism usually has four symptoms, including irrepressible cravings to drink and the inability to stop drinking once you start to imbibe. Alcoholics may also develop a physical dependence on alcohol, so that any effort to stop drinking is characterized by withdrawal symptoms such as nausea, sweating, shakiness, and anxiety. In addition, over time alcoholics develop a tolerance for alcohol, which means they need increasingly greater amounts of alcohol to achieve the "high" they seek.

An alcoholic's craving for alcohol is so strong that it overwhelms anything else that is happening in his or her life. Alcoholics will continue drinking even in the face of serious difficulties such as divorce, job loss, and financial struggles.

Even so, many alcoholics continue to deny that they have a problem, which in itself may be a symptom of alcoholism. Classic signs of alcoholism may include (but are not limited to) the following:

- Drinking alone or in secret
- Creating a ritual of drinking before, with, or after meals, and becoming irritated when the ritual is disturbed or questioned
- Forgetfulness
- Loss of interest in activities you once enjoyed
- Stashing alcohol in unlikely places
- Increasing irritability as the anticipation of drinking approaches
- Becoming distraught if alcohol is not available when the time to drink comes

People who abuse alcohol may behave in many of the same ways. But unlike alcoholics, they do not feel the strong urge to drink and usually don't suffer withdrawal when they don't drink.

## ¶¶¶ What to Eat

Alcoholism can put you at risk for malnutrition since the alcohol often displaces other healthy foods and drinks, says Christine Gerbstadt, M.D., R.D., a spokesperson for the American Dietetic Association. Alcohol is high in calories and low in nutrients, so you feel full even though you have not satisfied your body's nutritional needs. In fact, alcoholics may get as much as 50 percent of their day's calories from alcohol. Excess alcohol also impairs the body's absorption of important vitamins and minerals.

In particular, many alcoholics have low levels of thiamin, also known as vitamin B1. In fact, the higher your alcohol intake, the lower your thiamine levels. Good sources of thiamin include whole grains and enriched grains such as bread, pasta, rice, and fortified cereals. You can also get thiamin in asparagus, mushrooms, and pork.

Alcoholics are also at risk for zinc deficiency. Zinc is essential for tissue growth and repair, and the function of more than 200 enzymes. It is also involved in helping your body use carbohydrates, proteins, and fats. Good sources of zinc include meat, seafood, liver, eggs, and milk. It is found in wheat germ, whole grain foods, black-eyed peas, and tofu as well.

### FACT

*Unhealthy alcohol consumption goes hand in hand with unhealthy eating, according to a study in the* American Journal of Epidemiology.

In general, you should try to eat a healthy, well-balanced diet to replenish lost nutrients. That means eating plenty of fruits and vegetables, lean meats and fish, whole grains, and low-fat dairy foods, and drinking lots of water.

## What Not to Eat

If you are trying to overcome your alcoholism, you should obviously avoid any alcoholic beverage, even in small quantities. Also, avoid eating refined sugars, processed foods, and caffeine. Although you may want a quick energy boost with a cup of coffee or a sugary treat, these foods will only stimulate your cravings for alcohol. You should also steer clear of foods high in saturated fat and fried foods, which will tax an already-stressed liver.

## Supplements for Alcoholism

Individuals with alcoholism should take a multivitamin to restore missing nutrients and to strengthen their overall health on their path to recovery. Other supplements you may consider include zinc and a vitamin B complex.

### ZINC

As noted above, alcoholism puts you at risk for zinc deficiency. Make sure you're meeting your zinc needs without going over the tolerable upper intake of 40 mg/day for adults.

## Do You Have a Drinking Problem?

The National Institute on Alcohol Abuse and Alcoholism suggests asking yourself these questions, which are part of CAGE, a screening tool doctors use to diagnose alcoholism:

- **C:** Have you ever felt you should **cut down** on your drinking?
- **A:** Have people **annoyed** you by criticizing your drinking?
- **G:** Have you ever felt bad or **guilty** about your drinking?
- **E: Eye opener:** Have you ever had a drink first thing in the morning to steady your nerves or get rid of a hangover?

One "yes" answer suggests a possible alcohol problem. If you answered "yes" to more than one question, it is highly likely that a problem exists. In either case, you should talk to your doctor to find out whether you have alcoholism and what you can do about it.

Even if you answered "no" to all of the above questions, if you ever encounter drinking-related problems with your job, relationships, health, or the law, you should seek professional help. The effects of alcohol abuse can be extremely serious—even fatal—both to you and to others.

## B VITAMIN COMPLEX

A quality B vitamin complex will supply several B vitamins, including biotin, choline, folic acid, inositol, para-aminobenzoic acid (PABA), and the six "numbered" B vitamins: vitamin B1 (thiamin), B2 (riboflavin), B3 (niacin), B5 (pantothenic acid), B6 (pyridoxine), and B12 (cobalamin).

---

### TIP

*When it comes to alcohol, moderation is key. Men should have no more than two drinks a day, and women, just one. What's a drink? Five ounces of wine, 12 ounces of beer, or 1.5 ounces of 80-proof liquor.*

---

## Stay-Healthy Strategies

- **GET HELP FOR YOUR ALCOHOLISM.** Most people cannot overcome this disease without intervention from health care professionals and support groups.

- **CONSULT A NUTRITIONIST.** A registered dietitian can help you create an eating plan that sustains you through recovery.

- **TRY TO REDUCE STRESS.** Stressful situations can make it harder for you to give up alcohol.

- **ANTICIPATE RELAPSES.** The process of getting sober is just that, a process. When you do have a relapse, resolve to stop drinking again and do what you can to reinforce that goal.

# ALLERGIES

A CAT ENTERS THE ROOM AND YOU SNEEZE. When you mow the lawn, your eyes water. A thunderstorm sets off sneezing, congestion, and red eyes. If any of these ring true for you, chances are you have allergies.

An allergy is an overreaction of the immune system to a foreign substance such as pet dander, grass, dust mites, mold, or pollen that normally should not provoke a reaction. For people with allergies, the presence of these substances causes the body to produce several antibodies, including one called immunoglobulin E or IgE. IgE latches on to cells in the nasal passage that contain various chemicals, including histamine. When the cells burst, the histamines are released along with other chemicals, triggering sniffles, watery eyes, congestion, itching, and skin rashes—the symptoms we know as allergies.

Allergies are extremely common and affect approximately 20 percent of the U.S. population. Seasonal allergies alone afflict about thirty-five million people. No one knows exactly why one person reacts to a substance and another doesn't. But experts are certain that genetics play a role. A child with two allergic parents has a 60 to 70 percent chance of having allergies himself. A child with one allergic parent has a 25 percent chance.

Some allergies are seasonal, meaning that they occur during different times of the year when various plants are pollinating. With the exception of winter, seasonal allergies can occur any time. Other allergies are perennial, which means they can happen any time of year as a result of exposure to an airborne substance such as dust mites, pet dander, or mold. You might also be allergic to the touch of certain substances such as latex, nickel, or a particular dye or perfume, which can cause a condition called contact dermatitis. Other people are allergic to certain foods such as peanuts, wheat, dairy products, shellfish, and eggs.

Pinpointing the source of your allergies is important, because it will tell you which substances to avoid. The most common test is a skin test, which exposes your skin to potentially offending allergens. You may also be given a blood test that measures the amount of IgE produced when your blood is exposed to an allergen. To figure out a food or medication allergen, potentially allergenic foods or drugs are removed from the diet for seven to ten days, then gradually reintroduced while you look for a reaction.

Avoiding an allergenic substance is the obvious answer to preventing allergies, but some substances are so pervasive that it's nearly impossible to dodge them. Examples of these types of substances include mold, pollen, and grass. Some people simply suffer with the sniffles and watery eyes, but others may require medications or immunotherapy, injections that can help desensitize you to an allergen.

## 🔍 What It Looks Like

Allergies can trigger a range of reactions. Many people will experience difficulties breathing caused by congestion, wheezing, and sneezing. Your eyes may become red, watery, and itchy. Others may suffer headaches, hives, nausea, vomiting, diarrhea, and cramps. In some people, allergies are a mild nuisance, while in others, they can be extremely bothersome and disruptive.

The most severe reaction is anaphylaxis, a type of shock that causes your airways to constrict, making it difficult for you to breathe. Anaphylaxis is sudden and severe and involves a total-body allergic response to an allergen, such as a bee sting. Other symptoms include wheezing, hives, a rapid heartbeat, confusion, slurred speech, rapid or weak pulse, and anxiety.

Anaphylaxis always requires professional medical treatment, even if you're able to inject epinephrine, a hormone that helps quickly open up the airways. Always call 911 when you or someone with you experiences anaphylaxis.

## 🍴 What to Eat

Focus on eating a diet packed with fruits and vegetables, which are rich in immune-boosting antioxidants, says Fred Pescatore, M.D., author of *The Allergy and Asthma Cure*. Dark leafy greens, such as spinach, collard, and kale, are great choices and contain plenty of vitamins A, C, and E, as well as the mineral selenium. You should also eat apples, berries, and cherries, which contain quercetin, a bioflavonoid that acts like an antihistamine and can lessen inflammation.

Make sure to also include cold-water fish, such as tuna, salmon, and mackerel. These types of fish contain omega-3 fatty acids, which have been found to reduce inflammation. Other sources of omega-3s include walnuts and flaxseed.

Spice up your food with garlic and onions. Both foods can help tame inflammation. Also, drink plenty of water. The extra fluid will help thin the mucus caused by allergies.

### Fermented Veggies May Help Allergies

Studies have found that children who eat fermented vegetables have a lower incidence of allergies than peers who shy away from these foods. Choose fermented vegetables that contain live microorganisms that have not been killed off with excessive heat. Good sources include sauerkraut, kimchi, and pickles.

# What Not to Eat

If you think your allergies may be caused by something your diet, pinpoint food allergens by doing an elimination diet. Eliminate potential allergens, such as dairy products, eggs, peanuts, soy, wheat, and shellfish from your diet for seven to ten days, then gradually reintroduce them one at a time. Look for allergic reactions when you reintroduce the food, and ban those that seem to provoke symptoms.

You may find that you need to eliminate or cut back on dairy foods, which in some people, can stimulate mucus production. You may also need to avoid foods high in sugar, such as rich desserts and snack foods, and any foods that are fried or refined, including many fast foods.

Finally, consider avoiding foods that contain additives or preservatives, which are found in processed foods, dried or smoked foods, certain medications, and alcoholic beverages. Additives and preservatives such as sulfite, tartrazine, and benzoates can trigger allergy symptoms in some people. People with allergies may also benefit from following the Feingold Program, which is described in greater detail in the Attention Deficit Hyperactivity Disorder chapter on page 49.

# Supplements for Allergies

Start with a high-quality multivitamin for your essential nutrients. You may also want to consider taking some other supplements. Before you do, talk to your physician, since some of these remedies may have side effects. Possible supplements include the following:

### FISH OIL
The omega-3 fatty acids in fish oil can help reduce inflammation. But if you're on blood-thinning medication, talk to your doctor first, because fish oil may increase your risk for bleeding.

### VITAMIN C
This immune-boosting antioxidant may help to reduce spasms in the bronchial tubes and to decrease your symptoms. It also enhances overall immunity.

### MAGNESIUM
A major mineral, magnesium relaxes muscles and can lessen the severity of an asthma attack.

### QUERCETIN
Quercetin is a bioflavonoid that can help to reduce inflammation.

# Stay-Healthy Strategies

- **STEER CLEAR OF CIGARETTE SMOKE.** If you smoke, quit. If someone else in your house smokes, ask him or her to take it outside.

- **USE OVER-THE-COUNTER REMEDIES CAREFULLY.** Some, such as antihistamines, may cause drowsiness and interact with other medications and alcohol.

- **REDUCE STRESS.** Too much stress taxes the immune system, which is already under siege with allergies.

- **CONSIDER ENLISTING AN ALLERGIST/ IMMUNOLOGIST** if you have severe symptoms and need help determining your allergic triggers. These medical doctors are specially trained in treating allergies.

## Dodging Outdoor Allergens

You can't escape the great outdoors completely, even if you hibernate indoors all year. The following are some tips from the American Academy of Asthma, Allergy, and Immunology on how to reduce your exposure to bothersome outdoor allergens:

- Keep windows closed at night. If you're warm, use air conditioning.

- Avoid going outdoors in the early morning, when pollen levels are at their peak.

- Drive with car windows closed.

- Watch the weather. Stay indoors when pollen counts and the humidity level are high. Do the same on windy days, when dust and pollen are airborne.

- Get a reprieve. If possible, take a beach vacation during the peak of pollen season.

- Take your prescribed medications, but do not take more than prescribed.

- Ask someone else to mow the lawn. Mowing stirs up pollens and molds.

- Skip the raking, too, since this can stir up molds.

- Don't hang sheets or clothing out to dry, since they can collect pollens and molds.

# ALZHEIMER'S

WE CALL THEM SENIOR MOMENTS—those pauses in time when we can't recall a familiar word, lose our train of thought, or misplace an everyday item. Most of us have these mental lapses at one time or another, and they're perfectly normal.

These lapses become considerably more serious, however, when a person suddenly can't recall how a fork is used or a familiar route becomes a petrifying maze of confusion. People experiencing these issues may be on their way to developing Alzheimer's disease.

Alzheimer's is the most common form of dementia in people age 65 and over. Dementia is a type of brain disorder that causes changes in the way your brain functions. People who have Alzheimer's are slowly robbed of the ability to recall, think, and, eventually, perform the activities of daily living.

Here in the United States, approximately 4.5 to 5 million people have Alzheimer's. The disease affects about 3 percent of people between ages 65 and 74, but by age 85, nearly half of all people have it. In rare cases, Alzheimer's will emerge in adults in their 40s and 50s in a form known as familial Alzheimer's.

Increases in life expectancy have lead to significant increases in the numbers of people who have Alzheimer's. And while there is no known cure for the disease, there are several treatments for its symptoms. In addition, experts are increasingly convinced that our dietary habits can play a role in helping to prevent Alzheimer's.

## 🔎 What It Looks Like

The progress of Alzheimer's varies from one person to the next, but almost everyone will experience forgetfulness. Even healthy people will experience some degree of difficulty with recall as part of the normal aging process. But in people with Alzheimer's, the forgetfulness becomes more frequent and severe. Events that happened earlier in the day escape the mind more and more frequently. Lunch dates may go forgotten, utility bills unpaid.

Gradually, you lose judgment, the ability to learn new things, and your grasp of language. Some people become disoriented about the day and time, lose their sense of smell, become moody and irritable, and/or experience changes in their personality. Others become notably lethargic.

As the disease progresses, the confusion worsens. You may repeat stories and questions, behave inappropriately, and engage in repetitive activities such as pacing. In the final stages of the disease, you lose the ability to perform everyday tasks. You may lose the ability to eat, and your speech may be hard to understand. Walking may become difficult, even impossible, and you may suffer incontinence. Some people become bedridden. Eventually, Alzheimer's may lead to death. But often, a person with Alzheimer's is so weak that it's usually a deadly infection such as pneumonia that causes death.

## ⁂ What to Eat

Research shows that good nutrition can help prevent—or at least delay—Alzheimer's disease. Furthermore, studies show that being overweight or obese actually elevates your risk for Alzheimer's. People who weigh more are also more likely to have high cholesterol and blood pressure—two other factors that can raise your risk for Alzheimer's.

Even when the disease process is in motion, eating well can help you cope with the disease, lessen its symptoms, and prevent the onset of other illnesses, says Todd E. Feinberg, M.D., chief of the Yarmon Neurobehavior and Alzheimer's Disease Center in New York City and co-author of *What to Do When the Doctor Says It's Early Stage Alzheimer's*.

In short, any diet that helps keep your arteries clean will help reduce your risk for Alzheimer's.

That's because these strategies will promote blood flow to your brain, which in turn helps reduce the buildup of damaging plaques that are believed to be at the root of Alzheimer's. For starters, eat fish. Fish such as halibut, mackerel, salmon, and tuna are all rich in omega-3 fatty acids, which can help tame inflammation. In fact, a study by the Rush Institute for Healthy Aging looked at the fish-eating habits of elderly people between ages 65 and 94 and found that those who ate at last one fish meal each week were less likely to develop Alzheimer's.

It's also important to eat colorful fruits and vegetables. These foods are rich in antioxidants, such as vitamins A, C, and E, which can prevent oxidative damage to brain cells caused by disease-promoting free radicals. Good vegetables include spinach, broccoli, and red peppers. Good fruit choices include blueberries, strawberries, plums, and cherries. You might also want to drink fruit and veggie juices.

Another good food for reducing your risk for Alzheimer's is nuts, such as almonds, pecans, and walnuts, which also contain antioxidants. Although nuts do contain fat, most of the fat is monounsaturated—the healthy kind that can help lower cholesterol. Eating nuts can also fill you up, which will help rein in your appetite and prevent overeating.

# What Not to Eat

Since maintaining a healthy body weight may reduce your risk for Alzheimer's, it's important to eat foods that keep weight gain to a minimum.

To help prevent weight gain, limit your intake of fat and cholesterol. Saturated fat is found in whole-fat dairy products, meat, butter, and fried foods. Cholesterol—which does less damage than saturated fats and trans fats—is found in animal foods such as eggs, meat, fish, and dairy products. Too much saturated fat and cholesterol clogs the arteries, including those that lead to the brain, and raises the risk for Alzheimer's.

You should also limit your intake of processed foods, such as cookies, cakes, fast foods, snack foods, and candy. These foods are likely to contain trans-fatty acids, which have been linked to high cholesterol and heart disease.

# Supplements for Alzheimer's

Certain vitamins, minerals, and herbal supplements have been associated with brain health, but so far, the research is mixed. Before taking any supplement for brain health, remember to talk to your doctor.

## FISH OIL

Like fish, fish oil supplements provide omega-3 fatty acids that might help prevent or slow the progression of Alzheimer's disease. But older patients who already take blood thinners such as warfarin (Coumadin) should be cautious about taking fish oil, which could raise their risk for bleeding.

## HUPERZINE A

Huperzine A is an herbal supplement that has been used for centuries in China as a treatment for swelling, fever, and blood disorders. Recent clinical trials in China have reportedly shown that huperzine A also can benefit people with Alzheimer's disease. A clinical trial of huperzine A as a treatment for mild to moderate Alzheimer's disease is currently underway at the National Institute on Aging.

Experts believe that huperzine A functions much like cholinesterase inhibitors used to treat Alzheimer's, such as Razadyne (formerly known as Reminyl), Exelon, and Aricept. These drugs work by inhibiting the enzyme acetylcholinesterase and slowing the breakdown of acetylcholine, a neurotransmitter involved in the formation of memories, thoughts, and judgment. Note: if you're already taking one of these drugs, you should not take huperzine A.

### B VITAMINS

Some experts believe that taking B vitamins can slow the progress of Alzheimer's by lowering homocysteine levels. People with Alzheimer's disease typically have elevated blood levels of homocysteine. Supplemental doses of vitamins B6, B12, and folate can lower homocysteine levels and possibly improve cognitive functioning.

### CURCUMIN

Animal studies have found that curcumin, an ingredient found in the plant that gives us turmeric (a spice commonly used in curry), may disrupt the brain damage that causes Alzheimer's. Curcumin has anti-inflammatory and antioxidative properties, and it has been found to lower cholesterol. Some studies have shown it may help prevent certain cancers as well.

### VITAMIN C

It isn't clear whether vitamin C can help lower the risk for Alzheimer's, but eating foods rich in vitamin C seems to help. Vitamin C is an antioxidant, with the potential for slowing the damage caused by free radicals. One study in the *Archives of Neurology* found that combining 500 mg of vitamin C with 400 IUs of vitamin E may offer some protective benefits.

## Beware of Vitamin E

Not long ago, many doctors gave Alzheimer's patients vitamin E as part of their treatment regimen. Several studies had suggested that vitamin E could lower the risk for dementia by preventing oxidative stress caused by free radicals, highly reactive molecules that can damage brain cells and promote the development of Alzheimer's.

But in January 2005, a study published in the *Annals of Internal Medicine* found that taking more than 400 IUs of vitamin E each day slightly increased a person's risk for dying from all causes. In the aftermath of this alarming study, most physicians have stopped prescribing vitamin E for their patients.

# ANEMIA

ANEMIA IS A BLOOD DISORDER characterized by low amounts of all-important red blood cells, which transport oxygen-laden hemoglobin to body cells. When a blood test shows that you are deficient in these red blood cells, it's essential to find the cause of the anemia.

The most common form of anemia in the United States—and probably worldwide—is iron-deficiency anemia, which affects approximately 20 percent of all women, 50 percent of all pregnant women, and 3 percent of all men. Iron-deficiency anemia occurs when you don't have enough iron, a mineral needed to produce the oxygen-carrying hemoglobin.

Women who have heavy menstrual periods are vulnerable to this type of anemia because they lose so much blood each month. It can also occur if you have an ulcer, a polyp in your colon, or colon cancer—all conditions that cause slow, chronic blood loss. In some people, iron-deficiency anemia is the result of a diet low in iron. And in pregnancy, the iron needs of the fetus can sometimes deplete the mother's iron stores.

Anemia can also result from other nutritional deficiencies, specifically folate and vitamin B12. Not getting enough of these or the inability to absorb them can cause this kind of anemia. Vitamin deficiency problems typically cause megaloblastic anemias in which the bone marrow produces large, abnormal red blood cells.

Some people, especially older adults, may develop a condition called pernicious anemia, a deficiency of vitamin B12 as the result of a lack of intrinsic factor (a substance made in the stomach that is essential to B12 absorption). Older adults may also have atrophic gastritis, a condition that results in a decrease in stomach acids, making it hard to absorb B12. Treatment usually involves monthly injections of B12. Stomach bypass operations for obesity and other stomach surgeries or resections can also lead to vitamin B12 deficiency.

Many chronic health problems may cause anemia, including kidney disease, Crohn's disease, lupus, and rheumatoid arthritis. In addition, chemotherapy, environmental toxins, and certain medications, such as aspirin or nonsteroidal anti-inflammatory drugs, may cause anemia.

Whatever the cause, it's important to find out exactly what the problem is. Unless the cause of blood loss is obvious—heavy menstrual bleeding for instance—you should undergo a complete gastrointestinal evaluation. For example, patients with slow intestinal loss of iron from a colon polyp or cancer should not simply take iron to improve the anemia. Start your quest for answers by getting a blood test that measures your hemoglobin levels. Further tests may be needed to pinpoint the source of the problem.

## 🔍 What It Looks Like

Early on, people with anemia may have no symptoms at all. But as the condition worsens, it will become apparent that something is wrong. People who have anemia will notice they are frequently fatigued. They may also have chest pain and shortness of breath. Some may notice a rapid heartbeat, dizziness, fluid retention, and pale skin. Others may experience cognitive difficulties, numbness or coldness in the fingers and toes, and headaches.

All these symptoms occur because you don't have enough red blood cells, or your red blood cells aren't big enough to bring oxygen from your lungs to the rest of your body. Without adequate oxygen, body cells become starved for energy, which causes these feelings of tiredness.

## 🍴 What to Eat

If the source of your anemia is a nutritional deficiency, start by making sure you get enough iron-rich foods, says Marie Savard, M.D., author of *The Body Shape Solution to Weight Loss and Wellness*. Animal products provide what is called heme iron, which is much better absorbed than nonheme iron, the variety found in plant foods. Good sources of iron include liver, beef, pork, fish, leafy greens, fortified cereal, beans, and pumpkin seeds. Eating nonheme sources of iron

with a heme iron can boost absorption of the nonheme iron.

Eating foods rich in vitamin C enhances absorption of iron too. So it's always a good idea to eat or drink something with a lot of vitamin C when you're eating a food high in iron. For example, if you're eating a sirloin steak, have it with mustard greens on the side, or eat a bowl of strawberries with your peanut butter sandwich. The combination will ensure that you maximize your absorption of iron. When looking for sources of vitamin C, choose foods that are also high in fiber, since too much iron can cause constipation.

If your anemia is the result of a deficiency in B12 or folate, you will need to eat foods rich in these vitamins. Vegetarians in particular may not be getting enough vitamin B12, which is found primarily in animal foods such as meat, poultry, fish, milk, and eggs. It is also found in fortified cereals, vegetarian burger patties, and soy milk.

To make sure you get enough folate, eat lentils, spinach, peanuts, milk, and broccoli. Enriched grains are also a good source of folate.

## 🚫 What Not to Eat

Certain foods and minerals actually interfere with the absorption of iron, so it's best to not eat them with iron-rich foods if you're trying to improve your iron levels. Oxalic acid in spinach and chocolate, tannins in tea and coffee, and phytic acid in wheat bran and legumes all inhibit the absorption of iron.

You should also be wary of antacids and calcium supplements, which can disrupt stomach acids and interfere with the absorption of iron.

In addition, limit your intake of alcohol and caffeinated beverages such as soda, coffee, and tea. These beverages may interfere with the absorption of the nutrients that prevent anemia.

## The Spinach Conundrum

Yes, spinach is a good source of iron, delivering 3.2 mg per half-cup serving. And it has the vitamin C that can help promote absorption. But at the same time, spinach also contains oxalic acid, which binds to iron and impairs its absorption. Bottom line? Don't rely on spinach for boosting your iron stores.

## Supplements for Anemia

The supplements you need will depend on the type of anemia you have. Here are some you might take:

### IRON

Unless you know that you have iron-deficiency anemia, it's best to consult a doctor before taking iron supplements. Too much iron has been linked to various forms of heart disease. In people with a condition called hemachromatosis, the body can store too much iron, which can cause organ damage. Taking iron supplements will also cause your stool to turn black and can irritate your colon, leading to constipation or diarrhea.

Always take iron with a full glass of water. And if you take other medications, talk to your doctor or pharmacist about possible interactions.

For instance, iron can inhibit absorption of thyroid medication, so the two must be spaced four hours apart.

### B12

People who have anemia as the result of a deficiency in vitamin B12 may need to take supplements of this vitamin. B12 may be taken orally or given by injection.

### FOLIC ACID

If your anemia is the result of a folic acid deficiency, your physician may advise you to take folic acid supplements.

### VITAMIN C

Vitamin C will help promote the absorption of iron by creating an acidic environment in the stomach.

## Stay-Healthy Strategies

- **DO NOT SELF-PRESCRIBE SUPPLEMENTS OR FOODS** without first consulting a doctor. Remember, the key is to pinpoint the cause of your anemia.

- **USE CAST-IRON POTS AND PANS.** Food prepared in this type of cookware will absorb some of the iron.

- **DRINK LOTS OF WATER** if you increase iron intake. The extra fluids will help prevent constipation as you increase your iron.

- **FOLLOW UP WITH YOUR DOCTOR** if you have been diagnosed with anemia. A blood test can determine whether your treatments are making a difference.

# ANXIETY

EVERYONE IS FAMILIAR WITH THE JITTERS that come before a big exam, first date, or major presentation. It's normal to experience nervousness at these moments. But for some people, these anxious feelings are overwhelming and can interfere with daily life. These people suffer from anxiety.

Anxiety disorders are serious illnesses that affect about nineteen million Americans, according to the National Institutes of Mental Health. Someone who has an anxiety disorder feels nervous, uneasy, and fearful on a regular basis, without a real reason. These feelings can become so severe that they can significantly diminish your quality of life.

Women are more prone to anxiety than men. Anxiety also appears to have a genetic component, so that you're more likely to have it if you have a family history of the disease. In some cases, anxiety is the result of another illness, such as hyperthyroidism. It can also be brought on by stress and the challenges of coping with another illness.

Treatment for anxiety disorders often involves a combination of medications such as antidepressants or anti-anxiety drugs and psychotherapy. People who have anxiety disorders are also likely to have other conditions, such as depression or substance abuse. Treating these other conditions is essential to resolving the anxiety.

## A Family Affair

If you have a family member with an anxiety disorder, chances are, you're feeling the effects of their illness too. But getting well requires the support of the entire family. According to the Anxiety Disorders Association of America, you can help the recovery process by learning about anxiety. Lower your expectations of the person with anxiety and try to be flexible, while maintaining a routine. It also helps if you build your own support network to help you cope with the challenges of supporting a loved one with anxiety.

# 🔍 What It Looks Like

To understand the symptoms of anxiety, it helps to first distinguish the five distinct types of anxiety disorders:

- Generalized anxiety disorder (GAD) is chronic, exaggerated worry about everyday events that lasts at least six months. People with GAD always expect the worst possible outcome for no apparent reason.

- Panic disorder is characterized by recurrent panic attacks and extreme fear that often produce physical symptoms such as chest pain, nausea, and abdominal distress.

- Social phobia is an unrealistic fear about places, people, and things. People with social phobia often become obsessed with avoiding the focus of their fear, such as public gatherings or spiders.

- Post-traumatic stress disorder (PSTD) occurs after a stressful event such as rape, war, or abuse. People with PTSD may have nightmares, flashbacks, and depression.

People who have anxiety often experience heart palpitations, shortness of breath, trembling, headaches, muscle tension, and sleep problems. They may also have dizziness, sweating, and difficulties concentrating.

# 🍴 What to Eat

A diet high in vitamin B can help tame the symptoms of anxiety, says Janet Schloss, N.D., a naturopath and nutritionist in Brisbane, Australia. One of the most important B vitamins is B6.

Vitamin B6 helps the body convert tryptophan, an amino acid, into serotonin, a neurotransmitter that is involved in regulating mood and reducing depression. Good sources of B vitamins include brown rice, leafy greens, peanut butter, fortified cereals, and brewer's yeast. These vitamins are also found in lean meats such as turkey, pork, and chicken.

Anxiety accompanied by constipation or diarrhea may benefit from a high-fiber diet, which will promote regularity. Fruits, vegetables, and whole-grain foods are all good sources of fiber as well as other important vitamins and minerals.

People with anxiety may also benefit from eating foods rich in calcium, a mineral involved in nerve cell function and muscle contraction. Foods rich in calcium include milk, leafy greens, tofu, and yogurt. Another important mineral that can relieve anxiety is magnesium, which is also found in many of the same foods.

Finally, consider eating foods that contain glutamine, an amino acid found in high-protein foods that plays a role in numerous metabolic functions and helps produce GABA, a neurotransmitter that promotes relaxation. Good sources of glutamine include cottage cheese, ricotta cheese, and eggs.

# 🚫🍴 What Not to Eat

Certain foods can play a major role in your anxiety, and eliminating them can often help provide relief. For starters, anyone with anxiety should avoid caffeine, a stimulant that can cause nervousness, insomnia, and anxiety, even in people without an anxiety disorder. If you have anxiety, you should even steer clear of decaffeinated beverages because they still contain small amounts of caffeine.

It's also important to avoid alcohol. Alcohol may provide some temporary relief, but in reality, it makes you more vulnerable to stress. Drinking in excess can lead to difficulties with relationships, careers, and finances, which will only perpetuate your anxiety. Refined sugar should be avoided as well because it can cause blood sugar levels to rise and fall, resulting in bothersome mood swings. The low levels of blood sugar in particular will cause irritability and depression.

## 🦴 Supplements for Anxiety

Some people get relief from anxiety by taking certain supplements. Possible remedies to consider include the following:

### B VITAMIN COMPLEX

A quality B vitamin complex can help tame anxiety and will supply several B vitamins, including biotin, choline, folic acid, inositol, and para-aminobenzoic acid, as well as the six "numbered" B vitamins: vitamin B1 (thiamin), B2 (riboflavin), B3 (niacin), B5 (pantothenic acid), B6 (pyridoxine), and B12 (cobalamin).

### CALCIUM AND MAGNESIUM

Taking these two minerals can help relax the nervous system, relieve agitation, and prevent insomnia, which worsens anxiety.

## 📋 Stay-Healthy Strategies

- **FIGURE OUT WHETHER YOU HAVE A FOOD ALLERGY.** Allergies to food can trigger anxiety as well.

- **PRACTICE DAILY RELAXATION EXERCISES,** such as meditation, prayer, or deep breathing.

- **EXERCISE REGULARLY.** Getting physical activity every day can help relieve anxiety.

- **MAKE AN EFFORT TO GET ADEQUATE SLEEP.** Not having enough sleep on a regular basis can put you on edge and make anxiety worse.

---

### Eating Without Anxiety

The way you eat can sometimes trigger anxiety, says Janet Schloss, N.D., a naturopath and nutritionist in Brisbane, Australia. She recommends that you lower anxiety during meals with the following tips:

- Eat slowly. Chew your food at least 15 to 20 times.

- Do not eat on the run. Make each meal a time to pause and take a reprieve from your activities.

- Minimize your fluid intake to avoid over-diluting the stomach acids you need for proper digestion.

- Avoid eating to the point where you feel overly full and bloated.

- Eat small meals throughout the day. A steady supply of food will help keep blood sugar in balance and prevent it from falling, which can trigger anxiety.

# ARTHRITIS

MILLIONS OF PEOPLE IN THE UNITED STATES are familiar with the aches and pain associated with arthritis. Arthritis is an equal-opportunity joint disorder that occurs in more than one hundred different forms in people of all ages and races.

The most common form, osteoarthritis, tends to develop with advancing age, and according to the Arthritis Foundation, affects nearly twenty-one million people. Others forms include rheumatoid arthritis, gout, ankylosing spondylitis, and juvenile arthritis. When all forms are tallied, arthritis actually affects sixty-six million people. This chapter will focus primarily on osteoarthritis.

Osteoarthritis occurs when the cartilage that covers the end of your bones begins to erode and break away. Without this protective covering, bone grinds against bone, and the result is pain, swelling, and loss of motion of the joint. Over time, the joint may become misshapen, and small growths called bone spurs may start to grow on the edges of the bone. In some people, the bone or cartilage may break off and float in the joint space, which makes the pain even worse.

Every case of arthritis is different. Some people may develop symptoms rapidly. In others, it may occur gradually. While the exact cause of osteoarthritis is unknown, there are risk factors such as being overweight, advancing age, joint injuries, and excess stress on the joints. However, these risks don't guarantee that you'll have arthritis. For instance, not everyone who is eld-erly gets arthritis, and thin people may get the condition as well.

Some people with arthritis will experience significant lifestyle changes as a result of reduced mobility and flexibility. They may need to change jobs or give up a beloved sport or activity. Others may suffer depression as the result of these limitations. Treatment often requires a combination of medications, exercise, and lifestyle changes. Healthy eating is certainly a part of that multi-pronged strategy.

## What It Looks Like

No two people will have the exact same signs and symptoms of arthritis. In most cases, arthritis starts slowly with some mild soreness or stiffness that is barely perceptible. You may have some intermittent pain as well. Some people may remain in this stage for years.

Other people however, will experience a progression in their disease. After a while, the pain may intensify. The pain may also vary, often feeling less severe in the morning and more aggravating in the evening. Over time, some arthritis sufferers may notice that they are less coordinated and that they have difficulties walking or sustaining good posture. Other common symptoms include the following:

- Soreness in the joints after overuse or periods of inactivity.

- Stiffness after periods of inactivity that goes away when you resume movement.

- Morning stiffness that typically lasts no more than 30 minutes.

- Pain caused by weakened muscles surrounding the joint due to inactivity.

Arthritis can occur in any of several joints or in multiple joints. Common sites include the hips and knees, joints that get a lot of use and that must bear a lot of weight. It can also occur in the fingers, spine, and feet.

## ¶¶ What to Eat

According to Elizabeth Lipski, Ph.D., C.C.N., author of *Digestive Wellness*, people with osteoarthritis often have an acid-alkaline imbalance. Most people with osteoarthritis have too much acid, causing the body to use up essential nutrients and creating a deficit in these substances. To restore the imbalance, Lipski recommends eating an abundance of fruits and vegetables. These foods are also important for their antioxidant effects. Good choices include leafy greens, beans, broccoli, onions, rhubarb, grapefruit, pineapples, nectarines, and watermelon. Pineapple also contains bromelain, a natural anti-inflammatory. Other good foods to eat include eggs, yogurt, and grains such as oats, quinoa, and wild rice.

It's also important for people with arthritis to prevent weight gain. Extra weight taxes the joints and can increase your pain. To help meet that goal, make sure to eat a healthy diet that is rich in nutrients and low in empty calories.

Another food to include in your diet is fish, especially cold-water varieties that contain omega-3 fatty acids, such as salmon, herring, mackerel, lake trout, and tuna. Omega-3 fatty acids contain substances that can help ease the pain and inflammation sometimes associated with osteoarthritis.

## Some Facts on Arthritis

The incidence of arthritis or chronic joint problems is on the rise and a serious health problem. Here are some numbers from the Arthritis Foundation that prove it:

- In 1985, thirty-five million people had arthritis.

- By 2005, there were sixty-six million people with arthritis.

- More than half of those affected are under age 65.

- Arthritis is the nation's leading cause of disability among Americans over the age of 15.

- Arthritis affects nearly 300,000 children.

In addition, people with arthritis should get plenty of fiber. A diet rich in fiber will ensure regularity and help you feel full so you are less likely to overeat.

Finally, make sure to eat foods that contain sulfur, a major mineral that can help repair cartilage and boost immunity. Garlic, onions, beans, and cabbage are good sources of sulfur.

# What Not to Eat

Some people with arthritis notice improvements when they avoid nightshade foods, which are potatoes, tomatoes, peppers, and eggplant. To find out if that can help you, try doing an elimination diet by not eating these foods for a week, then gradually introducing them back and noting any physical changes.

To help prevent weight gain and reduce acid, it's best to steer clear of refined sugars and processed foods, such as crackers, packaged cakes, cookies, and desserts. It's also helpful to not eat foods high in sugar or saturated fat, such as red meat, eggs, and fried foods, which can promote weight gain.

# Supplements for Arthritis

People with arthritis should take a quality multivitamin to help ensure that they get adequate nutrients. On top of that, there are several supplements that may help relieve arthritis pain:

## GLUCOSAMINE AND CHONDROITIN SULFATE

These substances are found in small quantities in food and are also present in normal human cartilage. As supplements, glucosamine comes from crab, lobster, or shrimp shells, while chondroitin sulfate is derived from animal cartilage, such as shark.

Combined as an arthritis remedy, they can help repair cartilage and improve mobility. But some people have more success with these supplements than others. If you do try them, allow three months for the effects to kick in.

## VITAMIN C

Vitamin C is essential for the formation of cartilage and collagen, tissues that help enhance bone strength. It's also important for bolstering immunity and, as an antioxidant, helps combat free radical damage that leads to disease.

## B COMPLEX VITAMIN

Taken together, the B vitamins help strengthen connective tissue, such as muscles, bones, tissues, and joints.

## METHYLSULFONYLMETHANE (MSM)

MSM is high in sulfur and can help reduce pain and inflammation. It also aids in building and repairing cartilage. But be careful about taking too much, as it can cause diarrhea.

## BIOFLAVANOIDS

Bioflavanoids are substances in plants that influence bodily functions and reactions. Several may help tame arthritis pain by reducing inflammation, including quercetin, bromelain, curcumin, and turmeric.

## GINGER

The pungent spice is also a supplement that can help relieve pain and reduce inflammation. Take it in powdered form as a supplement, or use it in your food and tea.

## DEVIL'S CLAW

Devil's claw is an herbal remedy that may reduce pain and inflammation and allow you to reduce your dosage of nonsteroidal anti-inflammatory drugs. You should not take it if you are also taking antacids, diabetes medications, or blood-thinning drugs. You should also avoid devil's claw if you have gallstones, ulcers, or heart rhythm irregularities.

## Stay-Healthy Strategies

- **GET A DIAGNOSIS.** Pain, stiffness, or swelling around a joint that persists more than two weeks means it's time to see a doctor, according to the Arthritis Foundation. The earlier you're diagnosed, the quicker you're treated, and the less joint damage and pain you'll suffer.

- **MOVE!** Don't make the mistake of letting arthritis inhibit your physical activity. Exercise helps increase your range of motion and strengthens the muscles around the joints. It can also relieve pain and reduce inflammation. Even doing a little bit can help. If necessary, talk to a physical therapist about the best exercises for you.

- **CONSIDER CAPSAICIN.** Topical creams made of this fiery substance may help relieve your arthritis pain.

- **DITCH THE EXTRA WEIGHT.** Being too heavy will only worsen your arthritis by straining your joints. Do what you can to shed the additional pounds.

### What's Gout?

Gout is a form of arthritis that occurs primarily in men. It's extremely painful and occurs when you have a buildup of needle-shaped crystals of uric acid. Uric acid is formed in the breakdown of certain foods and, in excess, will lodge itself in connective tissues, the joints, or both. The result is swelling, redness, heat, pain, and joint stiffness.

Those with gout should avoid high-protein foods, which contain purine, a nitrogen-containing substance that is converted into uric acid. Foods high in purine include herring, organ meats, yeast, and anchovies. It is also found in asparagus, meat, fish, shellfish, spinach, eggs, and nuts. Do not drink alcohol, which speeds up the breakdown of purine into uric acid. In addition, try to maintain a healthy weight because excess weight contributes to increases in uric acid.

# ATHEROSCLEROSIS

EVERY MOMENT OF OUR LIVES, blood courses through our veins, transporting oxygen and vital nutrients through the body's intricate network of blood vessels to organs and cells. For some people, this process may become disrupted by the buildup of fatty deposits on the inner walls of these blood vessels—a substance called plaque. The plaque causes the blood vessel walls to thicken and narrow, causing a condition called atherosclerosis.

Atherosclerosis occurs gradually over a period of many years. It typically starts in childhood and worsens with age. But certain factors, including high cholesterol, high blood pressure, diabetes, and cigarette smoking, can speed up its development. People who eat a diet high in saturated fat are also more likely to get atherosclerosis.

Once the plaque is there, you are at greater risk for the formation of a blood clot. If the clot develops in an artery leading to the heart, blood flow to the heart is disrupted, resulting in a heart attack. If it occurs in an artery leading to the brain, blood flow to the brain is blocked, causing stroke. If the disruption occurs in the leg, it can cause difficulties with walking and eventually gangrene, which may require amputation.

It's hard to know exactly how many people have atherosclerosis. The disease typically causes no signs or symptoms. But in general, men are at greater risk for atherosclerosis, as are people with a family history of heart disease. In women, the risk increases after menopause, when they lose the protective benefits of estrogen.

The good news is that some of the other risk factors for atherosclerosis can be controlled. These risk factors include high blood pressure, high cholesterol, and high triglyceride levels. Giving up cigarettes and controlling blood sugars if you have diabetes will also help lessen the buildup of plaque. At the heart of managing any of these risk factors is a healthy diet.

## 🔎 What It Looks Like

Most people will have no indication that they have atherosclerosis. Instead, the disease occurs silently inside the arteries, where damage to the endothelium—the lining of the artery wall—starts the destruction known as atherosclerosis. Once damaged, the injured wall begins to allow fats, cholesterol, platelets, cellular waste, and other substances to accumulate in the artery wall, causing a buildup of plaque. The buildup is accelerated in people who have high blood pressure, high cholesterol, and high triglyceride levels, as well as in people who smoke.

As the plaque thickens, the diameter of the artery narrows, making it harder for blood to get through, which then reduces oxygen flow in the body. If this occurs in an artery leading to the heart, you may experience chest pain. If it occurs in an artery of the leg, you may feel pain in your leg. Some people may experience fatigue or high blood pressure. If a blood clot forms near this plaque and blocks the artery completely, there will be stoppage of blood flow.

## ¡¡¡ What to Eat

Because people generally don't know they have atherosclerosis, they should focus on eating a diet that is geared toward reducing its risk factors, namely high cholesterol, diabetes, and high blood pressure. So if you have any of these conditions, or if you're overweight, you smoke, or you are inactive, focus on eating a heart-healthy diet in order to lower your risk for heart attack and stroke, says Marie Savard, M.D., author of *The Body Shape Solution for Weight Loss and Wellness*. That means eating a lot of fruits, vegetables, whole grains, and legumes.

When choosing your fruits and vegetables, aim for color and variety so you'll get a lot of the antioxidant vitamins A, C, and E. Eating an abundance of fruits and veggies helps ensure you get adequate fiber as well. Soluble fiber, the kind that dissolves in water, is especially critical because it will help slow down digestion and keep blood sugar in check. It will also help lower LDL cholesterol (the bad or "lousy" cholesterol), triglycerides, and high blood pressure, while raising levels of HDL (the good or "healthy" cholesterol).

Both soluble and insoluble fiber can help minimize weight gain by making you feel full. Sources of soluble fiber include oats, kidney beans, peas, flaxseed, apples, oranges, and carrots. Insoluble fiber is found in whole-wheat foods, cauliflower, beans, spinach, peas, and apples. As you see, some foods supply both.

For protein, focus on chicken, fish, beans, and soy products. Soybean foods come in many forms including tempeh, tofu, edamame, soy milk, and soy burgers.

You should also try to eat fish that contain healthy omega-3 fatty acids, which may lower your risk for heart disease. Healthy fish include salmon, tuna, and mackerel. Omega-3s are also found in walnuts, flaxseed, and fortified foods, including peanut butter and breakfast cereal.

Try to get your fat intake from monounsaturated fats, which are healthier and less damaging than saturated fats. Good sources of monounsaturated fats include avocados, almonds, Brazil nuts, and pecans. Cook with olive or canola oil.

Consider using margarine-like spreads made of soybean extract (such as Benecol and Take Control), which contain plant stanols that have been found to lower cholesterol.

# 🚫 What Not to Eat

Steer clear of foods high in saturated fats and trans-fatty acids. Saturated fats occur primarily in animal products such as red meat, dairy products, and butter. Trans-fatty acids are often found in packaged foods such as candy bars, cookies, muffins, and crackers. Be on the lookout for any ingredient that is labeled "partially hydrogenated," which means the food contains trans-fatty acids. You should also avoid foods high in sugar, which can elevate insulin levels and cause an increase in cholesterol, triglycerides, and blood pressure.

If you already have high blood pressure, avoid foods high in sodium, such as canned soups, packaged meals, and deli meats. Approximately 30 percent of people are sensitive to the blood pressure effects of foods high in sodium.

Others foods to limit or eliminate include pastries, rolls, bagels, and creamy dressings. You should also steer clear of processed meats such as hot dogs, pastrami, and bologna; fried foods of any variety: and foods made with white flour.

## Should You Have Wine with That?

Whether or not to drink red wine for heart health is a nutrition question that's boggled health-conscious consumers for years. Several studies have suggested that wine may protect the heart and arteries from disease. But alcohol can also raise triglyceride levels and, in excess, can raise your risk for cancer, cirrhosis, and obesity. All alcohol is high in calories—seven calories per gram—compared with fats, which have nine calories per gram, and proteins and carbohydrates, which have four calories per gram.

If you do want to consider drinking red wine for heart health, talk to your physician first and make sure it's safe for you, especially if you're taking medications. People who take aspirin for instance, should not drink. If you choose to drink, however, do so in moderation (no more than one or two drinks a day).

## 🔬 Supplements for Atherosclerosis

Start with a quality multivitamin, which will give your body the basic nutrients you need to stay healthy and override those days when you don't eat as well. Other supplements to consider include the following:

### FISH OIL

Because omega-3 fatty acids are so beneficial to the prevention of heart disease, a fish oil supplement may be advantageous. But if you're on blood-thinning medication, talk to your doctor first because fish oil may increase your risk for bleeding.

### FOLIC ACID

Taking this B vitamin can help reduce levels of homocysteine, a substance that has been implicated in the development of heart disease. (Note: if your multivitamin contains folic acid, you may not need an additional supplement.)

### PSYLLIUM

Psyllium is a seed husk and a soluble fiber that can help with bowel regularity and lowering cholesterol. But if you have food allergies, you should talk to your doctor first because some people react to psyllium.

### ASPIRIN

Research has shown that one baby aspirin a day can prevent a heart attack in men and stroke in women. Talk to your doctor before starting on aspirin, which can cause a number of side effects including stomach irritation and bleeding.

## 📋 Stay-Healthy Strategies

- **TAKE PREVENTIVE MEASURES.** If you smoke, quit. If you have diabetes, make efforts to control your blood sugar. Preventing atherosclerosis is your best defense against it.

- **CHOOSE A TYPE OF PHYSICAL ACTIVITY YOU ENJOY.** Regular exercise can reduce your risk for atherosclerosis and the progression of the disease.

- **CHECK OUT THE AMERICAN HEART ASSOCIATION'S "DELICIOUS DECISIONS,"** an online cookbook that offers healthy recipes. (www.deliciousdecisions.org)

- **BE WARY OF FAD DIETS.** The healthiest diets incorporate foods from all the major food groups and stress moderation.

# ATTENTION DEFICIT HYPERACTIVITY DISORDER

ALL CHILDREN HAVE MOMENTS when they're fidgety, restless, and impulsive. Even adults can blurt out inappropriate comments, struggle to pay attention, and flit from one activity to another. But in kids—and even adults—who have attention deficit hyperactivity disorder (ADHD), these symptoms are frequent and severe, sometimes disrupting the child's academic performance and ability to get along with others.

ADHD affects 3 to 5 percent of children in the United States, or approximately two million kids. The condition was first described in 1845 by Dr. Heinrich Hoffman in a book called *The Story of Fidgety Philip*, about a little boy with ADHD. Today, ADHD is the most common psychiatric disorder in children.

Experts agree that the disorder is not the result of poor parenting, but rather a mix of genetics, biology, and environment. Children who have close relatives with ADHD are more likely to have it. There is also evidence that using cigarettes and alcohol during pregnancy may increase the risk for ADHD, and that exposure to certain toxins such as lead and aluminum may play a role as well. In addition, some experts believe that ADHD may be caused by allergies to certain foods and inhalants.

Many children with ADHD have coexisting disorders, including learning disabilities; oppositional defiant disorder, characterized by extreme obstinance, noncompliance, and belligerent behavior; and conduct disorder, a serious pattern of antisocial behavior characterized by violence, aggression, and possible criminal behavior. A smaller percent of children may have Tourette's syndrome, which is characterized by nervous tics, repetitive mannerisms, and odd twitches and grimaces. Some children with ADHD have anxiety and depression as well.

Treatment for ADHD is complex and always highly individualized. Children who take medications are usually given stimulants such as methylphenidate (Ritalin) or amphetamine (Adderall). Other possible remedies include tricyclic antidepressants, such as amitriptyline (Elavil), or antihypertensives, such as catapres (Clonidine). But medications aren't right for every child and must be carefully considered with a qualified doctor.

Other children undergo different types of therapy such as cognitive-behavioral therapy, which teaches new ways of thinking in order to help alter the behavior; psychotherapy, which works on boosting self-esteem in spite of ADHD; and social skills training. Parents of children with ADHD may attend special parenting classes to help equip them with the skills they need. Research has suggested that combining therapy with medication may work best, especially in areas such as social skills, academic performance, and parent-child relations.

But ADHD isn't just a childhood disorder. Many adults have symptoms as well but have never been formally diagnosed. Adults with ADHD often feel as if they simply can't get their act together. They're always running behind, highly disorganized, and unable to pay attention for extended periods of time. Many of them struggle just to get through the day. A diagnosis in adulthood is often a relief to those who have been suffering from ADHD for years and now finally have an answer to their daily struggles.

## What It Looks Like

ADHD is defined by three main symptoms: inattention, hyperactivity, and impulsivity. Inattentive children are easily distracted, have trouble listening, and struggle to complete tasks. They frequently lose things, make careless errors, and have difficulties remembering. Organizing their activities is extremely challenging, and as a result homework and chores are often incomplete.

Hyperactivity and impulsivity often result in rude and disruptive behaviors. Kids who are hyperactive or impulsive and can't sit still fidget constantly. They struggle to remain seated even in situations when they're expected to stay in their seats. They may blurt out answers inappropriately and have trouble playing quietly. Often, they are engaged in constant activity, such as running and climbing.

Not all children will have all these symptoms. Some may be simply inattentive or just hyperactive and impulsive. Others, however, may have a combination of the three.

### Is It Really ADHD?

It isn't always easy to distinguish normal behaviors from those of ADHD. According to the National Institute of Mental Health, ADHD behaviors start before age 7, last at least six months, and create a real problem in at least two areas of the person's life, such as at school or at social gatherings. A child who is overly active on the playground but who does well in the classroom is not likely to be diagnosed with ADHD.

The behaviors must also be excessive, long-term, pervasive, and occur more often than they do in other children the same age. In addition, the behaviors are continuous, occur in multiple settings, and are not just a reaction to a temporary situation.

## ¶¶ What to Eat

Eating a healthy, well-balanced diet that contains all the essential nutrients is critical for the child who suffers from ADHD, says Laura J. Stevens, M.S., author of *12 Effective Ways to Help Your Child with ADHD*. Such a diet will help eliminate the unhealthy foods that aggravate your child's condition.

Make sure your child eats plenty of complex carbohydrates, such as fruits, vegetables, and whole-grain breads and pastas. These foods are rich in important antioxidant vitamins and essential minerals such as iron and calcium. They also contain a lot of fiber, which will aid digestion and help prevent constipation.

For protein, focus on lean meats, poultry, fish, beans, nuts, and eggs. These protein sources often provide numerous other nutrients such as B vitamins. In addition, your child should get some protein from low-fat dairy products such as milk, yogurt, and cheese, which will supply him with calcium, essential for strong bones.

Finally, make sure your child gets plenty of fats in his diet, specifically the essential fatty acids omega-3s and omega-6s, which can prevent excessive thirst, dry skin, and frequent urination—symptoms that aggravate a child with ADHD. Good sources of omega-3s include cold-water fish, such as salmon, tuna, and mackerel, and walnuts and flaxseed. Also, get in the habit of cooking with healthy oils such as canola and soybean oils, which contain both monounsaturated and essential fatty acids. Certain beans, such as kidney, navy, pinto, red, and soy, are another good source of essential fatty acids.

## ⊘ What Not to Eat

Keep your child away from foods that set off allergies. If you don't know whether your child has food allergies, consider doing an elimination diet by cutting out potentially allergenic foods, then reintroducing them one at a time. (For specifics, check out the book *12 Effective Ways to Help Your ADD/ADHD Child*.) Common allergens include dairy, chocolate, artificial colorings, eggs, wheat, corn, citrus, and legumes.

It's best to steer clear of sugar, which in some kids, can set off hyperactive behaviors. If you choose to use artificial sweeteners, use these products sparingly. Some children experience an increase in hyperactive behavior after ingesting sweeteners as well. Sugar is also filled with empty calories—lots of energy with no nutritional value.

Cut back on saturated fats and trans-fatty acids. Saturated fats are found primarily in animal products such as red meat, whole dairy foods, and tropical oils. Trans-fatty acids are found in packaged foods such as crackers, cookies, and frozen breakfast foods, as well as shortening, most margarines, salad dressings, and mayonnaise. These foods promote unhealthy weight gain and heart disease and interfere with the metabolism of healthy essential fatty acids.

Finally, if your child has a history of taking numerous antibiotics for ear infections or suffered from extensive diaper rash, thrush, or conditions that required steroid treatment, check to see if he has a problem with yeast overgrowth, known as candidiasis. For more information, see the Candidiasis chapter on page 72. Your child may need to eat a diet free of yeast and sugar.

# ✿ Supplements for ADHD

Certain supplements may be helpful for your child with ADHD. It's always best to consult with a physician knowledgeable in nutrition (or a nutritionist who knows a great deal about ADHD) to help you figure out if supplements might benefit your child. Some you might consider include the following:

## VITAMIN C

Vitamin C is an antioxidant that can boost your child's immunity. It may also reduce the effect of some allergens.

## B VITAMIN COMPLEX

Some children benefit from the use of B vitamins, which are involved in the production of energy in the cells. A quality B vitamin complex will supply several B vitamins, which have been found to help children with ADHD. Large doses, however, may worsen some symptoms.

## ZINC

Studies suggest that this immune-boosting mineral may help relieve some symptoms of ADHD.

## MAGNESIUM

This major mineral may help calm a hyperactive child and promote healthy sleep. Combined with calcium, it may help relax the nerves.

## CALCIUM

Although most well known for bone formation, calcium also ensures the healthy function of the nervous system and helps maintain normal heart rhythms.

## PROBIOTICS

If your child has a yeast problem, a probiotic such as *Lactobacillus acidophilus* may help restore healthy bacteria for proper digestion.

# ☐ Stay-Healthy Strategies

- **BE PATIENT.** If your child is accustomed to a diet filled with sweets and void of healthy fruits and vegetables, make small dietary changes gradually.

- **EAT BREAKFAST.** A healthy morning meal gives your child a solid start for the day. But be wary of sugary cereals.

- **MODEL HEALTHY EATING.** Don't push fruits and veggies on your child but then grab a candy bar for yourself. Eat what you want your child to eat, and you'll both be healthier for it.

- **PINPOINT CHEMICAL SENSITIVITIES.** Exposure to certain chemicals can worsen inattentiveness and hyperactivity in children with ADHD. Figure out the ones that seem to bother your child and try to limit his exposure to them. Common ones include perfumes, cleaning products, and plastics.

## The Feingold Program

Over the years, some people with ADHD have benefited from a lifestyle program called the Feingold Program. The program was created by Ben Feingold, M.D., a pediatrician and allergist who first developed an eating plan in the 1960s for children with behavior problems. He is also the author of the book *Why Your Child is Hyperactive*, which was published in 1974.

The Feingold Program eliminates foods that contain certain additives that are believed to trigger symptoms of behavior and learning problems as well as some health problems such as headaches, asthma, and hives. These additives include artificial colorings, flavorings, and synthetic preservatives such as BHA, BHT, and TBHQ, as well as aspartame (NutraSweet). Food dyes can be found in ingredient listings and often appear as Red Dye #40 or Yellow #5. Eliminating these substances has been found to reduce hyperactivity, impulsivity, compulsive behavior, and emotional difficulties. Other potentially problematic substances include MSG (monosodium glutatmate), nitrites, sulfates, and benzoate.

The Feingold Program also eliminates synthetic fragrances found in non-food items. Salicylates, which are used in aspirin and found naturally in some foods, can also be a problem for some people. Surprisingly, the program does not ban all junk foods. For instance, the diet does allow Fritos but prohibits Cheetos. Similarly, the diet says Natural Doritos are acceptable but does not allow the regular ones. Check out www.feingold.org for more information.

# BACK PAIN

ALMOST EVERYONE EXPERIENCES at least an occasional bout of back pain at one time or another. A bad mattress, a car accident, and advancing age are all potential causes of back pain. The National Institutes of Health estimates that back pain will affect eight out of ten Americans during their lifetime.

Although back pain can affect anyone, certain factors do raise your risk for it. The condition is more likely as you get older and muscles weaken. The lack of regular exercise, a poor diet, and a job that involves heavy lifting can make you more vulnerable as well. People who have other medical conditions such as osteoarthritis or rheumatoid arthritis are at higher risk for back pain too. But even young, healthy people who work at low-risk jobs can suffer back pain. Simply sleeping on a bad mattress can trigger sore muscles in your back.

The best way to treat back pain is to prevent it in the first place. Prevention involves a healthy lifestyle that includes regular exercise. Activities that promote balance such as tai chi and yoga can help reduce your risk for falls that lead to back problems. Prevention also involves eating a healthy diet that minimizes weight gain. Being overweight stresses the body, and that includes the back.

## 🔎 What It Looks Like

Most people experience acute back pain, the kind that comes on suddenly, then goes away on its own. Acute back pain typically occurs as the result of an event, such as a fall, a bad maneuver on the tennis court, or straining the back from lifting something heavy. Acute back pain generally lasts from a few days to a few weeks. Symptoms may range from dull muscular aches to sharp, shooting pain. You may also experience limited flexibility and range of motion and feel incapable of standing up straight.

Chronic back pain is something that may come on gradually or suddenly but persists for more than three months. It may be hard to pinpoint the cause of chronic back pain, and the pain tends to become worse over time.

Treating back pain often involves taking over-the-counter pain relievers and applying heat or cold. Although bed rest may help, it's not recommended beyond a day or two. Instead, it's best to try and resume normal activities as soon as possible. Once you're well enough, it's a good idea to exercise and try to strengthen abdominal muscles that support the back. Chronic cases may involve physical therapy.

## ¡¦¡ What to Eat

Eat a diet that helps you maintain a healthy weight, says Milton Stokes, R.D., a spokesperson for the American Dietetic Association (ADA). A diet rich in fruits and vegetables can help do that and also supply your body with the fiber it needs to prevent constipation. Constipation can aggravate back pain. According to the ADA, adults should try to eat 20 to 35 grams of fiber per day. Good sources include fruits, vegetables, legumes, whole-wheat foods, oats, flaxseeds, and certain breakfast cereals. While boosting your fiber intake, you should drink a lot of water to make a high-fiber diet more tolerable and to flush out toxins.

Also, pay attention to portion sizes and to your true hunger cues. People who gain weight typically eat more food than their bodies really need. So get into the habit of eating in moderation. Resist the urge to take seconds. Eat only when you're hungry and stop eating the minute you feel satisfied.

## ⊘ What Not to Eat

If you suffer from back pain, the goal is to minimize weight gain. To do that, limit your intake of high-calorie foods that contain saturated fat, such as red meat, whole dairy products, and butter.

Go light on foods that contain trans fats, which are unhealthy fats produced in the hydrogenation of oils. These foods, such as baked goods, pastries, snack foods, and junk foods, tend to contain a lot of empty calories. Fat is high in calories (it has nine calories per gram, compared with proteins and carbohydrates, which each have four calories per gram). So even if you eat equal amounts of fat, proteins, and carbohydrates, you'll get more calories from the fat.

Cut back on or eliminate alcohol. All alcoholic beverages have seven calories per gram. Drinking in excess lowers inhibitions and stimulates appetite, which could lead to overeating. Too much alcohol also heightens your risk for falling, which could worsen back problems.

# 🔖 Supplements for Back Pain

The supplements you might take will depend on the cause of your pain. If you suffer from chronic back pain, supplements may help strengthen underlying weaknesses in muscles and bone. As always, consult with a physician before taking any supplements.

In addition to a quality multivitamin, you may want to ask your doctor about taking these:

### GLUCOSAMINE AND CHONDROITIN SULFATE

These substances are found in small quantities in food and also occur in normal human cartilage. As supplements, glucosamine comes from crab, lobster, or shrimp shells, while chondroitin sulfate is derived from animal cartilage, such as that found in sharks. People with allergies to shellfish, however, should avoid glucosamine.

Combined, glucosamine and chondroitin sulfate can help repair cartilage and improve mobility, especially if the source of your back pain is arthritis. Some people have more success with these supplements than others. But if you do try them, allow three months for the effects to kick in.

### CALCIUM

This bone-building mineral can help bolster any weakness in the bones of your back.

### MAGNESIUM

Combined with calcium, magnesium can act as a muscle relaxant. It also helps strengthen bones.

### GINGER

This spice is also a supplement that can help relieve pain and reduce inflammation. Take it in powdered form as a supplement, or use it in your food and tea.

### DEVIL'S CLAW

Devil's claw is an herbal remedy that may reduce pain and inflammation. You should not take it if you are taking antacids, diabetes medications, or blood-thinning drugs. You should also avoid devil's claw if you have gallstones, ulcers, or heart rhythm irregularities.

# 📋 Stay-Healthy Strategies

- **EXERCISE REGULARLY.** Activity has numerous benefits for back pain, including weight loss, improved flexibility and strength, and better posture. Regular activity, especially exercises that strengthen your abdomen, can also prevent any back pain.

- **LIFT CAREFULLY.** Bend at the knees, not at the waist. Stand close to the object. Use your leg muscles. And if it's too heavy, get help.

- **TRY TO AVOID STANDING FOR EXTENDED PERIODS OF TIME.**

- **IF YOU SMOKE, QUIT.** Smoking cigarettes aggravates back pain.

## The Power of Posture

What exactly is good posture? According to the American Physical Therapy Association (APTA), good posture in a standing position is when your body is straight and in vertical alignment from the top of your head through your body to the bottom of your feet.

Good posture supports the back and can help prevent not only back pain, but fatigue and muscle strain as well. It also gives you a more confident appearance.

Here are some tips on how to maintain good posture from the APTA:

- Keep your weight down. Excess weight exerts a constant forward pull on the back muscles and stretches and weakens muscles in the abdomen.

- Avoid staying in one position for extended periods; inactivity causes muscle tension and weakness.

- Exercise regularly. Exercise promotes strong and flexible muscles that keep you upright and in proper position.

- Sleep on a firm mattress and use a pillow under your head that's just thick enough to maintain the normal curvature of the neck. Don't use oversized or multiple pillows.

- Throughout the day, concentrate on keeping your three natural back curves in balanced alignment.

- Protect your back by using good body mechanics: Bend your knees when picking something up or putting it down and carry a heavy object by using two hands and keeping the load close to your waist.

- Wear comfortable and well-supported shoes. Avoid continuous use of high-heeled or platform shoes, which distort the normal shape of the foot and throw the back's natural curves out of alignment.

# BLADDER INFECTION

*See Urinary Tract Infections on page 314.*

# BULIMIA

MOST PEOPLE KNOW THE AWFUL FEELING that comes with overeating—and the subsequent guilt that comes with knowing that you've overdone it. Again. Some people may exercise a little more than usual to compensate for the extra calories they ingested. But in some people, mostly women, the cycle of overeating and compensation for it—often by purging—is taken to an extreme, causing an eating disorder known as bulimia.

Bulimia is characterized by a vicious cycle of bingeing and purging. People with bulimia gorge on large amounts of food in a short amount of time, then frantically look for ways to purge the food, either with vomiting, extreme exercising, or the use of laxatives. They may also become extremely restrictive about what they eat—all in an effort to prevent weight gain. Technically, a person is considered bulimic if she has two or more episodes of binge eating and purging per week for more than three months.

Unfortunately, bulimia is not uncommon. According to one U. S. report, bulimia affects about 6 percent of adolescent girls and 5 percent of college women. Approximately 1 to 3 percent of all women will experience bulimia in their lifetimes.

Bulimia takes a terrible toll on the body in numerous ways. People with bulimia are at risk for anemia, depression, stomach ulcers, dehydration, and irregular bowel movements. They may suffer from gum disease, erosion of tooth enamel, and injury to their esophagus. They may also be plagued with anxiety, guilt, shame, and poor self-esteem, knowing that what they are doing is unhealthy and dangerous and yet feeling powerless to stop it.

Although much of the toll is physical, many people develop bulimia as the result of psychological trauma or emotional difficulties. Many bulimics had difficult childhoods that left them with despair and a sense of helplessness that made them feel as if they had little control over their lives. Often, the act of binging and purging seems to help provide that sense of control.

In addition to the social and psychological components, bulimia may be influenced by genetics; women who have a mother or sister with an eating disorder appear to be at higher risk. Living in a culture that puts a premium on appearance and being thin may exacerbate the problem as well.

## 🔍 What It Looks Like

It isn't always easy to recognize bulimia in someone. Bulimics may be normal weight, underweight, or overweight. But people with bulimia often go to extremes to lose weight. You may suspect someone has bulimia if she goes to the bathroom immediately after she eats or if she exercises a great deal, even when she is sick, tired, or injured. She may also take diet pills or medications that promote urination or defecation.

Sometimes, a bulimic shows signs of throwing up. These include swelling in the cheeks or jaw area, frequent cuts and calluses on the back of the hands and knuckles, and teeth that look transparent. Some people with bulimia may withdraw from their friends and activities they enjoy. Some may become depressed.

Individuals suffering from bulimia frequently experience insomnia, poor concentration, and hints of depression. Bulimics often perform their rituals in secrecy, causing a sense of isolation. They may become obsessed with weight, food, exercise, and everything that surrounds it.

Physically, they may feel fatigued and exhausted as they become depleted of essential minerals such as zinc, potassium, magnesium, and sodium. They may also suffer from constipation, dehydration, osteoporosis, and infertility. In more extreme cases, they may experience seizure disorders, liver and/or kidney damage, and irregularities of the heart.

Diagnosis and treatment are essential to put a halt to the cycle and often include a combination of therapy, medications, and nutrition education.

The goal is to restore healthy eating patterns and to overcome the distorted thinking that underlies the disease.

### Bulimia Q&A

**Q.** Could you have bulimia and anorexia at the same time?

**A.** Yes. The condition is known as bulimerexia. The term describes someone who starts off with anorexia, an eating disorder characterized by an extreme obsession to be thin. After a long period of food deprivation and extreme exercise, the person succumbs to the desire to nourish her body, but then becomes fearful of weight gain and starts purging or overexercising to eliminate the excess caloric intake.

## 🍴 What to Eat

Focus on replenishing the vitamins and minerals that have been lost to purging. That means eating a diet rich in fruits, vegetables, and whole-grain breads and cereals, says Lynn Sutton, R.D., C.D.E., a registered dietitian in Albany, New York. Routine vomiting also puts you at risk for dehydration, so make sure to drink plenty of water—aim for more than eight glasses a day, Sutton says.

At meals, make sure to consume lean proteins such as chicken, turkey, and fish along with complex carbohydrates such as vegetables and whole grains. The combination will help stabilize appetite and energy levels and help restore deficiencies in tryptophan and serotonin, which may occur in bulimia.

Tryptophan is an amino acid found in many high-protein foods that is a precursor to serotonin, the feel-good hormone. People who experience tryptophan depletion may also experience reduced serotonin levels. Diminished amounts of serotonin may cause carbohydrate cravings that lead to binge eating. Good sources of tryptophan include cheese, meat, chicken, fish, turkey, yogurt, peanuts, and chocolate.

Choose foods that replenish lost minerals, such as potassium, zinc, magnesium, and sodium. Good sources of potassium include bananas, haddock, tomatoes, and turkey. Foods rich in zinc include lean ground beef, wheat germ, wheat bran, almonds, and tofu. For magnesium, consider spinach, peanut butter, and black-eyed peas. Sodium is found in almost all processed foods but should be eaten in moderation to prevent high blood pressure.

## What Not to Eat

Avoid foods that trigger binges, especially in the initial stages of recovery. Steer clear of the artificial sweetener aspartame, because it interferes with the uptake of serotonin.

Reduce your intake of refined sugar, which is found in cookies, cakes, snack foods, and other processed foods. Also, avoid drinking alcohol and caffeine, which can affect mood and reduce your efforts to avoid binge eating.

## Supplements for Bulimia

In general, supplements will do little to help treat bulimia, but they may play a role in restoring missing nutrients and in treating other symptoms associated with the disease, such as depression. Start with a high-quality multivitamin. Consult a registered dietitian about whether you need other supplements such as the following:

### ZINC
Studies have found that people with eating disorders may be deficient in this essential mineral, which ensures proper taste and smell.

### MAGNESIUM
Magnesium is an essential mineral that aids in the relaxation of muscles, reduces blood pressure, and helps stimulate the appetite.

## COENZYME Q10

CoQ10 is produced naturally by the body and used in the production of cellular energy. It also acts as an antioxidant.

## ST. JOHN'S WORT

For bulimics experiencing mild depression, St. John's wort may be able to help. But it should never be taken with other antidepressants, and it may interact with other medications as well.

## 5-HTP

5-HTP is similar to serotonin, a major neurotransmitter. Taking it at bedtime may help to promote sleep, and higher doses may relieve depression. But you should never take it if you're on antidepressants.

## Stay-Healthy Strategies

- **EAT SMALL MEALS AND SNACKS** throughout the day. By keeping blood sugar even, you'll avoid the ravenous hunger that could trigger binge eating.

- **GET PROFESSIONAL HELP.** Bulimia is a serious disorder that often needs intervention from health care professionals skilled in treating it. Do not hesitate to get help.

- **DO NOT DO OTHER ACTIVITIES WHILE YOU EAT.** The distraction will reduce your awareness of the sensations of eating.

- **WHEN EATING, FOCUS ON YOUR FEELINGS OF HUNGER AND FULLNESS,** as well as the way food tastes, smells, and feels. Becoming more aware of food will help retrain you to eat when you're hungry and to not eat when you're full.

# BURSITIS

Too much time in the garden. Lengthy rounds of tennis. Extended bike rides. These are the kinds of activities that can set you up for bursitis, a painful inflammation of the bursas, small fluid-filled sacs that lubricate and cushion the joints. Bursitis occurs when a joint is overused or repetitively stressed. It may also develop as the result of a bacterial infection or another preexisting condition such as rheumatoid arthritis or gout.

The human body has more than 150 bursas, but certain ones are more prone to bursitis, including the ones in your shoulders, elbows, hips, knees, and heels. Bursitis in the knees may develop if you spend too much time kneeling in activities such as gardening or scrubbing a floor. In the shoulder, bursitis may be the result of playing too much tennis. The buttocks may develop bursitis if you sit on a hard surface, such as a bicycle seat, for extended periods. In some cases, it may be hard to pinpoint the exact cause.

Most cases of bursitis can be treated at home. Resting the injured joint is often all it takes. Sometimes a splint can help support the joint and prevent excess use. A heating pad or a cold pack can relieve the pain and inflammation. Taking nonsteroidal anti-inflammatory drugs can help too.

But in some cases, you may need to see your physician if the pain persists or keeps recurring. Excess swelling, disabling pain, redness, fever, or sharp, shooting pain are all signs that you need medical attention. Severe cases of bursitis may require physical therapy to strengthen the surrounding muscles or injections of steroids to relieve inflammation.

## What It Looks Like

Bursitis causes intense pain that worsens when you try to move the affected joint. In some cases the pain comes on suddenly, but it can also develop gradually.

The affected area is typically swollen and red. Sometimes the bursitis can cause the area to jut out significantly. Some people may also experience a fever and warmth in the affected joint if there is an infection involved.

## ¶¶¶ What to Eat

People who suffer recurrent bursitis may be prone to inflammation and so should eat a diet that reduces inflammatory activity in the body, says Fred Pescatore, M.D., a New York City physician who uses nutrition to treat his patients and is the author of *The Hamptons Diet Cookbook*. To meet that goal, try eating cold-water fish, which contain omega-3 fatty acids. Omega-3 fatty acids contain substances that can help ease the pain and inflammation sometimes associated with bursitis. Good choices include salmon, herring, mackerel, lake trout, and tuna. Other sources of omega-3s include walnuts and flaxseed.

Also, focus on eating lots of fresh fruits and vegetables, which will enhance your immune function and help bring about healing.

If the cause of your pain is due to rheumatoid arthritis, see that chapter (page 277) for more information. If you have gout, check out the Arthritis chapter on page 41.

## ⊘ What Not to Eat

Steer clear of foods that may promote inflammation, such as processed foods and those that contain refined sugar. These types of food also promote weight gain, which may aggravate your pain. Some people notice a worsening of their bursitis when they eat nightshade vegetables, namely potatoes, tomatoes, peppers, and eggplants. Certain spices, such as cayenne, may also aggravate bursitis pain.

## ⁘ Supplements for Bursitis

Some people may want to try supplements to help relieve the inflammation caused by bursitis. Supplements you may consider include the following:

### GLUCOSAMINE SULFATE

Glucosamine is a popular arthritis remedy derived from crab, lobster, or shrimp shells. It can help support connective tissue.

### VITAMIN C

Vitamin C is essential for the formation of cartilage and collagen. It can help improve immunity and stimulate connective tissue repair, while also reducing inflammation.

### B COMPLEX VITAMIN

Taken together, the B vitamins help strengthen connective tissue, such as muscles, bones, tissues, and joints.

### BIOFLAVONOIDS

Bioflavonoids are substances in plants that influence bodily functions and reactions. Several, including quercetin, bromelain, curcumin, and turmeric may help reduce inflammation.

### GINGER

This pungent spice is also a supplement that can help relieve pain and reduce inflammation. Take it in powdered form as a supplement or use it in your food and tea.

## PROTEOLYTIC ENZYMES

These enzymes are best known for helping digestion, but they can also help tame the inflammation that accompanies bursitis.

## BROMELAIN

Bromelain is a type of enzyme found in pineapple juice that breaks down protein and that may relieve pain and inflammation.

## ARNICA

Derived from a plant found in Europe and Russia, arnica is a homeopathic remedy that, in a cream or pellet form, may help relieve pain and inflammation.

---

### FACT

*Bursitis is not arthritis. Arthritis is inflammation of the joint itself. Bursitis is inflammation of the bursas.*

---

## Stay-Healthy Strategies

- **DO YOUR BEST TO PREVENT BURSITIS.** Take breaks from lengthy activities. Cushion your knees. Strengthen your muscles.

- **AVOID PUSHING PAST THE PAIN.** As soon as you feel pain, stop the activity and rest.

- **STRETCH IT OUT.** If you do have bursitis, try stretching to improve your range of motion.

- **PRACTICE GOOD POSTURE.** Poor posture can make you vulnerable to bursitis and make the condition worse.

# CANCER

IN HEALTHY PEOPLE, BODY CELLS are in a constant state of flux—growing, dividing, then dying in a steady, orderly manner. In childhood, these body cells divide more rapidly. In adulthood, the process slows, so that cell division occurs only when old cells wear out or die, or when injuries occur.

Cancer is a disease that disrupts this normal process of cell division. The disease process begins with damage to DNA, the genetic material that exists in every single body cell and that directs all the cell's activities. Damaged DNA may be inherited—which explains why some cancers are genetic—but it can also be caused by exposure to something in the environment, such as tobacco smoke in lung cancer or ultraviolet radiation in skin cancer.

Usually, the body can repair this damage. But when cancer develops, the damaged DNA goes unrepaired and the cancer cells are allowed to replicate out of control. Over time, the cancer cells form a tumor, or mass of abnormal cells. These tumors can eventually overwhelm the ability of an organ to function properly.

Not all cancers result in tumors, and not all tumors are cancerous. Noncancerous tumors are considered benign. Those that are cancerous are considered malignant. In some cases, cancer cells can also travel to other parts of the body where they will start to grow and replicate, squeezing out healthy cells. The spreading of cancer is called metastasis.

The location of the cancer determines what type it is, and each form varies considerably depending on the location. But cancer can occur in virtually every part of the body.

Different types of cancer grow at different rates and respond to different treatments. The treatment you get depends on the location of your cancer, the stage that it's in, and whether it has spread elsewhere in the body.

According to the American Cancer Society (ACS), cancer is the second-leading cause of death in the United States, just behind heart disease. Half of all men and a third of all women in the United States will develop cancer during their lifetimes. As of 2001, there were approximately

9.8 million Americans still living who had a history of cancer.

The risk for developing cancer depends on many factors including family history and age, but also lifestyle factors that you can control, such as cigarette smoking, your diet, and your weight. But with all types of cancer, early diagnosis is the key. The sooner cancer is found and treated, the better your chances for prolonged survival.

A great deal of the prognosis depends on where the cancer is located, how early the cancer is detected and treated, and the success of any treatment protocol. Treatment of cancer can be rather rigorous, often involving a combination of chemotherapy (drugs), radiation, and surgery. For some people, the treatment is often worse than the disease itself. But trying to sustain a healthy diet during treatment is important. It is also important to deal with specific nutrition problems that arise while you're getting treated. Problems may include weight loss, nausea, lactose intolerance, and changes in taste and smell.

## What It Looks Like

Cancer is an insidious disease that may grow for years before there's a sign that anything is wrong. Many of the signs and symptoms may be vague and will vary depending on where the cancer strikes. People with cancers in the digestive tract for example, may suffer from inexplicable weight loss. Those with bone cancer may experience pain in the affected area. Changes in skin tone may be the result of any of several types of cancer.

According to the ACS, there are some symptoms that are common in certain types of cancer. Signs and symptoms that deserve medical attention include the following:

- Changes in bowel or bladder function, such as diarrhea, pain with urination, or blood in the urine or feces
- Sores that do not heal
- Unusual bleeding or discharge in any part of the body
- Unusual thickening or lumps in any part of the body
- Chronic difficulties with swallowing or indigestion
- Recent change in a wart or mole
- Nagging cough or hoarseness

None of these symptoms, by themselves or in combination, mean you necessarily have cancer, but it's always important to get them checked out if they persist for no apparent reason.

Keep in mind, too, that this list is incomplete—there are many other signs and symptoms that could indicate cancer. The key is to pay attention to the way your body functions and how you feel. If you notice something out of the ordinary, call your doctor and get it checked out. If it is cancer, you'll improve your odds for survival by getting it treated early.

## ¶¶¶ What to Eat

People who have cancer need a well-balanced diet of whole foods that includes at least five servings of fruits and vegetables a day, according to Michele Kearney, M.S., R.D., clinical nutrition coordinator at St. Barnabas Hospital, Bronx, New York. Make it your goal to eat a colorful diet and to include foods such as broccoli, tomatoes, sweet potatoes, apples, carrots, blueberries, and strawberries. These natural plant foods contain cancer-fighting antioxidants. By some estimates, the incidence of cancer could be decreased by 20 percent if all Americans ate at least five servings of fruits and vegetables a day.

If you can't get to the store often, consider eating canned or frozen fruits and vegetables. Sometimes frozen varieties are even healthier than fresh because they're usually ripe when they're first frozen, which seals in the nutrients. If you opt for canned fruits, make sure they are packed in 100 percent fruit juice or water rather than sugar-laden syrup.

Another benefit of fruits and veggies is the high fiber content. Fiber helps eliminate harmful substances from food in a more timely fashion, reducing the amount of contact these substances have with the intestines. In certain instances you might not want to eat too much fiber, however. After surgery for colon or intestinal cancer, or during radiation of this area or the pelvic area, a diet high in fiber may be irritating or make diarrhea worse. Ask your doctor how soon you can increase your fiber intake after these procedures.

# The Macrobiotic Diet

Some people believe that a macrobiotic diet, which is typically low in fat and high in fiber, can help cure them of cancer. The macrobiotic diet and lifestyle were developed by a Japanese philosopher named George Ohsawa. The diet was popularized in the United States by Michio Kushi, who opened the Kushi Institute in Boston in 1978. In addition to cancer, some people credit macrobiotics with healing arthritis, Crohn's disease, and hepatitis.

Macrobiotics is based on the principles of yin and yang in Chinese medicine. Proponents believe that achieving a balance between these two life forces can help promote health and healing. To do that, adherents are urged to eat plant foods, grains, beans, and sea vegetables such as seaweed—all foods that require less energy to produce. At the same time, the diet requires that you avoid animal products, refined sugar, tropical fruits, and soda, all of which require more energy to produce, transport, and store.

Besides outlining specific foods to eat, the macrobiotic diet encourages eating foods in your climate zone and choosing your foods according to what is in season. A macrobiotic diet also involves eating organic foods, preferably picked from your own garden and prepared in your kitchen over a gas stove. People who follow the macrobiotic eating plan generally do not use electric stoves or microwaves.

Not everyone, however, is in favor of following the macrobiotic diet to treat cancer. According to the American Cancer Society, "there is no scientific evidence that a macrobiotic diet is effective in treating cancer. It can lower fat intake and increase fiber, so it can provide general health benefits associated with low-fat/high-fiber diets. However, macrobiotic diets can lead to poor nutrition if not properly planned. Some earlier versions of the diet may actually pose a danger to health."

The prohibition against animal foods in the macrobiotic diet may be especially problematic. Before starting any diet plan, make sure to discuss it with your physician.

Make sure to also eat enough protein, which will help you maintain your strength and help repair healthy cells. Get your protein from lean meats such as chicken and turkey; fish; and legumes and beans. These protein sources are lower in fat and contain healthy nutrients.

Finally, eat plenty of whole grains, be it in the form of bread, pasta, or cereals. Whole grains are rich in fiber and many important vitamins, such as the B vitamins, which are essential for healing. (Again, note the aforementioned exceptions about fiber and certain cancers.)

## What Not to Eat

If you already have cancer, it's best to avoid alcohol, especially while you're undergoing treatment. Alcohol can actually increase the risk for some cancers, such as those of the mouth, throat, liver, breast, and esophagus.

Limit or eliminate completely foods high in sugar such as cakes, cookies, candies, muffins, and pies, which will cause rapid changes in your blood sugar. Avoid soda, sugary juices, and presweetened iced teas too. These foods can cause fatigue and often displace healthier options such as fruit.

Avoid eating a diet high in saturated fat. Too much saturated fat can stress your immune system and promote inflammation. Foods high in saturated fat include red meats, whole dairy foods, and butter, as well as most heavy desserts. If you like to eat meat, do so in moderation.

You should also restrict your intake of caffeine, which may disrupt your sleep. Caffeine is found in coffee, tea, chocolate, and many soft drinks and energy drinks.

Women who have breast or endometrial cancer should be careful about eating soy foods. Soy contains phytoestrogens that may act like the real hormone estrogen. In some cases, too much soy may actually promote the growth of breast and endometrial cancers.

Remember, each cancer is different, and treatments will vary considerably, even among people with the same type of cancer. People with cancers of the digestive tract, for instance, may need to avoid certain fruits and vegetables due to the irritation they might cause. Some treatments may cause diarrhea or vomiting, which may also restrict your food choices. That's why it's important to talk to a registered dietitian about the best foods for you to eat.

## Supplements for Cancer

Ask your doctor about high-quality multivitamins that will provide you with the essential nutrients you need. If your appetite is poor, a multivitamin will be especially important to ensure that you are getting the nutrients you need.

Some people take dietary supplements to enhance their health while battling cancer. Vitamin C, vitamin E, beta carotene, and selenium have all been touted as potent antioxidants that can destroy free radicals causing cell damage.

But during treatment for cancer, it's best to avoid taking supplements because some may interfere with treatment. If you are already taking a supplement—vitamins or herbal remedies—or you want to try a product, make sure to discuss it with your doctor first.

# 📋 Stay-Healthy Strategies

- **GET ENOUGH CALORIES.** Treatment for cancer can squash even the heartiest appetite and cause unhealthy weight loss. Make sure you're getting enough to eat. Try snacking frequently, or ask others for help with meal preparation if necessary.

- **AVOID FOODS THAT STRESS YOUR IMMUNE SYSTEM.** Treatment for cancer often weakens your immune defenses, so avoid foods that could stress your defenses even more. Also avoid aged cheese, undercooked meat, and any raw foods that could potentially harbor pathogens. Don't drink water from wells. Steer clear of anything unpasteurized.

- **GET SUPPORT.** Having cancer can rouse a host of emotions, which can then influence the course of your treatment. Find someone to talk with about difficult emotions. Tap into a social network that can help support you during these times. Or consider joining a support group with other cancer patients.

- **TAKE CONTROL OF STRESS.** Dealing with cancer is stressful enough without having to cope with other sources of anxiety in your life. Look for ways to manage stress in these areas and devote time to relaxation exercises that can help release your stress.

- **CONSULT WITH A REGISTERED DIETITIAN.** He or she can help you design a custom eating plan that addresses your health concerns and needs. Check out the American Dietetic Association Web site at www.eatright.org for a registered dietician near you.

# Preventing Cancer with Diet

The American Cancer Society (ACS) estimates that a third of all deaths from cancer are linked to poor diet and a lack of exercise. Wiser food choices and regular exercise could prevent approximately 186,000 cancer deaths each year, according to the ACS. In addition to exercising 30 minutes a day, most days of the week, the ACS recommends the following dietary strategies for cancer prevention:

- **EAT LESS FAT.** A diet high in fat, especially saturated fat, promotes cancer. So opt for lean meats and low-fat dairy foods. Substitute butter and lard with healthier vegetable oils. Eat fruit instead of high-fat desserts.

- **WATCH YOUR WEIGHT.** Being overweight is a risk factor for specific cancers such as those of the uterus, colon, breast, prostate, and kidneys. Getting regular exercise, limiting portions, and choosing your foods wisely will go a long way in helping you to maintain a healthy weight.

- **BOOST YOUR INTAKE OF FRUITS AND VEGGIES.** These natural foods are rich in phytochemicals, vitamins and minerals that can arrest the free radical damage to cells caused by oxidation. Make them the staple of your diet. You might even consider eating a few vegetarian meals every week.

- **EAT FIBER.** A diet rich in high-fiber foods speeds up transit time, the amount of time food spends in your digestive tract. Foods that linger for too long—typically the high-fat varieties—are given more time to wreak havoc on the body. Eating a lot of high-fiber foods will speed up the process and sweep out the bad foods before they can do too much damage.

- **LIMIT YOUR BARBECUES.** Everyone likes a good barbecue on a summer day, but enjoy these events sparingly. Grilling creates carcinogens that are potentially as harmful to the body as the toxins in cigarettes.

- **AVOID CERTAIN MEATS.** Ham, bacon, hot dogs, and pastrami are all meats that are high in nitrates and nitrites, substances linked to stomach cancer.

- **CRUNCH PICKLES IN MODERATION.** Pickling foods produces nitrates and nitrites, harmful toxins that boost your risk for cancer. People from countries like Japan and Korea, where pickled foods are a staple of the diet, typically have higher rates of stomach cancer.

- **WATCH YOUR WEIGHT.** The risk of dying from any form of cancer goes up as your weight increases, according to a 2003 study in *The New England Journal of Medicine*. The risk was especially pronounced in women. So watch your portions and choose your foods wisely.

- **EAT FOOD, NOT SUPPLEMENTS.** Studies have shown that some vitamins and minerals may offer protection from certain cancers. A diet rich in fruits and vegetables—many of which contain vitamin C, beta carotene, and other nutrients—has been associated with a reduction in oral, esophageal, stomach, pancreatic, cervical, rectal, breast, and lung cancers. But studies on supplements of vitamin C did not find the same protective benefits.

- **DRINK ALCOHOL IN MODERATION.** Excess drinking raises your risk for certain cancers, including those of the liver, esophagus, and throat. So if you do drink, limit it to one drink a day for women and two for men.

# CANDIDIASIS

WE ALL HAVE *CANDIDA ALBICANS* living in our bodies. This exotic-sounding yeast lurks in the gastrointestinal tract, mouth, women's vaginas, and even in parts of the skin. In healthy amounts, the yeast causes no harm. But when the yeast in your intestine grows unchecked, it may activate your immune system to cause a condition known as candida hypersensitivity syndrome, or candidiasis.

The yeast can grow out of control for numerous reasons. Excess use of antibiotics can wipe out the healthy bacteria that inhibit the growth of *Candida*. A diet high in carbohydrates can nourish the yeast and encourage overgrowth. Having diabetes or being pregnant makes you vulnerable to yeast overgrowth as well. You may also develop candidiasis if you have a weak immune system brought on by infections such as HIV. In addition, candidiasis is likely to occur in people who suffer from malnutrition, undergo chemotherapy, use birth control pills, or take steroids such as prednisone.

Any of these factors may allow the yeast to invade your tissues, which then triggers an immune reaction to the yeast. As the immune system breaks down the yeast, toxins are released, which get absorbed and circulated throughout the body. These toxins can interact with our bodies in a wide variety of ways, causing many different kinds of symptoms.

But candidiasis isn't always easily diagnosed, and many conventional doctors are not quick to consider yeast overgrowth as the source of illness. Some experts believe it plays a role in conditions such as fibromyalgia and chronic fatigue syndrome. Diagnosis is based on a combination of signs and self-reported symptoms, which can be extracted with a questionnaire that asks about food cravings, drug treatments, and symptoms. In addition, a blood test that looks for antibodies attached to yeast particles can be taken.

The goal in treating candidiasis is to reduce the yeast, says Michael McNett, M.D., owner and medical director of a multidisciplinary fibromyalgia treatment center in Chicago and co-author of *The Everything Health Guide to Fibromyalgia*. He says there are three strategies to treatment: starve the yeast by eliminating its food source (sugar) through diet, kill it with the use of antifungal drugs, and inhibit its growth with the aid of yeast-inhibiting bacteria.

The good news is that you don't have to live with candidiasis forever. Proper treatment for four to six months and a healthy diet that's sustained for the long run can eventually get the yeast under control. You can even resume eating a regular diet, with the exception of foods like refined sugar and white flour.

If you ever become ill or need treatments that may promote yeast overgrowth, such as antibiotics, you may need to resume taking antifungal drugs or become stricter with your diet for a while until the high-risk phase ends. In any case, keeping candidiasis in check will definitely involve a major overhaul of your eating habits.

## Healthy Avoidance

Some people are prone to yeast infections or candidiasis. If that's you, take steps to reduce the growth of yeast.

- **ASTHMATICS.** If you're on long-term steroids for the treatment of asthma, rinse your mouth after each inhalation.

- **BABIES.** If you have a baby prone to diaper rash, make sure to keep her diaper area clean, dry, and exposed to air.

- **WOMEN.** Look for another method of birth control if you're on oral contraceptives. If you get frequent vaginal yeast infections, don't use hygiene sprays and douches.

- **DIABETICS.** Try to get control of your blood glucose levels. Note: In some cases, candidiasis may be a sign of diabetes.

## What It Looks Like

The signs and symptoms of candidiasis are wide and varied. People with candidiasis are frequently fatigued and have low energy and motivation. They may also have pain, muscle aches, memory problems, depression, abdominal pain, loss of libido, and anxiety. Some people may experience numbness and tingling. Women may have menstrual irregularities, endometriosis, and vaginal burning, itching, or discharge. In addition, you may feel drowsy, irritable, and moody.

Other symptoms include sore throat, body odor, chest pain, indigestion, ear pain, and nasal congestion. As you can see, there are numerous symptoms for candidiasis, and they will differ considerably from one patient to the next. The severity of the symptoms also varies, and some people may experience symptoms intermittently.

People with candidiasis may notice, too, that they frequently crave sweets. They may have trouble sleeping and struggle with focus and concentration. For a complete listing of symptoms, ask your doctor for the candidiasis questionnaire (the questionnaire can also be found at www.yeastconnection.com).

## What to Eat

A high-quality diet is important for people with candidiasis. Focus on eating a diet filled with low-starch vegetables such as celery, cabbage, broccoli, cauliflower, leafy greens, brussels sprouts, squash, asparagus, radishes, onions, tomatoes, bell peppers, and green beans. Other good veggie choices that can be eaten in moderation include carrots, beets, peas, avocado, turnips, parsnips, and eggplant.

Try to eat a diet rich in whole grains, which will supply you with energy but not excess sugar. Good sources include brown rice, wild rice, millet, oatmeal, oat bran, barley, wheat, rye, and corn. Choose whole grain products, such as whole wheat pasta, over refined ones, such as ordinary pasta.

For protein, eat lean meats such as chicken, fish, and turkey, making sure to steer clear of the smoked and processed varieties. You can also eat legumes such as lentils, beans, and peas, which are rich in fiber and protein.

If you enjoy fruit, eat just two small servings a day at two separate times. This will minimize the amount of sugar (fructose occurs naturally in fruit) you ingest in one sitting.

Try to eat unsweetened yogurt regularly. Look for yogurts that contain *Lactobacillus acidophilus* cultures, healthy bacteria that help keep yeast in check. Some experts also advise drinking kefir, a cultured product made of milk that contains several strains of healthy bacteria as well as healthy yeasts that keep pathogens and parasites in check.

Finally, consider drinking pau d'arco tea, a type of tea derived from the inner bark of a South American tree. The tea acts as an antifungal and antibacterial remedy and may aid in your recovery.

## ⊘ What Not to Eat

Start by reducing your carbohydrates, especially the simple ones such as cookies, cakes, and other products that contain refined sugar. By eating fewer carbs, you starve the yeast and keep it from proliferating.

Do not eat anything with high concentrations of sweeteners, either natural or artificial. That means you should avoid anything made with refined sugar, artificial sweeteners (aspartame, sucralose, etc), dehydrated cane juice, honey, corn or maple syrup, molasses, and malt.

Steer clear of foods that contain yeast, including breads, pastries, pizza crust, beer and wine, vinegar, and anything that contains vinegar, such as ketchup, pickles, and certain salad dressings. In addition, you need to avoid foods that contain mold, such as aged cheese and mushrooms.

To enhance overall health, avoid eating fast foods, junk foods, and soft drinks, which are generally loaded with empty calories—energy with no nutritional value. The goal is to build up your health and immunity.

# The Specific Carbohydrate Diet

Some people have treated their candidiasis with help from the Specific Carbohydrate (SC) Diet, which was popularized by Elaine Gottschall, author of the book *Breaking the Vicious Cycle*. The SC Diet works by taming yeast and bacterial overgrowth. People who are on it eat few or no carbohydrates and instead focus on eating foods that contain monosaccharides, carbohydrates that are rapidly absorbed and more easily digested.

The SC Diet is based on the premise that sicknesses such as candidiasis, Crohn's disease, and ulcerative colitis are caused by an imbalance of intestinal flora. Too many of the wrong carbohydrates lure microbes to the intestinal tract. These microbes then digest unused carbs through the process of fermentation. This process results in the overproduction of lactic acid and unhealthy gases, which in turn, perpetuates the growth of harmful bacteria.

The SC Diet is intended to restore intestinal imbalance. More specifically, it requires that you eat fresh, raw, or frozen vegetables, legumes (only after symptoms stop, and they must be soaked for 10 to 12 hours before consumption), unprocessed meats, natural cheeses low in lactose, homemade yogurt, most fruits, and select oils including olive, coconut, soybean, and corn.

The diet also restricts many foods. It prohibits all flour, all sugars except honey and saccharin, and all starchy foods such as bread, potatoes, yams, and pasta. You must also avoid all milk products (except homemade yogurt fermented for 24 hours), canned vegetables, all grains (e.g., rice, wheat, corn, oats, etc), canola oil, mayonnaise, ice cream, candy, chocolate, and products that contain baking powder.

By following the SC Diet, proponents say, you can restore balance to your digestive tract and tame the bacterial overgrowth that is making you sick. Over time, the diet is believed to heal the gut, which will in turn relieve you of your symptoms. Check out www.scdiet.org or www.breakingtheviciouscycle.org for more details. For specific information on foods that are allowed and how to prepare homemade yogurt, pick up the book *Breaking the Vicious Cycle*.

## 🫛 Supplements for Candidiasis

Take a daily multivitamin to nourish your body with the essential nutrients you need for good health. Add a supplement that contains *acidophilus*, the friendly bacteria that helps inhibit yeast growth and restore balance to your body. After six months, you'll have significantly less yeast in your body.

In people who do not respond to antifungal medications such as nystatin, herbal remedies may be considered. Ones that are commonly used include the following:

### CAPRYLIC ACID

Caprylic acid is a fatty acid that has antifungal powers. It may lessen the ability of the yeast to grow and proliferate.

### UVA URSI

Uva ursi is an herbal remedy better known for combating urinary tract infections. It acts an astringent and can kill bacteria.

### BERBERINE

Berberine is an herbal treatment for yeast and fungus infections caused by *Candida*.

### GARLIC

This aromatic spice helps fight infection and enhances immunity. Look for supplements that contain allicin, the active ingredient.

### FRUCTOOLIGOSACCHARIDES

Fructooligosaccharides are sugars that feed *acidophilus* and may help promote healthy bacteria.

## 📋 Stay-Healthy Strategies

- **TAKE TIME OUT FOR YOURSELF.** Stress exacerbates candidiasis, so it's important to relax and reduce stress.

- **EXERCISE REGULARLY.** Getting some activity every day will help build your energy.

- **ELIMINATE FOOD ALLERGENS,** which can aggravate candidiasis and weaken immunity. If necessary, follow an elimination diet by removing potentially allergenic foods from your diet, then gradually reintroducing them

- **STEER CLEAR OF ANTIBIOTICS**—they're a leading cause of candidiasis. Ask your doctor not to prescribe them to you unless they are absolutely necessary.

# CANKER SORES

ANYONE WHO HAS EVER HAD A CANKER SORE can tell you how much they hurt. Tiny as they may be, these shallow sores inside the mouth can cause incredible pain for their sufferers, especially if there are several sores at once.

Unlike cold sores, which tend to appear on the lip, canker sores occur inside the mouth. They may develop inside your lips, on the insides of your cheeks, under your tongue, or at the base of your gums. And unlike cold sores, which are caused by a virus, canker sores are the result of inflammation.

Canker sores can occur in anyone at any age, but they seem to be more common in women, especially younger women in their teens and 20s. They also occur in children. Experts estimate that about 50 percent of all people get canker sores at one time or another.

The cause of canker sores is a mystery, but some experts suspect the immune system plays a role. There may also be a genetic link, so that children whose parents get canker sores may be prone to getting them too. Stress, poor nutrition, food allergies and sensitivities to certain foods, and menstrual periods appear to be possible triggers.

Most canker sores go away without any treatment. Adults with severe ulcers may be prescribed tetracycline or a topical anesthetic to relieve pain. You can also try applying hydrogen peroxide diluted with water, ice chips, or milk of magnesia to the sore to reduce pain. Ultimately, the best treatment is the passage of time.

## What They Look Like

Canker sores are usually round with a red edge and a white interior that resembles a crater. Some people may notice a tingling or burning sensation shortly before the sore appears. Others may develop a canker sore after burning or biting the area where the sore appears.

Once they appear, canker sores hang around for about seven to ten days before they start to heal. Complete healing can sometimes take as long as a month, depending in part on the size of the canker sore. As they heal, the sores may develop a grayish hue.

In rare cases, canker sores may be accompanied by fever, malaise, and swollen glands. These other symptoms may or may not be related to the canker sore, and you may want to consult your physician if you notice them.

## 🍴 What to Eat

Boost your intake of foods that support the immune system, such as fruits and vegetables, which contain plenty of vitamin C, says Fred Pescatore, M.D., author of *The Allergy and Asthma Cure*. Good choices include leafy greens, broccoli, red peppers, and cantaloupe. Make sure you're eating foods that contain vitamin B6, vitamin B12, and folic acid—all essential B vitamins that may be lacking in people vulnerable to recurrent canker sores. Good sources of vitamin B6 include brewer's yeast, whole grains, and nuts. Vitamin B12 is found in lean meats such as chicken and pork, and also in fish and soybean products. Healthy sources for folic acid include whole grains, spinach, and wheat germ.

Eat foods rich in iron to restore a possible deficiency. Iron is found in red meat, chicken, and pork, and also in bran and whole-grain foods. You should also eat yogurt, which contains *Lactobacillus acidophilus*, a healthy bacteria that supports immunity.

## 🚫 What Not to Eat

Stay away from highly acidic foods such as tomatoes, citrus fruits, and coffee. You should also avoid milk and spices such as chili pepper, pepper, paprika, cayenne, nutmeg, and cinnamon. In addition, do not eat foods high in nitrates, which occur in higher amounts in processed meats. Bacon, sausage, and ham, for instance, are all high in nitrates. You should also eliminate wine since it contains nitrates as well.

Consider doing an elimination diet to pinpoint any food allergies that may be involved in the development of canker sores. Try eliminating foods that contain gluten—namely wheat, rye, barley, and oats—from your diet, then gradually reintroducing them.

## 💊 Supplements for Canker Sores

Start with a high-quality multivitamin, which will ensure you get enough of the essential nutrients. You might also talk to your doctor about taking some other supplements including:

### VITAMIN C

Vitamin C is an antioxidant that will help bolster the immune system.

### B COMPLEX VITAMINS

Studies have found that people prone to canker sores are often deficient in several B vitamins, including folic acid, thiamin, pyridoxine (B6), and B12. A quality B complex vitamin will promote healing and help reduce stress.

### IRON

Find out whether you have an iron deficiency, then add an iron supplement to your diet. Some people with canker sores may be deficient in this mineral. Note: Men and postmenopausal women should talk to a physician before taking iron because too much iron in these populations can cause organ damage.

## LYSINE

Although best known for its benefits for cold sore sufferers, lysine may also help prevent outbreaks of canker sores.

## DGL

Deglycyrrhizinated licorice (DGL) is derived from licorice, but does not contain glycyrrhizic acid. In one study, DGL caused improvements in canker sores in just one day.

## Stay-Healthy Strategies

- **AVOID TOOTHPASTES THAT CONTAIN SODIUM LAURYL SULFATE (SLS).** Toothpastes that contain SLS may dry out the mucous lining in the mouth and raise the risk for canker sores.

- **MINIMIZE STRESS.** Stress may make you vulnerable to canker stores, so look for ways to avoid stressful situations or do relaxation exercises that help control it. Consider taking up yoga or meditation to relieve stress.

- **DON'T EAT FOODS THAT ARE HARD, CHEWY, OR CRUNCHY.** Avoid chewing gum too. All these substances may cause trauma to your mouth.

- **COVER THEM UP.** Over-the-counter remedies such as Anbesol or Orabase provide a protective sealant that can make it easier to eat and drink with a canker sore.

> ### TIP
>
> *Practice good oral hygiene. Brushing and flossing regularly do more than protect your teeth. These habits can also help you avoid canker sores. So brush after meals and floss once a day. Use a soft toothbrush so you don't irritate your gums or an active sore.*

# CELIAC DISEASE

MANY PEOPLE TODAY ARE ACCUSTOMED to reading food labels to find out the amount of nutrients they're getting. But for the millions of people who suffer from celiac disease, careful scrutiny of a food label is essential for survival.

Celiac disease is an autoimmune and intestinal disorder in which the body cannot tolerate gluten. Gluten is a protein found in wheat, rye, and barley. It is the substance that gives kneaded dough its elasticity—the ingredient that makes soft pretzels, pizza dough, and bagels so delightfully chewy. But for people with celiac disease, gluten can be as toxic as a poison.

In someone with celiac disease, gluten damages the villi in the lining of the small intestine and inhibits the absorption of critical nutrients. Villi are the fingerlike protrusions that help enable the proper absorption of nutrients from food. But in people with celiac disease, consuming gluten disrupts this process. As a result, the person with undiagnosed or untreated celiac disease becomes malnourished and will experience a range of symptoms.

According to the National Institute of Diabetes and Digestive and Kidney Diseases (NIDDK), approximately two million people in the United States suffer from celiac disease. The condition may start in infancy or childhood but is most likely to begin in adulthood. The condition has a strong genetic component: If you have celiac disease, about 5 to 15 percent of your first-degree relatives (siblings, parents, children) will also have the condition. Celiac disease is also more common among people with type 1 diabetes and Down syndrome.

There is no cure for celiac disease. The only treatment is to eat a gluten-free diet, which can be enormously challenging. But strict adherence to such a diet is also quite successful at relieving sufferers from the pain and discomfort associated with celiac disease. In addition, adhering to the diet will allow the intestine to heal and to start absorbing nutrients normally again.

## What It Looks Like

Celiac disease resembles many other health conditions, which is one reason why it can be hard to diagnose. To make matters worse, symptoms vary widely and can fluctuate. Many people endure years of testing and doctor visits before being properly diagnosed.

According to the NIDDK, symptoms may include one or more of the following:

- Gas
- Abdominal bloating and pain
- Chronic diarrhea
- Constipation
- Pale, foul-smelling, or fatty stool
- Weight loss or gain
- Fatigue
- Joint pain
- Bone pain
- Behavioral changes
- Tingling numbness in the legs
- Muscle cramps
- Absence of menstruation
- Failure to thrive in infants
- Delayed growth in children
- Infertility or recurrent miscarriage
- Sores inside the mouth
- Tooth discoloration or loss of enamel

Over time, celiac disease may result in other medical problems. Some people become anemic and have a low red blood cell count. Others will develop osteoporosis (low bone density) or osteopenia (low bone mass). Some people develop an itchy skin rash called dermatitis herpetiformis, a condition that confirms you have celiac disease. Many people become lactose intolerant.

The key to obtaining an accurate diagnosis is getting a blood test that looks for certain autoantibodies, substances in the blood that attack the body's own healthy tissues. Unlike antibodies, which defend the body against invaders such as viruses and bacteria, autoantibodies can be the cause of disease. Your doctor may also do a biopsy of the small intestine to examine it for damage.

As serious as it is, celiac disease can be successfully managed through diet. Avoiding foods that contain gluten can actually help reverse the damage and prevent symptoms from recurring.

## ￦ What to Eat

Because celiac disease is treated entirely with diet, it's essential that you consult a registered dietitian for guidance, says Lola O'Rourke, R.D., a spokesperson for the American Dietetic Association (ADA). A registered dietician can help you find new sources of foods that provide the nutrients you still need, even as you give up foods that contain gluten.

The key is looking for foods that are gluten-free. In general, fruits, vegetables, fish, rice, beans, and meat are safe, provided they are not served with any sauces or dressings that may contain gluten. Make sure to select condiments, seasonings, and sauces that are gluten-free.

Safe grains include products made from corn, rice, potato, and whole bean flours. That means products such as rice noodles, puffed corn, rice cakes, corn tortillas, and popped corn are all safe.

All dairy products, including milk and yogurt are okay, too, unless they contain gluten additives. Any lactose intolerance is likely to go away once you start eating a gluten-free diet.

# What Not to Eat

Become a vigilant label reader and steer clear of any foods that contain gluten. The list of foods that contain gluten is quite extensive and includes foods you may not suspect, such as egg substitutes and beer. You must also avoid anything made with wheat, rye, and barley, all which contain gluten. It's also important to avoid oats. Although oats themselves do not contain gluten, they are typically grown and/or processed in close proximity to wheat and other grains, raising the risk for cross-contamination. It wasn't until recently that some growers started ensuring that their oats are gluten-free, but these are only now becoming available.

## Eating Away from Home

For someone with celiac disease, eating on the road can be tricky. Even grabbing a sandwich in the office cafeteria can be hazardous. When you eat out, be diligent. Ask your server if he can find out how a food is prepared or what it contains. Find out if the restaurant offers a gluten-free menu. When in doubt, stick with the plainer version of a food.

If you're going to a party, consider bringing your own food. Explain that you have to eat your own food for health reasons. You might also consider eating something beforehand so you're less apt to eat mindlessly.

Of all the foods to avoid, wheat is probably the toughest to escape. Wheat is a primary ingredient in numerous foods and products, including breakfast cereals, crackers, pasta, and baked goods. Wheat derivatives are found in less obvious foods such as soy sauce and texture enhancing products. But it's essential for anyone with celiac disease to ban wheat from her diet.

The only way to know if a food contains gluten is to check the ingredient list on the label. Certain ingredients are a tip-off to the presence of wheat. According to the ADA, these are just a few ingredients to avoid:

- Malt or cereal extracts
- Malt flavoring
- Thickeners that contain wheat
- Emulsifiers
- Stabilizers
- Food starch and modified food starch that come from wheat
- Hydrolyzed vegetable protein derived from wheat
- Enriched flour

In addition to label reading, remember the importance of consulting a registered dietitian, who can equip you with the skills it takes to identify foods that contain gluten.

## Supplements for Celiac Disease

The supplements you might take for celiac disease vary depending on the nutrients you may be missing since you've had celiac disease. To find out which ones you need, consult your doctor or dietitian for advice.

## Stay-Healthy Strategies

- **GET SUPPORT.** Celiac disease can be overwhelming. To help make it more bearable, consider getting in touch with a support group through the Celiac Disease Foundation (www.celiac.org) or the Celiac Sprue Association (www.csaceliacs.org).

- **CONSIDER COOKING MORE OFTEN,** instead of eating out. Try picking up a gluten-free cookbook and experimenting with a new recipe.

- **IF YOU DON'T HAVE TIME TO COOK, EXPLORE AN ETHNIC CUISINE, SUCH AS MEXICAN OR ASIAN—** these cuisines often offer many delicious gluten-free options.

- **BE WARY OF MEDICATIONS.** Certain drugs may contain gluten. Always ask the pharmacist before taking a new drug.

- **INVOLVE YOUR FAMILY.** Teach them about your condition and how you now have to eat. Try to familiarize them with the foods you eat so that you aren't always preparing extra dishes at every meal.

- **CONSIDER THE SPECIFIC CARBOHYDRATE DIET,** described on page 75. The plan involves eating few or no carbohydrates while emphasizing foods such as fresh and frozen vegetables, and natural cheeses and yogurt.

# CHRONIC FATIGUE SYNDROME

ALMOST EVERYONE SUFFERS FROM FATIGUE at one time or another. But chronic fatigue syndrome (CFS), also called chronic fatigue and immune deficiency syndrome (CFIDS), is much more destructive than the normal tiredness that comes with not getting enough sleep. People with CFS suffer from a fatigue that is strong, persistent, and debilitating, often making you too weak to perform everyday tasks. With CFS, you're tired even after a good night's rest.

According to the U.S. Centers for Disease Control and Prevention, approximately 500,000 Americans, mostly women, suffer from CFS. When the condition first emerged in the 1980s, CFS was called the "yuppie flu" because most sufferers were young, upper class professionals, or yuppies. These women were typically in their 30s and 40s, very well-educated, and ranked among the middle and upper socioeconomic classes. Today, we know that anyone of any age and background can be affected by CFS.

The cause of CFS, however, remains a mystery. Some studies have suggested that a chronic, low-grade viral infection may be involved. And because there are no blood tests or clinical signs that distinguish CFS, diagnosis can be difficult. A doctor must rely on the patient's description of the symptoms, and some people—medical professionals included—are skeptical that CFS even exists. Often, the condition is diagnosed after other conditions such as hypothyroidism, depression, and fibromyalgia are first ruled out. But CFS can also coexist with these conditions.

## Mixed Up with Fibromyalgia

It isn't always easy to distinguish chronic fatigue syndrome (CFS) from fibromyalgia. Even doctors can't always separate the two conditions. Patients with CFS often experience some pain, while those with fibromyalgia are frequently fatigued. In some cases, it may simply depend on the doctor you see and the level of expertise he has in one condition or the other.

But subtle differences do exist. Fibromyalgia is often linked to an injury or trauma. CFS typically starts off like a bad bout of flu. People who have CFS typically don't have tender points, sensitive spots on their bodies that hurt when pressed. And in research, people with CFS are less likely to have high levels of substance P, a chemical that has been associated with greater levels of pain in people with fibromyalgia.

Unfortunately, there is no treatment for CFS or CFIDS at the current time. The goal, rather, is to make lifestyle modifications that can help lessen the symptoms. Eating a balanced diet, getting an adequate amount of sleep (strive for at least 8 hours per night), and exercising regularly can all help do that.

## 🔎 What It Looks Like

Fatigue is the predominant symptom in CFS. According to criteria established by a scientific panel of experts and published in the *Annals of Internal Medicine*, you may be diagnosed with CFS if you have severe chronic fatigue that has lasted longer than six months without the presence of any other medical conditions. At the same time, you must have at least four of the following symptoms:

- Substantial impairment in short-term memory or concentration
- Sore throat
- Tender lymph nodes
- Muscle pain
- Joint pain in several joints without swelling or redness
- Headaches that seem different in severity, type, and pattern than those you've experienced in the past
- Unrefreshing sleep
- A feeling of malaise after exertion, lasting more than twenty-four hours

Some people may also experience fever, abdominal cramps, allergies, weight loss, rapid pulse, chest pain, night sweats, rash, and chest pain. However, if you have another documented illness that can cause these symptoms and chronic fatigue, such as cancer or hepatitis, your doctor will not diagnose you with CFS.

## 🍴 What to Eat

Consider eating a vegan diet for three months, then transitioning to a vegetarian diet, says Lisa Dorfman, M.S., R.D., a spokesperson for the American Dietetic Association and author of *The Tropical Diet*. Vegan diets contain no animal products at all, meaning you do not eat fish or dairy products. A vegetarian diet, on the other hand, may include these foods.

A vegan diet will improve your immunity, lower your body-mass index, and reduce any pain and stiffness. It may also help improve the quality of your sleep. Good foods to eat include uncooked vegetables, berries, nuts, fruits, seeds, and sprouts. These foods have high levels of carotenoids and vitamins C and E, which help reduce joint stiffness.

## 🚫 What Not to Eat

Avoid highly processed foods, which are often limited or deficient in magnesium and manganese, two important minerals. Magnesium is involved in the energy production of body cells. Manganese aids in the metabolism of energy-producing nutrients. Also, be wary of eating foods rich in vitamin B1 (thiamin). Thiamin can sometimes cause pain in people with CFS. Foods that contain B1 include whole-grain breads, rice, and pasta; fortified cereals; liver, beef, and pork; and beans and legumes.

Steer clear of high-fat foods as well. A diet that contains too much fat, especially the saturated variety or trans fats can promote weight gain and worsen pain and stiffness.

## Supplements for CFS

According to Dorfman, no supplements have been proven beneficial to patients with CFS, contrary to many claims you might read. However, you may want to consider taking a quality multivitamin to make sure you're getting the essential nutrients. Other supplements you may want to consider include the following:

### VITAMIN C

This immune-boosting antioxidant may help strengthen immunity and decrease pain.

### VITAMIN E

Vitamin E provides the same benefits as vitamin C. But be careful to consult a physician first and to limit your intake of vitamin E because too much may be harmful.

### B VITAMIN COMPLEX

A quality B vitamin complex may help boost flagging energy levels.

### MAGNESIUM

This essential mineral can help in the production of cellular energy.

### FISH OIL

Taking fish oil can sometimes reduce the pain and inflammation that occurs in people with CFS. Be careful of taking fish oil, however, if you are taking a blood-thinning medication such as warfarin (Coumadin) or aspirin.

## Stay-Healthy Strategies

- **MAKE A SERIOUS EFFORT TO EXERCISE.** Studies have found that even moderate amounts of exercise can reduce symptoms in most people with CFS.

- **CONSULT WITH A REGISTERED DIETITIAN** to assess dietary patterns and look for factors that might cause CFS symptoms and deficiencies.

- **TAME YOUR STRESS.** Avoid doing too much and practice strategies for managing stress, such as meditation or tai chi.

- **RESORT TO MEDICATIONS IF NECESSARY.** Some people find relief with low-dose tricyclic antidepressants such as Elavil or selective serotonin reuptake inhibitors such as Prozac, which improve sleep quality and decrease fatigue.

- **GET SUPPORT.** Talk to friends and family about your frustrations. Consider joining a support group. If necessary, consult with a mental health professional.

# Do You Need a Detox Diet?

Detoxifying your body may help some people overcome some of the symptoms of chronic fatigue. The basic idea behind a detox diet is to purge your body of chemicals, toxins, and additives that are causing uncomfortable symptoms such as fatigue, headaches, pain, or congestion.

According to Elson Haas, M.D., author of *The New Detox Diet*, eating a non-toxic diet involves eating organic foods whenever possible, focusing on fruits, vegetables, whole grains, legumes, nuts and seeds, fresh fish, organic poultry, and certain low-fat dairy foods. Eating non-toxic also involves avoiding over-the-counter, prescription, and recreational drugs, and replacing them with natural remedies such as herbal supplements and homeopathic treatments. In addition, detoxing requires that you drink filtered water, avoid alcohol, coffee, saturated fats, refined foods, sugar, salt, canned foods, coffee, and all red, cured, and organ meats.

Other variations of detoxification involve eating nothing but fresh fruits, a diet of just fresh fruits and vegetables, a raw foods diet, or liquid cleanses or fasts. In each form, water plays an essential role in the daily diet.

Not everyone can benefit from a full-blown detox diet, and each detox should be customized for individual circumstances. For example, some people should limit their detox to just three days, while others may need supplements to supply essential nutrients. Before attempting any of these detox programs, you should consult a supportive health professional who can advise you on the best detox diet for you.

# CHRONIC OBSTRUCTIVE PULMONARY DISEASE

IT'S A FRIGHTENING MOMENT when you can't catch your breath. You gasp. Your heartbeat quickens. Perhaps you start to panic. For people who have chronic obstructive pulmonary disease (COPD), everyday breathing can be constant a challenge.

COPD is actually a combination of two distinct diseases of the lungs: chronic bronchitis and emphysema. Both conditions are characterized by obstruction to airflow, making it hard to breathe normally. Often, people who have one condition also have the other one.

Here in the United States, approximately twelve million adults over the age of 25 have been diagnosed with COPD. Another twenty-four million adults have impaired lung function. Symptoms may be mild, but they can also be debilitating, making it hard to perform everyday tasks. COPD is the fourth-leading cause of death in the United States.

In recent years, COPD has started to take a greater toll on women than on men. Between 1980 and 2000, the number of women who died from COPD doubled and in 2000 surpassed the number of men who died from the condition. According to the American Lung Association, female smokers are nearly thirteen times more likely to die from COPD than women who have never smoked. Male smokers are twelve times as likely to die as men who have never smoked.

The primary cause of COPD is smoking. The condition is also influenced by air pollution, secondhand smoke, and a family or childhood history of respiratory infections. People who

work in jobs that expose them to industrial pollutants are at greater risk for COPD as well.

What exactly are the two conditions that compose COPD? Chronic bronchitis is the inflammation and scarring of the lining of the bronchial tubes, the tubes that lead to each lung. The inflammation makes it harder for air to flow to and from the lungs, causing a buildup of heavy mucus or phlegm. Eventually, the lining becomes thickened and the airflow is permanently restricted, causing scarring in the lungs. The irritation in the bronchial tubes also paves the way for bacterial infections, which further impedes air flow.

Emphysema, on the other hand, occurs when the air sacs, also called the alveoli, in the lungs are damaged. The air sacs play a vital role in our breathing—they're the site where oxygen, which the body needs, is exchanged for carbon dioxide, which the body is trying to eliminate. Over time, less oxygen is transferred into the bloodstream, causing shortness of breath. The damage eventually results in the lungs becoming increasingly stiff. The stiffness makes it hard for the airways to remain open, and exhaling becomes difficult too.

COPD develops slowly, and quality of life gradually diminishes. Breathing becomes increasingly difficult, and eventually, people with COPD may require supplemental oxygen. COPD also interferes with the individual's ability to engage in everyday activities and can make it difficult to sleep.

Unfortunately, there is no cure for COPD, only the management of symptoms. Drugs that relax and open the airways to the lungs are critical to managing air flow. For some people, lung transplants become an option.

Many people live for years with COPD. Quitting smoking, taking the right medications, and making efforts to lead a healthy lifestyle can help ensure that. And while there is no dietary cure for COPD, a healthy eating plan can make you feel better and improve your quality of life.

## What It Looks Like

In its earliest stages, COPD causes no symptoms. But even without any obvious signs or symptoms, the damage in the lungs is slowly developing. Eventually, people with COPD will experience wheezing, which often sounds like a whistle or a squeak; shortness of breath, especially during any kind of exertion; and fatigue. Even simple activities of daily living, such as taking a bath, may cause difficulties with breathing. Most people also develop a cough that may or may not produce mucus.

Many people with COPD experience inexplicable weight loss. That's because they expend extra calories just trying to breathe. They may also battle frequent and long-lasting bouts of lung infections such as the flu and pneumonia. In addition, COPD can sometimes cause swelling as the lack of oxygen begins to affect the heart's ability to effectively pump blood.

## What to Eat

Many people with COPD frequently suffer from malnutrition, says Christine Gerbstadt, M.D., R.D., a spokesperson for the American Dietetic Association. The extra exertion required for breathing can lead to being underweight and nutritionally deficient. That's why eating a healthy diet is critical for people with COPD. A healthy diet will also help prevent infections, especially lung infections, which are common in people with COPD.

Start by making sure to eat plenty of foods rich in antioxidant vitamins. These foods are also abundant in fiber, which will help with digestion and prevent constipation. Good sources of these foods include whole grain breads and cereals, fruits, and vegetables. But choose your vegetables and fruits wisely, and limit those that might promote gas. Too much gas can put pressure on your diaphragm and make breathing more difficult.

People with COPD are often short of breath and lack the stamina for preparing a meal. If you're suffering from lack of energy, eat healthy foods that require little or no preparation. Good foods include fresh fruit, dried fruit, cereals, eggs, cheese, yogurt, and sandwiches.

If you have COPD and are taking diuretics to reduce swelling, you may need to eat more potassium. Good sources of potassium include bananas, asparagus, potatoes, and tomatoes.

Consider eating small meals throughout the day. Digesting one big meal requires more energy, and therefore oxygen, which can be a strain on someone with COPD. While eating, sit up straight and eat small bites. Chew slowly and breathe steadily while you eat. Drink your beverages at the end of the meal, so that you don't fill up on liquids at the expense of food.

If you are underweight, talk to a registered dietitian or your physician about how to gain weight. You might need to eat more high-calorie snacks and to eat more frequently.

## What Not to Eat

Avoid foods and beverages that cause gas, such as apples, avocados, beans, broccoli, cabbage, cauliflower, melons, corn, peppers, and onions. You might also want to avoid carbonated drinks, greasy foods, and spicy foods.

Limit your salt intake. Read nutrition labels and avoid foods that contain more than 300 mg of sodium per serving. Too much sodium can cause water retention, which will make it harder to breathe. If you want to use a salt substitute, consult a registered dietitian or physician first. Certain substances in salt substitutes can also cause water retention.

## Supplements for COPD

Taking a quality multivitamin can help ensure that you get the nutrients you need, but most people with COPD will not benefit from other supplements. People who are having trouble eating and sustaining their weight, however, may need to consult a registered dietitian about taking specific nutritional supplements with ample calories and nutrients.

## Stay-Healthy Strategies

- **TRY TO MAINTAIN A CLEAN ENVIRONMENT.** Do not allow anyone to smoke in your house, car, or work site. Try to reduce dust and fumes in your living space. Use air conditioning in your car instead of opening the windows.

- **EXERCISE REGULARLY.** Activity will strengthen your chest muscles, stimulate appetite, and help improve sleep and mood.

- **LEARN RELAXATION.** Getting a handle on stress and practicing relaxation skills such as meditation can help keep you calm and prevent shortness of breath.

- **AVOID PEOPLE WITH RESPIRATORY INFECTIONS, COLDS, AND FLUS.** Get an annual flu shot to help you stay well during flu season.

# Quit the Habit

Cigarette smoking is the leading cause of preventable death and disease in the United States. Yet, approximately forty-six million people smoke. According to the American Lung Association (ALA), the habit is fully responsible for 80 percent of all cases of COPD.

For someone with COPD, giving up cigarettes is critical to survival. Even so, it isn't easy to quit. Here are some strategies from the ALA:

- Join a stop-smoking program like Freedom from Smoking® from the ALA. Check out www.lungusa.org to learn more. The organization also offers many self-help tools, including Freedom from Smoking® guidebooks, videotapes, and audiotapes.

- Pick a good time to quit. Don't attempt quitting when you're stressed out or around a holiday.

- Exercise every day. The regular activity will reduce your stress, boost your mood, and help you prevent weight gain.

- Get enough sleep, eat a balanced diet, and drink lots of water. These healthy habits will support your efforts.

- Enlist family, friends, and coworkers. A walking companion or a friend to chat with can help get you through those tough moments.

- Anticipate setbacks. Some smokers need to practice quitting before they actually do. The key is not giving up.

- Consider nicotine replacement therapy. Smoking can cause true addiction to nicotine. Combining nicotine replacement therapy with a behavior change program can improve your chances of quitting.

You might also want to consider using bupropion (Wellbutrin/Zyban), says Christine Gerbstadt, M.D., R.D., a spokesperson for the American Dietetic Association. Wellbutrin is a prescription drug used to treat depression that has also been approved for the treatment of nicotine addiction.

# COLD SORES

COLD SORES ARE SMALL, BOTHERSOME BLISTERS that appear on the lips in tiny bunches or as one larger blister. They are also sometimes called "fever blisters." In spite of the name, you don't need to have a cold or a fever to develop a cold sore.

What you do have is infection by the herpes simplex virus (HSV). Most cold sores are caused by HSV-1, though HSV-2 can also cause them. HSV-2 is generally responsible for genital herpes. The herpes virus is extremely common, and many people may have it without any signs or symptoms. But once you've had a cold sore, the virus never goes away. Instead, the virus lies dormant until it is reawakened by things such as stress, illness, menstruation, or sun exposure.

Cold sores are transmitted through contact with someone who is already infected and can be transmitted even before the sore surfaces. Kissing or sharing towels, drinking glasses, and lip balms are all ways that the virus can be spread.

Most cold sores go away on their own a week or two after they first emerge. In the meantime, while they're active, you can relieve the pain by taking over-the-counter analgesics or using topical ointments. Applying hot or cold compresses can also relieve the pain.

## What It Looks Like

A cold sore typically starts with a tingling or itchy sensation on the lips. For those who have had cold sores before, they know what's about to come. And usually within a day or two a sore will appear.

Cold sores are red or purplish blisters, which may be just one large bump or a cluster of tiny bubbles. They generally appear on or near the lips. At first the cold sore may just be a bump, but once it starts healing, it may develop a crust and turn into a darker scab.

## ¶¶ What to Eat

Boost your immunity by eating a lot of fresh, unprocessed foods such as fruits, vegetables, and whole grain foods, says Fred Pescatore, M.D., a New York City physician who uses nutrition to treat patients and author of *The Hamptons Diet Cookbook*. Make sure to include foods that are rich in L-lysine, an amino acid that may block the activity of the herpes virus. L-lysine occurs in beans, fish, red meat, and dairy products.

### Hygiene Counts

Good personal hygiene habits can make all the difference when it comes to staying free of cold sores and preventing their spread. When you have an active cold sore, it's important to avoid activities that will pass the virus along to others. That means you should avoid kissing, oral sex, and even intercourse (if you can't resist kissing), as well as the sharing of glasses, utensils, and other items. And while the cold sore is active, make sure to wash your hands frequently. Avoid touching your eyes or genitals, which may be vulnerable to the virus.

## ⊘ What Not to Eat

Stay away from foods that contain arginine, an amino acid that helps promotes the replication of the herpes virus. These foods include peanuts, almonds, raisins, nuts, and seeds, as well as anything with chocolate.

Do not drink caffeine or alcohol and try to avoid foods rich in sugar. Some experts also believe that highly acidic foods may aggravate cold sores, so avoid grapefruit, oranges, and tomatoes for the time being.

## ⊶ Supplements for Cold Sores

Take a high-quality multivitamin to ensure overall health and well-being. You might also consider taking the following:

### L-LYSINE

L-lysine has long been regarded as a treatment for cold sores and other forms of herpes. It works by inhibiting replication of the herpes virus.

### ZINC

Some studies have suggested that zinc may help reduce the duration and severity of cold sores. You might also ask your doctor about topical creams that contain zinc.

## NATURAL ANTIVIRAL REMEDIES

Certain plants contain substances with antiviral properties that may help reduce cold sores and prevent their recurrence. Among them:

- Lemon balm. This herb contains terpenes and tannins, substances in plants that may have antiviral properties.

- Lauric acid. This fatty acid occurs naturally in human milk and coconut milk and is available in a supplement called monolaurin.

- Olive leaf extract or oil.

- Oregano oil.

## Stay-Healthy Strategies

- **REDUCE STRESS.** Chronic stress can weaken immunity and make it more likely for cold sores to appear. So make time to relax with practices such as meditation, deep breathing, or yoga.

- **GET YOUR SLEEP.** You're more vulnerable to a herpes outbreak when you're not well rested. Get into the habit of getting enough sleep every night.

- **USE SUNBLOCK.** Liberally apply sunblock to your lips and face whenever you spend time outdoors. Sunshine can trigger an outbreak of cold sores.

- **CONSIDER MEDICATION.** If you're prone to cold sores, keep medications handy for those unexpected outbreaks.

# COLIC

ALL NEW PARENTS EXPECT THEIR BABIES TO CRY, and certainly some babies will cry more than others. But when unrelenting wails of a newborn become a nightly occurrence, your baby may be suffering from colic.

Colic is a frustrating and distressing condition that describes a pattern of excessive crying for no apparent reason. The condition is quite common and affects up to 10 percent of all babies. Colic typically starts a few weeks after birth, peaks at about six weeks of age, then gradually improves somewhere between the third and fifth month.

Your pediatrician needs to rule out reflux and allergies to milk proteins, both of which can cause colic. Beyond that, the most probable cause of colic is swallowing too much air. The excess air causes abdominal distention, a condition in which internal pressure causes the belly to expand and become uncomfortable. Some babies may also have increased sensitivity to pain.

Dealing with colic can be extremely difficult, especially for first-time parents who can't calm their baby's screams and are at a loss for what to do. To make matter worse, most new parents are already exhausted and sleep deprived. The combination makes for a frustrating experience. The mom's diet (if she's nursing) and the way the child is fed might make a difference but do not guarantee relief from the crying.

## What It Looks Like

Many babies go through fussy spells in the late afternoon and early evening, which is why pediatricians are often reluctant to label these bouts of crying as colic.

True colic starts between the second and fourth weeks after birth. Colicky babies may cry around the clock but worsen in the early evening. The crying is inconsolable and often accompanied by the baby extending or pulling up his legs. During the crying jag, the baby may pass gas and his stomach may be enlarged or distended by gas. Fortunately, the crying does dissipate eventually.

## What to Eat

If your baby is using formula, consider switching brands, says Mary Ann LoFrumento, M.D., a pediatrician and author of *Simply Parenting: Understanding Your Newborn and Infant.* A study in the journal *Pediatrics* found that babies who ate a hypoallergenic infant formula made with whey hydrolysate, a type of protein, decreased the amount of daily crying in colicky infants by 63 minutes.

## What Not to Eat

If you're nursing, consider cutting out foods that might promote gas, such as beans, broccoli, and cabbage. Consider also eliminating spicy foods, caffeine, and high-fiber foods, all of which can irritate your baby.

Nursing moms might also want to consider giving up cow's milk. One older study looked at sixty-six moms of breastfed infants who were put on a diet free of cow's milk. The study, which was published in the journal *Pediatrics*, found that the colic disappeared in thirty-five infants, but reappeared in twenty-three of the infants when cow's milk was reintroduced.

Other food allergens may be involved too. A separate study in the same journal looked at the effects of a maternal diet low in food allergens. Moms in that study eliminated highly allergenic foods such as cow's milk, eggs, wheat, peanuts, tree nuts, soy, and fish. Babies whose moms ate the low-allergen diet experienced a reduction in the duration of their crying spells.

## Supplements for Colic

There are no supplements recommended for the colicky infant or a nursing mom.

## Stay-Healthy Strategies

- **FEED YOUR BABY WHENEVER SHE'S HUNGRY.** Babies are generally less fussy when they have a full tummy.

- **TAKE CARE OF YOURSELF.** Colic can be exasperating. Enlist help from family and friends who can provide you with a brief reprieve.

- **SOOTHE HER IN OTHER WAYS.** Sing to your baby. Walk her around the room to soft music. Massage your baby's abdomen or cover it in a warm washcloth.

- **MAKE SOME NOISE—WHITE NOISE.** The hum of a dryer or a vacuum cleaner can help settle some colicky infants. But be careful where you put the baby if you use a dryer. Never place the baby on top of a dryer, only beside it.

- **TRY TO AVOID FEEDING YOUR BABY LATE IN THE DAY,** which can worsen gas and abdominal distension. You also need to avoid overfeeding.

- **DO NOT GIVE YOUR BABY A PACIFIER,** which increases the swallowing of air.

- **IF YOUR BABY DRINKS FORMULA,** use a bottle that reduces air intake. Good choices are the bottles that use plastic bags, which allow you to squeeze the air out.

- **GIVE HER SIMETHICONE DROPS TO RELIEVE GAS,** if necessary.

# COMMON COLD

APTLY NAMED, THE COMMON COLD afflicts everyone at one time or another. Every year, there are about a billion colds in the United States, with children getting an average of three to eight colds a year. They're the number-one reason why children wind up at a doctor's office.

Colds are upper respiratory infections caused by any of more than 200 viruses. These viruses invade the nasal passages, triggering the symptoms we know as the common cold. Viruses are highly contagious microorganisms that travel quickly, especially among children.

Colds are most common during cooler months when people spend more time indoors in dry air, giving viruses ample chance to spread. The germs may be passed along in the air when someone coughs or sneezes. It's also possible to catch a cold when you touch a surface contaminated by the virus, then touch your finger to your eye, nose, or mouth. Once you come in contact with a cold virus, it takes about two to three days before the symptoms appear.

Most colds don't require a doctor's treatment, and they certainly won't respond to antibiotics, which work only on bacterial diseases. In fact, there are no medications to treat the common cold, only remedies to relieve the symptoms. The best care, however, is plenty of rest and fluids.

## 🔍 What It Looks Like

Most colds start with a scratchy throat or stuffy nose and a feeling that you're just not well. From there, most people develop congestion, a runny nose, and coughing. There is often a great deal of mucus, which may even be green or yellow. Other symptoms may include muscle aches, headaches, fatigue, and decreased appetite.

Children may have a fever, though a fever in adults is more likely to mean you have the flu. In children who have asthma, colds often trigger asthma symptoms. In young children, colds often lead to ear infections.

Although uncomfortable, most colds do not last long and will usually go away without treatment in about a week. Many people confuse the cold with the flu, which is also a respiratory illness, but one that is caused by a different virus. Colds are generally milder, less likely to cause a fever, and disappear more quickly. And unlike the flu, colds don't tend to cause muscle aches.

## 🍴 What to Eat

It may sound like an old wives' tale, but chicken soup may be one of the best nutritional remedies for someone who is suffering from a cold, says Fred Pescatore, M.D., a New York City physician who uses nutrition to treat patients and co-author of *The Hamptons Diet*. Chicken soup has been used since the twelfth century as a way to relieve colds and is celebrated as a favorite remedy among moms. In 2000, scientists offered up some proof when researchers at the University of Nebraska found that chicken soup actually contains substances that can help reduce the inflammation in the upper respiratory tract.

In addition to chicken soup, it's important to drink plenty of fluids, preferably water, hot tea, or broths. Staying hydrated will prevent the mucus from becoming too thick and worsening your congestion.

Ignore the adage, "Starve a cold and feed a fever." Your body requires nutrients to strengthen immunity. When you do eat, choose foods that are light, such as steamed vegetables or fruit, which contain immune-boosting antioxidants such as vitamin C. Foods rich in vitamin C include oranges, grapefruit, kiwi, and papaya. Try to eat foods that contain selenium and zinc, minerals that are also antioxidants. Good sources of both include chicken, eggs, and whole-grains.

## 🚫 What Not to Eat

Avoid eating large amounts of sugar, even the natural kinds such as honey and maple syrup. If you like to drink fruit juices, dilute them with water to reduce your sugar intake. Steer clear of dairy products, which in some people can increase the production of mucus. You should also avoid drinks that can cause dehydration, including alcohol and caffeinated beverages.

## 💊 Supplements for the Common Cold

In the throes of battling the cold, make sure to take a quality multivitamin. You may also consider taking certain supplements. Possible supplements to consider include the following:

### VITAMIN C

Boost your intake of vitamin C, which will help strengthen your immunity while you're sick.

### ZINC

Some studies have suggested that zinc may help lessen the severity of the common cold and shorten the cold's duration. But others have shown no difference. The best way to use zinc, Pescatore says, is to apply it topically to the mucous membrane of the nose. Simply taking a zinc supplement will not do anything.

### ECHINACEA

Although once believed to be potent against the common cold, some studies have since refuted these claims. Still, some experts believe that Echinacea can shorten the duration of the cold and lessen its symptoms.

## AHCC

Active hexose correlated compound is a Japanese medicinal mushroom extract that may strengthen the immune system and has been found to decrease the duration of colds and flus.

## Stay-Healthy Strategies

- **PREVENT COLDS THROUGH FREQUENT HAND WASHING.** Encourage children to wash for at least 15 seconds and scrub with soap and water. Do it each time you return home and before every meal. Alternatively, you can use an alcohol-based hand sanitizer.

- **DIMINISH THE SPREAD.** Practice coughing and sneezing into your elbow or a tissue and teach your children to do the same. Wash your hands every time you cough or sneeze and change towels frequently.

- **GIVE YOURSELF TIME TO REST AND RELAX.** Rest will help your body recover more quickly from a cold. Staying away from others will help prevent its spread.

- **LIMIT YOUR USE OF OVER-THE-COUNTER REMEDIES.** Decongestants, analgesics, cough medicines, and cold remedies provide only temporary (if any) relief and may cause side effects such as drowsiness, dizziness, and upset stomach.

## The Stats on Colds

According to the National Institute of Allergy and Infectious Diseases, Americans suffer as many as a billion colds a year. Here are some other intriguing numbers on our most common ailment:

- Each year, twenty-two million school days are lost annually because of the common cold.

- In families that have children in school, the number of colds per child can be as high as twelve per year.

- Adults get an average of two to four colds a year, although the range varies widely for individuals.

- Women, especially those in their 20s and 30s, have more colds than men, possibly due to their closer contact with children.

- On average, people older than 60 have less than one cold a year.

# CONSTIPATION

ALMOST EVERYONE HAS AN OCCASIONAL BOUT of constipation. A poor diet, the lack of exercise, and even a weekend trip can cause your bowel movements to decrease and become more dry and sluggish.

Constipation is one of the most common medical complaints in the United States and affects approximately four million people on a regular basis. But most cases are temporary and not serious. The condition is more common in women and in adults over the age of 65. All told, Americans spend about $725 million a year on over-the-counter laxatives to resolve the problem, according to the National Institute of Diabetes and Digestive and Kidney Diseases.

Constipation occurs when waste products from the food you eat move too slowly through the colon. The slowdown causes the stool to become hard, dry, and difficult to pass. In some people, the strain of trying to eliminate the hardened stool causes hemorrhoids, in which the veins around the anus or lower rectum become swollen and inflamed. During defecation, anal fissures, or tears in the skin around the anus, may also result.

Most people develop constipation as the result of a poor diet that lacks fiber and fluids. But certain diseases can cause constipation too, including diabetes, hypothyroidism, multiple sclerosis, lupus, and colon cancer. You can also develop constipation if you have functional problems in your colon, rectum, and intestines. Medications such as antidepressants, beta blockers, diuretics, and painkillers can cause constipation, as can iron tablets and calcium supplements.

## 🔎 What It Looks Like

Some people think they are constipated if they do not have a bowel movement every day. That is not true. Some people may defecate only once a week and feel perfectly fine, and have no trouble with elimination.

In truth, the frequency of bowel movements varies a great deal, but constipation is technically defined as having a bowel movement fewer than three times a week. In people who are constipated, the stools are usually hard, small, dry, and difficult to eliminate. Defecating is often painful, and you may find yourself straining to eliminate the stool.

Some people may experience short spells of constipation for no apparent reason. These brief bouts of constipation are quite normal and affect almost everyone at one time or another.

## ♟ What to Eat

People who have constipation need to add more fiber into their diet, says Fred Pescatore, M.D., a New York City physician who uses nutrition to treat patients and co-author of *The Hamptons Diet*. Fiber is an indigestible carbohydrate that has many health benefits, including the prevention and treatment of constipation.

As you may know, fiber comes in two forms. Both play a role in preventing constipation. The soluble type dissolves in water and acts as a gel in the intestines, while the insoluble variety absorbs water and helps soften the stool. Soluble fiber is found in oats, kidney beans, peas, flaxseed, apples, oranges, and carrots. Insoluble fiber—also known as roughage—is found in whole-wheat foods, cauliflower, beans, spinach, peas, and apples.

Other good sources of fiber include whole grains such as brown rice, bulgur wheat, and quinoa as well as legumes such as chickpeas, kidney beans, pinto beans, and black beans. Prunes, figs, and flaxseeds are also helpful for constipation.

When you do start eating more fiber, do so slowly. Most Americans get far less than the 25 to 30 grams per day recommended by the American Dietetic Association. Adding too much fiber to the diet too quickly can cause gas. That's why you should boost your fiber intake gradually and while consuming additional fluids.

Drinking more fluids is important for constipation itself. Liquids lubricate the colon and add bulk to the stools, making them softer and easier to eliminate. Water is the best option, but all-natural fruit juices are also a good choice. Aim for eight 8-oz. glasses of fluid a day. If you're overweight, you should drink even more than that.

Some experts also believe that eating lacto-fermented vegetables, such as sauerkraut and kimchi, can relieve constipation. Fermented foods are those that have been soaked and preserved in salty brine but not heated above 110°F. Not only do these foods provide fiber, but they also help re-establish a healthy balance of intestinal microorganisms that can aid digestion, improve immunity, and prevent constipation.

## ⊘ What Not to Eat

Most foods do not cause constipation unless they displace other foods that are rich in fiber, Pescatore says. For instance, cheese can be binding, but not if you drink enough water and eat plenty of fiber. The same is true for saturated fats, which in large amounts can slow digestion and cause stools to be harder. Saturated fat is found primarily in animal products such as red meat, whole dairy foods, and butter. But it is also common in fried foods, which may aggravate constipation.

Avoid drinking excessive amounts of coffee, tea, and alcohol when constipated. Although caffeine is a stimulant that can provoke a bowel movement in many people, too much of it can be dehydrating and will rob the body of vital fluids. Some people become constipated from consuming dairy products, which may need to be eliminated from the diet as well.

Certain supplements can also cause constipation. Iron and calcium supplements, for instance, can sometimes lead to constipation, as can excessive amounts of vitamin D.

## 🫘 Supplements for Constipation

Constipation can be eased with the help of the following supplements:

### PSYLLIUM

Psyllium is a seed husk and a soluble fiber that can help regulate bowels and lower cholesterol. Talk to your doctor first before taking psyllium, especially if you have food allergies, because some people react to psyllium. The same is true of laxatives such as Metamucil, which contain psyllium.

### PROBIOTICS

Healthy bacteria such as *Lactobacillus* and *Bifidobacteria* may help relieve constipation.

### SENNA

Senna is an herb that may be considered as a short-term remedy for constipation. It can be taken in the form of a capsule, tablet, or tincture, or used in a tea.

### FLAXSEED OIL

Flaxseed oil helps soften the stool and lubricate the colon, making it easier to pass the stools.

## 🗒 Stay-Healthy Strategies

- **EXERCISE REGULARLY.** Physical activity can help prevent constipation, especially among the elderly.

- **PAY ATTENTION TO THE NEED TO DEFECATE.** People who try to ignore the need to have a bowel movement may stop having the sensation, which can lead to constipation. Always go when the urge strikes.

- **SEEK MEDICAL ATTENTION IF CONSTIPATION PERSISTS.** According to the American Society of Colon and Rectal Surgeons, get treatment if it lasts more than three weeks. If there's blood, get to a doctor immediately.

- **USE LAXATIVES WITH CAUTION.** Mild constipation does not call for treatment with laxatives at all. If you do need them, use them only for a limited time. Laxatives can be addictive.

# Laxatives

Laxatives are medications that can help resolve constipation, but there are actually several types:

- **Bulk-forming.** Also known as fiber supplements, these work by absorbing water into the intestine and softening the stool. Common brands include Metamucil, Citrucel, and Fiberall.

- **Lubricating.** Lubricants are oils that soften the stool, which makes it easier for the stool to get through the intestines. The most common kind is mineral oil.

- **Stool-softening.** These laxatives soften the stool by adding moisture to it. The active ingredient is usually docusate. These are often given to women shortly after giving birth or patients after surgery.

- **Stimulating.** Stimulants work by inducing contractions in the intestines, which in turn provokes a bowel movement.

- **Saline-containing.** Saline laxatives contain minerals and ions that draw water into the intestines, thereby softening the stool and causing more pressure in the intestines. The added pressure then causes a bowel movement.

- **Osmotic-containing.** Osmotic agents help the colon retain water, which stretches out the bowel and causes more contractions.

Not all laxatives are safe for everyone, and not all types will always work in every patient. Also, most people should limit their use of laxatives to a short period of time. The best thing to do is to consult a doctor before taking any laxative.

# CROHN'S DISEASE

CROHN'S DISEASE IS AN INFLAMMATORY BOWEL DISEASE, an uncomfortable and chronic disorder that has been linked to an abnormality in the immune system. The condition is named after a physician named Burrill B. Crohn, who in 1932 published a paper describing the symptoms that we know today as Crohn's disease.

Crohn's can involve any area of the gastrointestinal tract from the mouth to the anus, but it tends to affect the small intestine and/or colon. It is most likely to occur in the lower part of the small intestine, called the ileum. The disease is sometimes known as ileitis or enteritis.

No one knows exactly what triggers the inflammation in Crohn's disease, but experts believe it is an autoimmune response, in which the body's immune system mistakes healthy substances in the intestine for foreign invaders or germs. The immune system then launches an attack, which summons protective white blood cells to the intestines, causing chronic inflammation that damages the lining of the intestines and ulcers and injury to the bowel. What remains unknown is what sets off the improper immune reaction.

Crohn's disease affects approximately 500,000 people in the United States and occurs equally in men and women. The condition tends to emerge in adolescence and young adulthood but can arise in late adulthood or childhood as well. The disease appears to have a genetic link: Approximately 20 percent of people with Crohn's disease have a relative with some form of inflammatory bowel disease (IBD). Crohn's is more common among people of Jewish descent and less common among African-Americans. It is sometimes confused with another type of IBD called ulcerative colitis.

## What It Looks Like

Crohn's disease is painful and causes persistent diarrhea, abdominal pain, and rectal bleeding. Some people may also experience weight loss, skin problems, fever, and arthritis. If the bleeding is severe, Crohn's can lead to anemia. In children, severe cases can result in delayed development and growth problems.

If the anus and rectum are involved, you may develop fistulas, tunnels that inappropriately link loops of the intestines or connect the intestines to the bladder, vagina, or skin. You may also develop small tears called fissures in the lining of the anus, which can cause pain and bleeding. Some people may experience blockage of the intestines as the intestinal wall swells and thickens. Crohn's also puts you at greater risk for malnutrition because proper absorption of nutrients may be impeded.

To diagnose Crohn's disease, your doctor may administer blood tests and obtain stool samples, which can rule out infectious causes of diarrhea. In addition, your doctor may do a sigmoidoscopy to view the lower end of the colon and the rectum or a colonoscopy to view the entire colon. While doing these procedures, she will look for ulcers, inflammation, and bleeding.

Keep in mind that Crohn's disease fluctuates. Most people go through periods in which the disease is active and periods of remission. Most people, with proper treatment and a healthy lifestyle, are able to lead normal, productive lives.

## TIP

*You may want to consider the Specific Carbohydrate Diet. Some people with Crohn's have experienced relief with this diet, which permits most fruits and vegetables, select processed meats, and natural cheeses, while prohibiting all grains, starchy foods, canned vegetables, pasta, and sugars (except honey). The diet plan is believed to especially benefit people with digestive disorders, including Crohn's. For more information, see page 75 or visit www.scdiet.org to learn more.*

## ¶¶ What to Eat

No special diet works for everyone with Crohn's disease, but experts agree that a healthy, well-balanced diet is helpful for staying well, says Jeannie Moloo, R.D., a nutritionist in Sacramento, California, and co-author of *The No-Salt Lowest Sodium* cookbook series. In general, you should try to eat fresh, unprocessed foods, such as fruits and vegetables, and lean proteins, including chicken and fish.

But choose your fruits and vegetables wisely. Certain ones, especially cruciferous veggies like cabbage and broccoli, may cause gas that makes your symptoms worse. To make veggies more tolerable, try steaming, stewing, or sautéing them rather than eating them raw.

Be sure to drink plenty of fluids as well. Any disease that causes diarrhea puts you at greater risk for dehydration. When you drink, practice sipping rather than gulping, which can introduce air into your system and create discomfort.

Finally, some experts recommend eating fermented foods, particularly those that nourish the body with live bacteria, says Sandor Katz, host of the web site www.wildfermentation.com and author of *Wild Fermentation*. These foods include unpasteurized sauerkraut, miso, yogurt, and quality kefir. Because they have not been heated above 110°F, they contain living organisms that can improve digestion and strengthen immunity.

## Keep Up Your Appetite

It's not uncommon for people with Crohn's to lose their appetite. Abdominal pain, changes in taste, and nausea are enough to squelch the heartiest of eaters. But if eating loses its appeal, you put yourself at risk for malnutrition and excess weight loss. Some people may require high-calorie nutritional supplements to replenish their deficiencies and ensure a healthy weight.

If you think you're at risk, talk to your physician. Malnutrition is a serious health condition: It can cause growth problems in children, cause menstrual irregularities in women, and make some medications less effective.

# What Not to Eat

To figure out which foods aggravate your symptoms, consider doing an elimination diet, which involves keeping a food diary that tracks the foods you eat and any symptoms you experience. A written record will help you pinpoint the foods that are most bothersome, which you should then remove from your diet.

In general, it's best to avoid foods that aggravate your digestive tract during a flare-up of Crohn's. These include spicy foods, bulky grains, alcohol, and milk, which can increase diarrhea and cramps. Cut back on fried and greasy foods as well as heavy creams, butter, and margarine.

These heavy fats can cause diarrhea and gas if they're not properly absorbed.

Avoid any high-fiber foods that can create gas and aggravate your symptoms, such as raw fruits and vegetables, beans, seeds, and nuts.

# Supplements for Crohn's

People with Crohn's disease are at risk for malnutrition, so it's important to take a quality multivitamin to make sure you're getting the essential nutrients. Nutritional deficiencies may require supplementation but will depend on the severity and location of your particular case. You should talk to your doctor about supplements you might need, such as the following:

### VITAMIN B12

If the disease affects your lower ileum, you may be deficient in this essential vitamin. Some people need shots of B12 to correct it.

### VITAMIN D

According to the Crohn's and Colitis Foundation of America, as many as 68 percent of people with Crohn's are deficient in vitamin D. A supplement to replenish vitamin D will ensure good bone health.

### CALCIUM

This bone-building mineral may be reduced in people with Crohn's because of poor absorption, limited intake, or the long-term use of steroids such as Prednisone.

### IRON

Some people with Crohn's are iron-deficient, due to blood loss from inflammation and ulceration. Note: Taking iron may cause the stool to blacken.

### POTASSIUM

Diarrhea and vomiting can result in a potassium deficiency, which can be restored with a supplement.

### MAGNESIUM

A deficiency in magnesium can also be blamed on diarrhea and vomiting.

### SELENIUM

Some people may benefit from supplements of this antioxidant mineral, which is often deficient in Crohn's sufferers.

### FISH OR FLAXSEED OIL

These oils are rich in omega-3 fatty acids, which might help reduce the inflammation in Crohn's and may aid in healing irritated membranes.

### PROBIOTICS

Efforts to heal the digestive tract may benefit from the use of healthy bacteria such as *Lactobacillus acidophilus*.

## Stay-Healthy Strategies

- **WORK CLOSELY WITH A PHYSICIAN YOU LIKE AND TRUST.** Getting quality care will ensure you get the best treatment for your condition.

- **MAKE TIME TO RELAX EVERY DAY.** Stress doesn't cause Crohn's, but it can aggravate it. So find activities that help you unwind.

- **WATCH FOR DEPRESSION.** Living with Crohn's disease can be difficult, and it's not unusual to feel sad about it. Seek professional help if the depression becomes severe.

- **TRY TO EXERCISE.** Physical activity will help keep bones and muscles strong and also boost energy levels and mood. Consult your physician first before starting a program.

---

### TIP

*Eat small, frequent meals. Large meals can be harder to digest and may worsen your symptoms.*

---

# CYSTITIS

*See Urinary Tract Infections on page 314.*

# DEPRESSION

EVERYONE SUFFERS FROM AN OCCASIONAL bout of the blues, but for some people, these spells of sadness are actually depression, a serious mental illness that can cause tremendous pain and suffering. Depression is the leading cause of disability in the world, according to the World Health Organization.

Distinguishing depression from a periodic case of sadness isn't easy. It's entirely normal to feel unhappy when someone you love dies, you lose a job, or you're going through a difficult time with your finances. The unhappiness you feel is a normal response to a downturn in life.

But in some people, these feelings last considerably longer. Others may feel inexplicably blue without a change in circumstances. These people may be suffering from depression.

Almost nineteen million people in the United States (9.5 percent of the population) suffer from a depressive illness in a given year, according to the National Institutes of Mental Health. Twice as many women are affected as men.

What makes depression so hard to detect is that many of the signs and symptoms are subtle and easily blamed on stress, fatigue, and a hectic lifestyle. As a result, depression often goes unrecognized and untreated, and can potentially weaken your immune system and worsen other health problems such as arthritis or asthma. Worst of all perhaps, undetected depression can keep you from being as happy as you really can be, and can also negatively affect your relationships with loved ones.

## What It Looks Like

The signs and symptoms of depression can be subtle. After all, it's perfectly normal to have bad days when you're distracted, irritable, and just plain tired. The key is in the intensity of these bad feelings and how long they last. They also shouldn't interfere with the way you get through your day or how you get along with others. Also, it isn't normal if you stop taking pleasure in activities you once really enjoyed.

The following is a checklist of symptoms for depression:

- Frequent sadness, often accompanied by crying

- Feelings of hopelessness, helplessness, and worthlessness

- Loss of interest in things that normally bring you pleasure

- Irritability

- Difficulties getting along at work and at home
- Trouble concentrating and forgetfulness
- Unexplained physical complaints such as headaches and stomach pains
- Changes in appetite
- Changes in the amount of sleep you get
- Thoughts of suicide

You don't need to exhibit all of these symptoms to have depression. But if any one of these problems persists for two weeks or more and starts to affect your functioning, consider getting professional help.

Also, be on guard for other conditions that can sometimes accompany or lead to depression, namely generalized anxiety disorder and substance abuse.

## ⫴ What to Eat

Many people with depression crave carbohydrates, which trigger the release of the feel-good neurotransmitter serotonin, says Lisa Dorfman, M.S., R.D., a licensed psychotherapist and spokesperson for the American Dietetic Association. When choosing your carbs, however, make sure to eat a lot of complex carbohydrates such as fruits, vegetables, and whole grain foods. These foods are rich in nutrients and will help you feel full longer than simple carbs such as bagels and pasta.

Make sure to also select foods rich in folate, a B vitamin that may be deficient in people with depression. Good sources include spinach, lentils, and peas.

Another important nutrient is tryptophan, an essential amino acid that aids in the production of serotonin. Good sources of tryptophan include poultry, bananas, dairy products, and peas.

You should also eat cold-water fish such as salmon, tuna, and mackerel, which are rich in omega-3 fatty acids. These healthy fats are important for proper brain function. Some studies have found that these healthy fats may help relieve depression.

Make sure to balance out any carbohydrates with some protein, which will help prevent lethargy. For instance, spread peanut butter on a bagel, or add grilled chicken to your whole-wheat pasta. The combination will help you feel fuller and prevent the highs and lows that come with eating carbs alone.

## ⊘ What Not to Eat

Reduce your intake of foods high in saturated fats, such as red meat, cheese, butter, and rich desserts. Although depression can cause cravings for these comforting foods, they ultimately make your body feel sluggish and fatigued.

The same goes for all kinds of sugar, even the natural variety. Foods high in sugar give you a quick jolt of energy—popularly known as a "sugar high"—but then cause a resounding crash that depletes energy and causes fatigue, the last things you need when you have depression.

Some individuals should also avoid aspartame, the artificial sweetener commonly known as Equal or NutraSweet. Studies have found that aspartame may affect the proper function of serotonin, a neurotransmitter involved in regulating mood. If you find that after consuming a product with aspartame it triggers a headache or feelings of lethargy, anxiety, or generalized fatigue, discontinue its use.

Finally, limit or eliminate your intake of alcohol and caffeine. Alcohol is a depressant that also causes dehydration, which can lead to fatigue. Caffeine is a stimulant, but in excess, it can cause anxiety, irritability, and exhaustion.

## Supplements for Depression

Start by taking a quality multivitamin, which will ensure you're getting the essential nutrients you need. Before taking any supplement talk to your doctor. Some remedies may interact with antidepressant medications. Possible supplements include the following:

### SAM-E

SAM-e, or adenosylmethionine, is a natural substance that may relieve depression and fatigue. It helps produce and regulate hormones that affect mood. But any benefit requires very high doses, and it can be quite expensive.

### ST. JOHN'S WORT

Although highly regarded in Europe as a treatment for depression, experts in the United States say it is effective only for mild depression. And be careful: St. John's wort should never be taken with other antidepressants, and it may interact with some medications.

### 5-HTP

5-HTP is a form of tryptophan that can help boost levels of serotonin. Taking it at bedtime may help promote sleep, and higher doses may relieve depression. But it should never be taken if you're on antidepressants.

### B COMPLEX VITAMIN

The B vitamins are involved in the healthy metabolism of neurotransmitters. Some of these vitamins may be deficient in people with depression.

### FISH OIL

Fish oil supplements contain omega-3 fatty acids, which may help with proper brain function.

---

### TIP

*If there's any chance that you are experiencing depression, get help immediately. Treating depression is critical, not only to your state of mind, but also to your health. Studies show that depression can raise your risk for serious illnesses such as heart disease, Alzheimer's disease, and stroke as well as minor ailments such as colds. Besides being an independent risk factor for disease, depression can worsen existing health problems and make recovery more difficult. For instance, cancer patients with a history of depression are 160 percent (2.6 times) more likely to die than those who have not experienced depression.*

# Stay-Healthy Strategies

- **TALK TO A DOCTOR ABOUT DEPRESSION.**
Depression is a serious medical condition that may warrant professional treatment such as psychotherapy or antidepressant medications.

- **CONSULT WITH A REGISTERED DIETITIAN** about your food habits and eating behaviors. A nutrition expert can evaluate your diet patterns, assess nutritional excesses and deficiencies, and identify interactions between foods that trigger depression.

- **GET ENOUGH LIGHT.** Some people suffer from seasonal affective disorder (SAD), a form of depression that occurs when exposure to sunlight is minimal. Staying in bright rooms or going outside during daylight hours can sometimes help people with SAD.

- **EXERCISE REGULARLY.** Physical activity is a natural mood booster, so be active every day.

- **PAMPER YOURSELF.** It might be hard to muster the energy to do anything when you're depressed. But look for small ways to treat yourself well, be it time spent with friends, a manicure, or a movie.

## Depression: Not Just One Type

One reason depression is hard to detect is that there are actually two different types. Most people are familiar with major depression, the kind that makes it hard to get out of bed, take care of your family, or do your job. Even doing simple everyday tasks can seem monumental to someone with major depression. The condition can last as little as two weeks, but it can also go on for months, or even years.

Dysthymia is a less severe, but chronic form of depression that persists for at least two years. People with dysthymia are never truly happy, but they are not incapacitated. They're still able to do their jobs, socialize with friends, and tend to their families, but they suffer from an undercurrent of unhappiness. Left untreated, dysthymia can last a lifetime and may result in bouts of major depression.

One way to distinguish dysthymia from major depression is through the individual's awareness of their negative feelings. People who have dysthymia are still able to realize that their bad feelings are out of proportion with reality—they know that they have a good life and that they really have no reason to despair. Those with major depression, however, lose that objectivity and can no longer appreciate the positive aspects of their lives.

# DIABETES

TOO MUCH FOOD. TOO LITTLE EXERCISE. For many people, this deadly combination has added up to a condition called diabetes. Diabetes is a metabolic illness, a condition that occurs when your body is unable to convert the glucose from food into energy for your cells. The malfunction is the result of a problem with insulin, a hormone made in the beta cells of the pancreas that helps convert glucose into energy.

Diabetes actually occurs in two forms. Most people with diabetes (90 to 95 percent) have type 2 diabetes, an increasingly common condition that develops when the body no longer responds to insulin or has stopped making insulin completely. The other form, type 1 diabetes, is an autoimmune disease that occurs when the immune system attacks the beta cells in the pancreas. Type 1 usually presents itself in childhood or young adulthood and cannot be prevented.

Left untreated, the excess glucose lingers in your bloodstream, wreaking havoc throughout your body and damaging organs. The complications of unchecked diabetes can be devastating and include heart disease, blindness, kidney failure, and the loss of limbs.

In the United States, and even around the world, diabetes has started to reach epidemic proportions. Approximately 7 percent of all people in the United States—nearly twenty-one million—are living with diabetes, according to the American Diabetes Association (ADA). Another forty-one million people between the ages of 40 to 74 have a condition called prediabetes, elevated blood sugars that aren't quite high enough to be considered diabetes, yet are sufficiently high to demand medical attention. Even more alarming these days is the surge in the numbers of children who now have diabetes. The ADA estimates that 33 percent of all children born in the year 2000 will develop diabetes in their lifetime. Among minority children, that number rises to 50 percent.

Unlike many other health conditions, the cause of type 2 diabetes is known. The condition has a genetic link and it is also highly influenced by lifestyle factors. People who are overweight or obese, do not exercise, and do not eat a healthy diet are at a significantly higher risk for diabetes. Giving birth to a baby that weighs more than nine pounds also increases your risk, as does having gestational diabetes, a condition that occurs during pregnancy. In addition, diabetes is more common among ethnic minorities and in older people.

Experts believe that 80 percent of all cases of type 2 diabetes can be prevented with simple lifestyle changes. As evidence, they point to the famous Diabetes Prevention Program, a three-year clinical trial that compared the benefits of moderate exercise and weight loss with Metformin, a diabetes drug. The study found that people with prediabetes could lower their risk for developing type 2 diabetes by 58 percent just by doing 30 minutes of moderate exercise five days a week and losing 5 to 7 percent of their body weight.

## What It Looks Like

Early on, as your blood sugars start to rise, you may not notice anything. But gradually, as the amount of glucoses continues to increase, you'll notice you're urinating more frequently, always with a full bladder. Excessive urination is the result of your kidneys working overtime to rid the body of glucose, a process that involves soaking up water throughout your body. The absorption of water perpetuates your thirst, and you'll notice that you're frequently and extremely thirsty. Even drinking gallons of water doesn't satiate your thirst.

Many people also experience changes in their weight. Some people will start losing weight for no apparent reason. The weight loss is actually the result of the body breaking down muscle for energy because cells can't get the energy from food. In others, there may be weight gain as your appetite increases because your body cells are starved for energy.

The lack of energy in your cells produces fatigue, and you may notice you are frequently tired and weak, even after getting a lot of sleep. If the amount of glucose in your blood is high enough, you may develop blurry vision, slow-healing cuts and infections, numbness and tingling from nerve damage, and, in women, more frequent yeast infections.

People with type 1 diabetes may experience flu-like symptoms such as fever; nausea; deep, rapid breathing; and loss of appetite. These symptoms are the result of a condition called diabetic ketoacidosis, in which your urine has elevated levels of ketones. Ketones are toxic chemicals produced by the breakdown of fats for energy. If this condition goes untreated, it can be fatal.

## What to Eat

Knowing what to eat for diabetes involves working closely with a registered dietitian or certified diabetes educator, a health professional trained in working with people who have diabetes, says Melvin Stjernholm, M.D., F.A.C.E., co-author of *What to Do When the Doctor Says It's Diabetes*. With their help, you can design a customized eating plan that matches your blood sugar patterns, medications, and lifestyle. Over time, you'll become more familiar with how the foods you eat affect your blood sugar levels.

But there are different types of nutritional tools that can help people with diabetes determine their best strategy.

- **CARBOHYDRATE COUNTING.** Tallying up the carbohydrate content of foods at each meal and snack works especially well for people who use insulin. The glucose in your blood comes primarily from carbohydrates, which includes everything from fruits and vegetables to pasta and bread and dairy products. Carbs can be counted by adding up servings or grams.

If you choose to do carb counting, the key is to eat a balanced meal with about 50 percent of your calories coming from carbohydrates. Try to get those carbs from healthy sources such as fruits, vegetables, and whole grains.

- **EXCHANGE SYSTEM.** This system of eating involves using lists of six food groups—fruit, starch/bread, meat and meat substitutes, vegetables, fat, and milk. The foods are assigned a serving size that contains roughly the same amount of carbohydrates, protein, fat, and calories. The person with diabetes can then create menus by exchanging one food for another on the same list and meeting guidelines for servings from each category.

- **GLYCEMIC INDEX.** This index involves rating foods according to how quickly they raise blood glucose levels. Although helpful for determining how foods affect blood glucose, the index is imprecise and doesn't take into account how the food was prepared and served and whether it's eaten with other foods—all factors that can affect the change in your blood glucose levels.

In general, people with diabetes should keep carbohydrate intake the same from one day to the next to avoid fluctuations in blood glucose. It's also essential to keep portions in control, especially if you're trying to lose weight.

When choosing your carbs, try to focus on eating fruits, vegetables, and whole grains, which not only contain more vitamins and minerals but are also rich in fiber. Soluble fiber, in particular, is important for diabetes because it can lower your blood sugar levels and reduce your need for insulin or medications. It appears to work by delaying the absorption of glucose into the bloodstream. Good sources include dried beans and peas, apples, oats, and carrots.

## What Not to Eat

Pass up foods high in saturated fats, such as red meat, butter, and whole dairy products. These foods can raise your risk for heart disease by boosting cholesterol levels and causing weight gain. Being overweight makes your body less sensitive to the effects of insulin.

Other fats to avoid are trans-fatty acids, which are produced when oils are hydrogenated or partially hydrogenated. These types of fats have been linked to high cholesterol and heart disease. They're typically found in processed foods such as frozen waffles, granola bars, snack foods, cookies, crackers, and more. They also occur in margarine and shortening.

Diabetics also need to avoid eating diets high in protein, especially if they have any signs of kidney disease. Too much protein can tax the kidneys and promote kidney failure. In addition, excess protein in the body is stored as fat.

If you like to drink alcohol, do so in moderation, but only if your blood sugar is well controlled and if you are free of complications such as nerve damage, diabetic eye disease, or high blood pressure. When you do drink, make sure to do so with food. Drinking on an empty stomach can cause blood sugar to plummet. You should also avoid alcohol after exercising, which naturally lowers blood sugar.

Finally, if you're trying to lose weight, avoid diets that restrict carbs or fats. Your body requires both nutrients, along with protein, for overall health. The best strategy for weight loss is to count calories and to watch your portions.

## Tools for Weight Loss

Getting to a healthy weight is critical for anyone, but especially people with diabetes. Losing weight can make your body cells more sensitive to insulin, lower your need for medications and insulin, and improve your lipids, or cholesterol levels. Best of all, it can mean a better quality of life.

- **MEASURE YOUR PORTIONS.** Take out your measuring cups and get in the habit of figuring out exactly how much you're eating. After a while, you'll have a better handle on your food intake.

- **LEARN TO READ LABELS.** Nutrition labels are chock full of important information that can help you lose weight. Always check the serving size, too, to make sure you're not overdoing it.

- **EAT ONLY WHEN YOU'RE HUNGRY.** Many people eat in response to emotional triggers such as boredom, anger, stress, or sadness. Ask yourself if

you're truly hungry when you feel the urge to grab a bite. Or try taking a short walk first to see if the hunger is real.

- **ANTICIPATE CHALLENGES.** You know you'll want to sit by the appetizers at the company party, so what can you do to prevent that from happening? Look for ways to avoid eating traps before you're in them. For instance, you might want to eat some fruit before you head out.

- **KEEP A FOOD DIARY.** A written record of what you eat will help you see what you're really eating and give you a better picture of what changes you need to make.

- **DON'T DEPRIVE YOURSELF.** Banning favorite foods from your eating plan won't make losing weight any easier. Instead, devise ways to include these foods in moderation.

## Supplements for Diabetes

Beyond taking a quality multivitamin that ensures you get all your essential with nutrients, people with diabetes do not need to take supplements to address their condition. However, if you have another condition or would like to try taking a supplement for a complication, consult your doctor or a registered dietitian first. Some supplements may interact with diabetes medications.

## Stay-Healthy Strategies

- **GET REGULAR EXERCISE.** Physical activity is one of the best things you can do for your body. It naturally lowers blood sugars and helps with weight loss and maintenance. Look for an activity you enjoy and that you'll do regularly.

- **LEARN AS MUCH AS YOU CAN ABOUT DIABETES.** Regardless of the type of diabetes you have, knowledge is critical. Good self-care requires that you know what affects your blood sugars and how you can get them to a healthy level.

- **BE ON THE LOOKOUT FOR DEPRESSION.** Having a chronic disease like diabetes, which affects virtually every aspect of your life, can take a heavy toll on you emotionally. But depression can affect how well you care for yourself. If you think you're depressed, talk to a health care professional about getting treatment.

- **KEEP STRESS IN CHECK.** Too much stress can elevate blood glucose levels, so do what you can to manage it, either by adopting new habits, altering your perspective, or getting help from others. A daily relaxation exercise such as yoga or meditation can help too.

- **MONITOR YOUR BLOOD GLUCOSE.** It may not be easy at first, but regularly monitoring your blood glucose is critical to diabetes care and can help you prevent complications later on. If necessary, talk to your doctor about ways to make it less painful.

# DIARRHEA

ALMOST EVERYONE HAS SUFFERED the unpleasant experience of diarrhea. Whether it results from a bout of food poisoning, a viral infection, or a parasite picked up during international travel, diarrhea is a common medical problem that usually resolves on its own.

In most people the diarrhea is acute, the result of an infection caused by a virus, bacteria, or a parasite. But it can also occur in someone taking certain medications or who is going through extreme stress and anxiety. In some people, diarrhea may be a more chronic condition, which is usually a sign of something more serious such as Crohn's disease or irritable bowel syndrome.

Diarrhea occurs when the digestive system is exposed to a toxic substance. In an effort to eliminate it, the digestive system secretes extra fluid to neutralize the toxin and then increases its contractions. The result is loose, watery stools and more frequent trips to the bathroom. In most cases, the diarrhea lasts just a day or two and goes away on its own without treatment.

## ⚲ What It Looks Like

Some people with diarrhea will experience abdominal pain, cramps, bloating, nausea, or an urgent need to have a bowel movement. Depending on the cause of the diarrhea, the condition is sometimes accompanied by a fever or blood in the stools.

Short-term diarrhea, the acute kind, usually lasts just a few days and not more than four weeks. Chronic diarrhea, which lasts more than four weeks, is often related to a more serious medical condition and, in some cases, may come and go. In people with irritable bowel syndrome, it may even alternate with bouts of constipation.

Diarrhea can occur in anyone at any age, and the greatest risk is dehydration, especially in infants and newborns. The focus for treating anyone with diarrhea is to make sure they remain hydrated.

## 🍴 What to Eat

Since preventing dehydration is your primary concern, look for mild fluids that can help you stay hydrated, says Lynn Sutton, R.D., C.D.E., a registered dietitian in Albany, New York. Try drinking water, broth, electrolyte drinks, or weak tea. You might also try eating foods that are high in fluids, such as sherbet, pudding, yogurt, or gelatin.

When your appetite returns, go easy with your food choices. Start with bland foods such as crackers or foods in the BRAT diet (bananas, rice, applesauce, and toast). Consider adding oatmeal or another hot cereal. Slowly reintroduce others foods, such as cooked vegetables, plain turkey or chicken, and sherbet.

## 🚫 What Not to Eat

Avoid dairy products, which can unsettle the stomach. Some people may actually have a condition known as lactose intolerance, in which they cannot digest lactose, a sugar found in dairy products. Lactose intolerance can cause diarrhea.

Steer clear of greasy, fried, and high-fat foods, which aggravate the digestive tract. You should also avoid sugar, because a bacterial infection will thrive on sugar. In addition, do not ingest foods or drinks that contain caffeine. Caffeine promotes urination and the further loss of fluids.

If the diarrhea persists, consider doing an elimination test to figure out if certain foods are causing the diarrhea. An elimination test involves cutting out allergenic foods for seven to ten days, then reintroducing them back one at a time to see if they provoke symptoms. Common culprits include eggs, gluten (which could indicate celiac disease), nuts, and dairy.

## 💊 Supplements for Diarrhea

People with diarrhea may become deficient in certain nutrients, especially if the diarrhea lasts for many weeks or months. To ensure you get the nutrients you need, start with a quality multivitamin. If you do want to try taking a supplement, discuss it with your doctor first. Some supplements you might consider taking include the following:

### VITAMIN A
Chronic diarrhea can cause deficiencies in vitamin A, an antioxidant.

### PROBIOTICS
Diarrhea can deplete the digestive tract of healthy bacteria such as *Lactobacillus acidophilus*, which may be replenished with supplements.

### GOLDENSEAL
Goldenseal is an herb that contains a compound called berberine, which can kill bacteria. It may also help promote immunity.

### PSYLLIUM
Psyllium is a seed husk and soluble fiber that can help stabilize any bowel irregularities. Talk to your doctor first before taking psyllium, especially if you have food allergies, because some people react to psyllium.

## 📋 Stay-Healthy Strategies

- **WATCH FOR DEHYDRATION.** Look for signs in young children, such as the absence of tears, dark or infrequent urination, dry mouth, irritability, and rapid heartbeat. Adults may experience excessive thirst, dry mouth, little or no urination, and severe weakness, dizziness, or lightheadedness.

- **BEWARE THE USE OF ANTIDIARRHEAL DRUGS** such as Imodium A-D and Kaopectate. These drugs slow intestinal motility and provide relief, but some experts think it's best to let the diarrhea resolve on its own.

- **SEE A DOCTOR IF THE SYMPTOMS PERSIST,** if you have a fever, or if you suspect dehydration. You should also get checked out if the symptoms worsen or you cannot tolerate food or drink after a few days.

## Prevent Travelers' Diarrhea

People who venture to foreign countries are at risk for travelers' diarrhea (TD), the most common illness to affect travelers. TD occurs in 20 to 50 percent of international travelers.

According to the Centers for Disease Control and Prevention (CDC), high-risk destinations are the developing countries of Latin America, Africa, the Middle East, and Asia. People who are at greatest risk include young adults, those with suppressed immunity, people with inflammatory bowel disease or diabetes, and anyone taking H-2 blockers or antacids. The main source of infection is food or water that has fecal contamination.

To avoid TD, do not eat foods or drinks purchased from food vendors or any place that appears to be lacking in hygiene. Stick with bottled waters, hot tea, or coffee. Don't eat raw or undercooked meat or seafood. Avoid eating raw fruits and vegetables that you did not peel yourself. Also, become familiar with risks in specific regions.

For more information, check out the traveler's health page at www.cdc.gov/travel/ on the CDC Web site.

# DIVERTICULITIS

AS YOU AGE, IT ISN'T UNUSUAL to develop pouches that jut out from the wall of your colon. These pouches are called diverticula, and the condition is known as diverticulosis. Most cause no problems, and you probably have no idea they're there. Approximately 10 percent of all people over age 40 have this condition.

In some people, however, these diverticula become inflamed or infected. This condition is known as diverticulitis. Those suffering from the condition may experience abdominal pain, often in the lower left side. If the cause is an infection, fever, nausea, chills, diarrhea, constipation, and cramping may result.

Most experts believe that diverticulitis is the result of a diet low in fiber. The condition became more common in the early 1900s, at the same time processed foods arrived on the scene. The disease is more prevalent in developed countries such as the United States and England but less common in places where high-fiber diets are the norm, such as Asia and Africa. The condition is also more likely in older adults. Experts believe that the lack of fiber causes constipation, which in turn leads to straining during a bowel movement. The straining creates pressure in the colon that causes weak areas of the colon to bulge and form pouches.

Treatment for diverticulitis involves eating a high-fiber diet and, sometimes, taking a pain medication. In some people, diverticulosis may be discovered during a routine digital rectal exam or a colon cancer screening. Knowing you have diverticulosis can help you avoid diverticulitis if you start eating more fiber. But if diverticulitis is left untreated, it can lead to bleeding, perforations, tears, infections, and blockages.

## What It Looks Like

While diverticulosis causes no symptoms, diverticulitis can result in abdominal pain, especially in the lower left side of the abdomen. As mentioned above, you may also experience constipation, diarrhea, bloating, fever, nausea, vomiting, and, less commonly, bleeding from the rectum.

## What to Eat

The most important strategy for diverticulitis is to boost your fiber intake, says Fred Pescatore, M.D., a New York City doctor who uses nutrition to treat patients and co-author of *The Hamptons*

*Diet Cookbook.* Most American get far less than the 25 to 30 grams recommended by the American Dietetic Association (ADA).

Fiber is a carbohydrate that occurs naturally in plant foods and comes in two forms. The soluble type dissolves in water and acts as a gel in the intestines, while the insoluble variety absorbs water and helps soften the stool. Good sources of soluble fiber include oats, kidney beans, peas, flaxseed, apples, oranges, and carrots. The insoluble kind—fondly known as roughage—is found in whole-wheat foods, cauliflower, beans, spinach, peas, and apples.

Fiber is also found in whole grains, such as brown rice, bulgur wheat, and quinoa, as well as legumes, such as chickpeas, kidney beans, pinto beans, and black beans. Prunes, figs, and flaxseeds contain fiber too.

When you do start increasing your fiber intake, do so slowly. Too much too soon can cause gas. To reduce gas, make sure to drink enough fluids, which are also helpful for diverticulitis.

Fluids lubricate the colon and add bulk to the stools, making them easier to eliminate and resulting in less pressure on the diverticula. The best fluid to drink is water. Aim for eight 8-oz. glasses of fluid each day. If you're overweight, you should drink even more than that.

During an acute attack, don't eat solid foods until the diverticulitis clears up. Instead drink clear liquids such as broth and water.

## Fiber Superstars

Eating more fiber is the best way to treat diverticulitis. But what exactly constitutes a high-fiber food? On food labels, high fiber means there are 5 grams or more in a single serving. A good source means there are 2.5 to 4.9 grams. Having "more or added fiber" means each serving has at least 2.5 grams more fiber per serving than the traditional version of the food. Here are just a few fiber powerhouses:

| | |
|---|---|
| Apple (1 medium) | 3.7 g |
| Dried plums (5) | 3.0 g |
| Dried figs (3) | 5.2 g |
| Pear (1 medium) | 4.0 g |
| Raspberries ($\frac{1}{2}$ c) | 4.2 g |
| Broccoli ($\frac{1}{2}$ c) | 2.8 g |
| Raw carrot (1 medium) | 2.2 g |
| Peas ($\frac{1}{2}$ c) | 4.4 g |
| Sweet potato (1 medium) | 3.4 g |
| Lentil beans ($\frac{1}{2}$ c) | 7.8 g |
| Vegetarian baked beans ($\frac{1}{2}$ c) | 6.3 g |
| Barley ($\frac{1}{2}$ c) | 4.3 g |
| 100% bran cereal (1 oz) | 9.7 g |
| Bran flakes (1 oz) | 4.7 g |
| Whole wheat bread (1 slice) | 2.0 g |

*Source: American Dietetic Association*

## 🍽 What Not to Eat

Most doctors used to discourage patients from eating nuts, seeds, and fruits and veggies with small seeds because they thought these foods could get lodged in the diverticula and cause an attack of diverticulitis. But these days, the guidelines are less rigid. While some foods such as popcorn, nuts, and sunflower seeds are still apt to get caught in the diverticula, many of the smaller seeds in strawberries, tomatoes, and raspberries are now believed to be harmless.

The truth is that the rule on nuts and seeds may vary with individual patients. Not every patient will be hurt by these foods, but some may experience problems. The best thing to do is to cut back your intake of these foods during an attack and to eat them in small amounts when you're healthy.

## 💊 Supplements for Diverticulitis

Start by taking a high-quality multivitamin to ensure you get all the essential nutrients, especially if you have diarrhea. Some other supplements you might consider include the following:

### PSYLLIUM

If you're having a hard time tolerating a high-fiber diet, you might want to take psyllium, a soluble fiber. Talk to your doctor first before taking psyllium, especially if you have food allergies, because some people react to psyllium. The same is true of laxatives, such as Metamucil, which contain psyllium.

### FISH OIL

Taking fish oil, which contains healthy omega-3 fatty acids, can greatly improve the overall health of your colon. But always consult your doctor first because fish oil can cause the blood to become thinner and raise your risk for bleeding.

### GLUTAMINE

Glutamine is an amino acid that occurs naturally in the body. As a supplement, it can help strengthen the lining of the intestinal tract.

## 📋 Stay-Healthy Strategies

- **DON'T HOLD IT.** When you feel the urge to defecate, don't wait too long to go. Resisting a bowel movement can harden stool and cause constipation that may lead to diverticulitis.

- **EXERCISE REGULARLY.** Physical activity helps the bowels to function properly.

- **COMMIT TO EATING A HIGH-FIBER DIET FOR LIFE.** Once you have diverticula, you have them for good. Eating plenty of fiber will help prevent the attacks of diverticulitis.

- **GIVE THE COLON TIME TO RECOVER.** If your doctor recommends that you stay in bed for a while, by all means, do it. Adequate bed rest is critical to your recovery.

# EAR INFECTIONS

ANYONE CAN GET AN EAR INFECTION, but most cases occur in infants and toddlers. In fact, 90 percent of all children will have an ear infection before they attend school, according to the American Academy of Pediatrics.

Acute otitis media, the most common type of ear infection, is an infection of the middle ear. It typically results from an upper respiratory infection such as a cold and may occur in one or both ears. When the Eustachian tube inside the ear becomes swollen due to the cold, fluid pools in the middle ear. If the fluid becomes infected with bacteria, pus builds up behind the eardrum, causing pain. If the fluid builds up but is not infected, it is called otitis media with effusion.

Ear infections are more common in young childhood for several reasons. The Eustachian tubes in the ear are wider, shorter, and more horizontal in children than those in adults, which makes it harder for the fluid to drain from the middle ear but easier for bacteria and viruses in the back of the nose and throat to infect the ears. In addition, children don't have fully developed immune systems until age seven. A less mature immune system makes them more vulnerable to infections, especially upper respiratory viral infections that frequently put them at risk for ear infections. Children who are exposed to cigarette smoke and those who are bottle-fed or attend day care are generally at greater risk too.

In the past, pediatricians were quick to give antibiotics to children with ear infections. But these days, with people becoming increasingly resistant to antibiotics, that thinking has changed. According to the Centers for Disease Control and Prevention, it's best to start with a wait-and-see approach. Many infections, especially the ones caused by viruses, clear up on their own without any treatment. But if the infection is still present after a few days, your child may then need antibiotics. Your doctor may want to see the ear again after 48 hours to see if the infection is worsening or improving.

Some children suffer from recurrent ear infections. These children may require the surgical insertion of small ventilation tubes to allow the fluid to drain out and normal air pressure to return to the ear. And some may need a small dose of antibiotics to keep the fluid from getting reinfected while the body works to reabsorb the fluid. But in most kids, ear infections are a temporary nuisance that they will outgrow as the Eustachian tube matures.

## What It Looks Like

The symptoms of an ear infection vary widely. Some children may experience severe pain; others just have a vague sense that something is bothering them in the ear. Babies may cry inconsolably, while toddlers may tug at the ear and behave more irritably. An older child may complain that his ear hurts. The pain may make it hard for your child to lie down, chew, or suck, so you may notice he is not eating as much or is having problems sleeping. In addition, some children may experience fever, nausea, vomiting, and dizziness.

In some cases, the fluid buildup can block sound and you may notice your child has trouble hearing. If there's severe pressure from the fluid, a small part of the eardrum may open up and allow the pus and fluid to drain from the eardrum (and often out of the ear). Some people refer to this as a "ruptured" eardrum, although the eardrum actually remains intact. This releases the pressure behind the eardrum, usually bringing relief from the pain.

## What to Eat

Encourage your child to eat a healthy, well-balanced diet that bolsters his immune system, says Mary Ann LoFrumento, M.D., pediatrician and author of *Simply Parenting: Understanding Your Newborn and Infant*. Make sure he gets plenty of fruits and vegetables, which contain nutrients such as antioxidants that can help combat. The same advice applies to adults.

Also, be sure to offer plenty of healthy fluids, such as water. Drinking a lot of fluids will help thin any mucus secretions that may develop from a cold.

If your child is bottle-fed, try switching him to a formula that does not contain any cow's milk protein. This might help in some cases. Note, too, that prolonged breastfeeding appears to have a protective effect against ear infections, while children who are bottle-fed seem more prone to them.

## What Not to Eat

If you suspect that your child has increased mucus from food allergies or sensitivities, try eliminating all allergenic foods from your child's diet. These foods could be the culprit behind the ear infection. If necessary, do an elimination diet that removes common allergenic foods from the diet, including dairy products, eggs, wheat, peanuts, and citrus foods. After a few days, gradually reintroduce the potential allergen into the diet. If you notice that allergic symptoms or an ear infection develops, eliminate that food from your child's diet for good.

Cut back or eliminate refined carbohydrates such as cookies, muffins, cakes, and breads. These foods are rich in simple sugars that provide few nutrients and weaken immunity.

## 💊 Supplements for Ear Infections

Give your child a multivitamin to make sure he's getting all the essential nutrients he needs. Before giving him any other supplements, consult your physician. Other supplements you may consider include the following:

### VITAMIN C

This antioxidant vitamin can help bolster immunity. But never give more than the recommended daily dosage for a child because in excess it can cause diarrhea.

### ZINC

Zinc is a major mineral that supports the body's immune function.

## 📋 Stay-Healthy Strategies

- **RELIEVE YOUR CHILD'S PAIN WITH AN OVER-THE-COUNTER PAIN RELIEVER** such as acetaminophen or ibuprofen.

- **ENCOURAGE OLDER CHILDREN TO SIT UP** as much as possible because that can help relieve the pressure.

- **ELEVATE THE HEAD OF THE MATTRESS** by rolling a towel underneath it or prop up an older child with extra pillows. The slight incline can also help ease the pressure.

- **LOOK FOR WAYS TO KEEP YOUR CHILD HEALTHY** if he's prone to ear infections. Strategies to prevent colds will help him avoid having ear infections. So wash hands frequently and stay away from other children who have colds.

## Preventing Ear Infections

It's not always possible to prevent your child from getting an ear infection. But some strategies can help.

- **BREASTFEED RATHER THAN BOTTLE-FEED YOUR INFANT.** If you do bottle-feed your baby, keep her in a slightly vertical position when feeding. Don't give her the bottle when she's lying down.

- **KEEP HER AWAY FROM CIGARETTE SMOKE.** If anyone in your household smokes, encourage him or her to quit. Contact the American Lung Association to find smoking cessation programs in your area. They're at 1-800-LUNG-USA. Ban smoking in areas where your child spends a lot of time.

- **CHOOSE HER DAY CARE SETTING WISELY.** Try to find one with fewer children and in a setting where the caregivers do not smoke. Although ear infections themselves are not contagious, the upper respiratory infections that cause them are.

# ECZEMA

MOST PEOPLE ARE FAMILIAR with the occasional bout of dry, itchy skin. But for approximately fifteen million Americans, this condition is a chronic problem, one that leads to embarrassing red patches and unsightly crusts on the skin. These people suffer from a skin disorder called eczema.

Eczema, also called atopic dermatitis, is an inflammation of the skin that often begins in infancy. It is a common skin disorder characterized by dry, red, itchy skin. Children who can't resist the urge to scratch often get caught up in a vicious cycle of itching and scratching that only leads to more redness, swelling, and cracking. Sometimes the patches of affected skin develop blisters that may "weep" a clear fluid. Eventually, the skin may thicken and crusts may form.

According to the National Institutes of Health, eczema accounts for 10 to 20 percent of all visits to dermatologists. The disease affects males and females equally, with approximately 65 percent of all cases beginning in the first year of life. Ninety percent of patients experience their first symptoms before age five. After age 30, eczema is uncommon and more likely the result of exposing the skin to harsh or moist conditions.

No one knows exactly what causes eczema, but it's most likely a combination of genetics and environment. Children with parents who suffer from allergies, asthma, or other allergic conditions are more likely to develop eczema than children whose parents do not have these conditions. Although eczema is a chronic condition, it does sometimes go away with age. Unfortunately,

however, children with eczema may go on to develop allergic conditions such as asthma. Experts also believe that eczema is a disorder of the immune system.

Treatment often involves the use of topical corticosteroid creams, which can help calm the inflammation. When these are not effective, you may be given a systemic steroid. In more severe cases, people may need drugs that suppress the immune system.

## What It Looks Like

Eczema causes the skin to appear red, swollen, and cracked. With excessive scratching, the skin may excrete a clear fluid. Eventually, crusty patches may develop, as well as some scaliness. Prolonged scratching may lead to secondary infections.

The effects of eczema typically vary over time. Stress, humidity, the presence of pets, hormones, and molds are all factors that can affect the severity of your eczema.

Another form of eczema is allergic contact eczema (dermatitis). This type of eczema results from contact with an allergen, a substance the immune system treats as a foreign invader. Examples of allergens that trigger allergic contact eczema include poison ivy, lotion, soaps, or laundry detergent. People with this type of eczema will experience the same symptoms as those with atopic dermatitis.

## ¶¶¶ What to Eat

Make sure to include foods rich in omega-3 fatty acids in your diet, says Elizabeth Lipski, Ph.D., C.C.N., a clinical nutritionist and author of *Digestive Wellness*. Good choices include cold-water fish such as tuna, salmon, sardines, and halibut. You can also get these healthy fats from flaxseed.

In addition, eat foods rich in vitamin C, which can strengthen the immune system. These foods include citrus fruits, blueberries, leafy greens, broccoli, red bell peppers, and asparagus.

If you're pregnant and suffer from allergies and/or eczema, consider breastfeeding your baby. Studies show that babies who are breastfed are less likely to develop eczema than infants who are formula-fed.

## What Not to Eat

Many people with eczema suffer from food allergies that can trigger inflammation. So consider doing an elimination diet that helps you pinpoint the problematic food. Eliminate all potential allergens from your diet, then gradually reintroduce them and look for symptoms. Possible culprits include soy, peanuts, milk, eggs, and wheat.

Because inflammation is involved in eczema, it's also a good idea to avoid—or at least cut back on—foods high in fats, refined sugars, and anything that is highly processed. These types of food are more likely to cause inflammation that will aggravate the eczema.

### The Skin Cure Diet

Kathleen Waterford suffered from eczema for years. Then she decided to stop eating all carbohydrates, except fresh green vegetables and small amounts of pumpkin, sunflower, and sesame seeds. She even shunned complex carbs such as brown rice and quinoa for six weeks, and slowly reintroduced them after that. She also limited her protein to mostly fish and chicken.

Over the next three months, her skin improved. When the diet regimen helped her get rid of her lifelong battle with eczema, she became so convinced of the power of diet that she wrote a book, *The Skin Cure Diet*.

## When Your Child Has Eczema

It's hard enough to stop yourself from scratching a bothersome itch. But try telling that to your three-year-old who feels overwhelmed by the itchy sensation.

According to the American Academy of Dermatology, there are ways you can help your child get relief. Start by keeping his skin moist. Rub unscented lotion on his body within minutes after his bath to retain the moisture. Use gentle soaps and wash his clothes in mild detergents. Dress him in loose, breathable fabrics. Try to keep his bedroom clean and free of dust. And of course, avoid foods that are potentially allergenic.

## Supplements for Eczema

Start with a quality multivitamin, which will provide all the nutrients needed for good health. Choose a vitamin that is free of common allergens. In addition, you may consider taking these other supplements:

### VITAMIN C

As a potent antioxidant, vitamin C may help improve immune function and reduce the severity of your symptoms.

### PROBIOTICS

Healthy bacteria such as *Lactobacillus* may help improve digestion of foods you don't realize are allergenic.

### EVENING PRIMROSE OIL

This oil contains gamma linolenic acid, a type of fatty acid that may help reduce inflammation and boost immune function.

### FLAXSEED OR FISH OIL

These oils contain omega-3 fatty acids, which are often deficient in people with eczema. Omega-3s help lower inflammation. But talk to your physician before using them, because these oils have a thinning effect on the blood and may promote bleeding.

### QUERCETIN

Quercetin is a bioflavonoid that has an anti-inflammatory effect. It may also help control allergic reactions.

### CHAMOMILE OR LICORICE ROOT CREAMS

These substances may be applied topically to affected skin for temporary relief. Licorice root triggers the production of prostaglandins, natural substances involved in healing and taming skin inflammation.

## Stay-Healthy Strategies

- **KEEP YOUR HOUSE CLEAN.** Vacuum and dust regularly to minimize exposure to allergenic dust mites, mold, and pet dander.

- **CONSIDER USING AIR PURIFIERS.** These can help reduce the allergens in your house.

- **LIMIT YOUR USE OF CHEMICAL IRRITANTS** found in household cleaning products. People with eczema may be sensitive to these substances.

- **PRACTICE STRESS REDUCTION** with relaxation, meditation, or another form of therapy. Regular exercise can also help alleviate stress.

# ENDOMETRIOSIS

INSIDE EVERY WOMAN'S UTERUS is a lining called the endometrium. Every month, this lining thickens in anticipation of a fertilized egg. When fertilization does not occur, the lining is shed through menstruation. The monthly repetition of this process is known as the menstrual cycle.

For some women, the endometrium grows outside the uterus. It may turn up on or under the ovaries, behind the uterus, or in the pelvic areas that support the uterus. Sometimes the tissue grows on the bowels or the bladder. And in rare cases, it may even grow in the lungs or behind the knees. This is a chronic condition known as endometriosis.

Although the tissue is displaced, it continues to be affected by the monthly cycle. So when a woman has her monthly period, the displaced tissue will also thicken and bleed. But unlike the lining and blood that is shed in menstruation, the blood from this tissue has nowhere to go. Trapped in a foreign place, the tissue may develop growths, which are called tumors or implants. These growths can cause severe pain, infertility, and heavy bleeding. Patients may also experience inflammation and a buildup of scar tissue.

According to the American College of Obstetrics and Gynecology, endometriosis affects 7 to 10 percent of U.S. women. Among women who are infertile, endometriosis is believed to affect somewhere between 7 and 38 percent of women. Some experts believe five to six million women of childbearing age have endometriosis. The condition affects women of all races, socioeconomic backgrounds, and ages. The disease has been diagnosed in girls as young as age nine and in postmenopausal women, according to the Endometriosis Association.

No one knows exactly what causes endometriosis, but theories abound. Some experts believe it is caused by exposure to toxins. Others think it is a backup of menstrual tissue in the fallopian tubes into the pelvic cavity. Still other experts think endometriosis is the result of a malfunction of the immune system. Other theories suggest that endometriosis involves metaplasia, the changing of normal tissue into another type of normal tissue; lymphatic or vascular spread, in which endometrial tissue travels through the blood to distant sites; and family history, in which the disease is passed on through genetics.

Treatment for endometriosis varies and may involve pain relievers and/or hormone treatment. In severe cases, surgery may be necessary to remove extensive amounts of tissue or to relieve severe pain.

## ⌕ What It Looks Like

Four out of five women with endometriosis don't even know they have the disease. The most common symptom of endometriosis is pain in the abdomen, lower back, and pelvic areas. But the severity of the pain does not reflect the severity of disease. Some women may have no pain, even if they have scarring and widespread disease. Other women may have severe pain though the disease is limited to just a few areas.

Typical symptoms of endometriosis include the following:

- Pain before and during menstruation that may be extreme, even disabling. The pain may worsen over time.

- Pain during or after sex

- Chronic pelvic pain that is also felt in the lower back

- Intestinal pain and gastrointestinal symptoms such as diarrhea, nausea, and constipation

- Painful bowel movements or urination during monthly periods

- Heavy bleeding during menstruation

- Spotting or bleeding between periods

- Fatigue

Confirming whether you have endometriosis requires a visit to an obstetrician/gynecologist, who will do imaging tests to look for abnormal growths or tissue.

## ꗋꗋꗋ What to Eat

A healthy, well-balanced diet of whole, unprocessed foods can help women with endometriosis experience fewer symptoms, says Thomas Lyons, M.D., medical director of the Center for Women's Care and Reproductive Surgery in Atlanta and co-author of *What to Do When the Doctor Says It's Endometriosis*. Eat an abundance of fresh fruits and vegetables, which will fortify your immune system with disease-combating antioxidants. These foods are also rich in fiber, which will help prevent and ease gastrointestinal problems.

Make sure to eat foods rich in B vitamins. The B vitamins help the liver metabolize estrogen, and keeping estrogen in balance can help relieve the symptoms of endometriosis.

Maintaining a healthy weight is also important to someone with endometriosis. So watch your portions and calorie intake. Excess fat cells promote estrogen, which can worsen symptoms.

# What Not to Eat

Avoid dairy products, which contain prostaglandins that can worsen pelvic pain and cramps. Instead get your calcium from other sources, such as leafy greens, fortified cereals, and supplements.

Do your best to eat less saturated fat. These fats also contain prostaglandins. In animal products, fat is a storehouse for dioxins, toxic chemicals that may be involved in promoting endometriosis.

In addition, beware of foods rich in sodium. Too much salt will promote premenstrual bloating and worsen the symptoms of endometriosis.

Also steer clear of alcohol, caffeine, and sugar. These substances promote inflammation and can worsen your pain. In addition, alcohol stresses the liver and, in excess, can cause nutrient deficiencies that you can't afford.

## The Diagnosis Challenge

Many women wait years before they're correctly diagnosed with endometriosis. In fact, it may take as many as nine years for a diagnosis for some women.

Why the difficulty? Pain is a vague, subjective symptom, and women's tolerance for it can vary significantly. Many women are told the pain is normal with menstruation and to simply ignore it. But in reality, your monthly period should cause only mild discomfort, not excruciating pain.

Other women are too embarrassed to discuss certain symptoms such as pain with sex or painful bowel movements during menstruation. It's also easy to confuse the symptoms of endometriosis with other disorders such as chronic fatigue syndrome or irritable bowel syndrome, which may coexist with endometriosis but are distinct and separate disorders.

If you think you may have endometriosis, be assertive about getting checked, even if that means finding a new doctor. But don't be shy about it. A correct diagnosis will lead to the proper treatment and relief from your suffering. So don't delay. Your health is worth it.

## ♔ Supplements for Endometriosis

Start by taking a quality multivitamin to make sure you get all the essential nutrients. Other supplements you might want to consider taking include the following:

### B VITAMIN COMPLEX

The B vitamins help the liver metabolize estrogen. In particular, vitamin B6, or pyridoxine, may help relieve premenstrual syndrome and heavy menstrual bleeding.

### VITAMIN C

This potent antioxidant builds your immune system and may help relieve cramps and bloating.

### EVENING PRIMROSE OIL

This herbal remedy contains the essential fatty acid gamma linolenic acid, which helps relieve the symptoms of endometriosis.

### PROGESTERONE CREAM

The topical use of progesterone can sometimes counteract any excess estrogen and promote greater hormonal balance. Do not use this cream without consulting your doctor first. Evidence suggests that the effectiveness of this therapy varies among women.

## ▭ Stay-Healthy Strategies

- **FIND SUPPORT.** Endometriosis is a chronic condition that can affect your life in many ways. Strengthen your ability to cope with help from family, friends, or a support group.

- **GET EDUCATED.** Learn as much as you can about endometriosis. Knowledge is your greatest ally and can help you better deal with your condition.

- **ENLIST A DOCTOR YOU TRUST.** A good physician can help you wade through all your options and give you the stamina to live well with this disease.

- **EXERCISE REGULARLY.** Physical activity reduces the stress of having a chronic condition and may even lower a woman's risk for endometriosis. Consider doing a meditative form of exercise such as yoga or tai chi, which can help relieve stress.

# EPILEPSY

IN HEALTHY PEOPLE, NERVE CELLS IN THE BRAIN are constantly firing off tiny electrical charges to the rest of the body. In someone who has epilepsy, this pattern of activity is disrupted by bursts of energy that are more intense than normal, causing the person to have seizures.

Epilepsy is a neurological disorder characterized by repeated seizures. Some children are born with epilepsy, but others may develop the condition later on as the result of injury, trauma, or infection. Diseases that affect the way the brain functions such as meningitis or encephalitis, for instance, can lead to epilepsy. Exposure to toxins such as lead can also result in epilepsy. Although most cases begin in childhood, the condition can actually occur at any time, even in later adulthood.

According to the Epilepsy Foundation, epilepsy and seizures affect 2.7 million Americans of all ages. Approximately 200,000 new cases are diagnosed each year. Most cases occur under the age of two and over the age of 65. The condition occurs slightly more often in males than females. Ten percent of all Americans will experience a seizure in their lifetime.

Some people experience partial seizures in which the abnormal bursts of energy occur in just one part of the brain. In others, these unusual surges of energy happen throughout the brain, producing generalized seizures. Some people may have a single seizure as the result of severe illness.

A single seizure doesn't mean you have epilepsy. Rather, the condition is diagnosed after you've had recurrent seizures. Doctors use special diagnostic equipment such as the electroencephalograph (EEG) to record brain waves during or between seizures to detect patterns that reveal epilepsy.

Treatment for epilepsy involves anti-epileptic medications, surgery, diet, or vagus nerve stimulators (VNS). With VNS, a battery-like device is implanted in the chest and programmed to send electrical energy to the brain via the vagus nerve, a large nerve in the neck. VNS therapy is used to prevent seizures in older children and adults who have not responded to medications or surgery.

## ⌕ What It Looks Like

The sight of someone having a seizure can be frightening, especially when it's the first time in a small child. During a seizure, the person may have jerky movements and muscle spasms. There may be intense staring involved, and some people may become disoriented or confused. Still others may lose consciousness.

The symptoms of a seizure vary depending on the type of seizure involved. A generalized tonic-clonic seizure–commonly known as a grand mal seizure–for instance, affects both sides of the brain and produces loss of consciousness. A myoclonic seizure is also a generalized seizure but only produces brief, rapid contractions of bodily muscles.

Partial seizures–the most common kind–affect just one part of the brain and may be simple or complex. A simple partial seizure causes uncontrolled muscle movements, odd sensations in all five senses, and intense emotional reactions, most often fear and impending doom, but also anger or elation. A complex partial seizure involves a loss of control over actions, emotions, and speech. There may be a blank stare or trance-like appearance, and even a loss of consciousness.

When a person you're with is having a seizure, it's important to stay calm. Here are some more tips from the Epilepsy Foundation:

- Reassure other people who may be nearby.
- Don't hold the person down or try to stop his movements.
- Time the seizure with your watch.
- Clear the area around the person of anything hard or sharp.
- Loosen ties or anything around the neck that may make breathing difficult.
- Put something flat and soft, like a folded jacket, under the person's head.
- Turn him gently onto one side to help keep the airway clear. Do not try to force the mouth open with any hard implement or with fingers. A person having a seizure cannot swallow his tongue. Efforts to hold the tongue down can injure the teeth or jaw.
- Don't attempt artificial respiration except in the unlikely event that the person does not start breathing again after the seizure has stopped.
- Stay with the person until the seizure ends naturally.
- Be friendly and reassure the person as consciousness returns.
- Offer to call a taxi, friend, or relative to help the person get home if he seems confused or unable to get home by himself. Be sure, however, that you don't need to call 911 or an ambulance instead (see page 136 for more information).

## 🍴 What to Eat

Controlling epilepsy with diets is not a new approach, with the most popular strategy being the ketogenic diet, according to Carl E. Stafstrom, M.D., Ph.D., a pediatric neurologist at the University of Wisconsin. The ketogenic diet is a high-fat, low-carb diet that forces the body to burn fat for all its energy needs.

It starts with a twenty-four-hour fast, which forces the body to burn up its reserves of glucose. After that, the diet is comprised of 80 percent fat, with protein and carbohydrates making up the remaining 20 percent. Each meal is carefully measured, and the child must finish the entire meal for the ketogenic diet to be successful.

Close adherence to the ketogenic diet can prevent seizures, especially in children. In fact, research has found that at least half of patients who do the ketogenic diet experience a 50 percent or more reduction in seizure frequency. The patient typically remains on the diet for about two years, and then is gradually weaned off of it. Although the diet may elevate cholesterol levels during that time, cholesterol generally returns to normal when the diet is discontinued.

Some people may also benefit from following the Atkins diet, the popular weight loss plan that restricts carbohydrates but allows for high-fat foods. Unlike the ketogenic plan, the Atkins diet doesn't restrict calories, and it also allows for a higher intake of protein. But studies are preliminary, and more research is needed.

Researchers are also just beginning to consider other nutrition strategies, such as restricting calories or increasing polyunsaturated fatty acids, the kinds found in vegetable oils. In the meantime, try to eat a healthy well-balanced diet, and be sure to consult a nutrition expert if you want to try the ketogenic diet.

If you're taking anti-seizure medications, make sure to also get plenty of calcium and vitamin D,
says Marie Savard, M.D., author of *The Body Shape Solution*. Many anti-seizure medications can lead to osteomalacia, a softening of the bones. As seizures put you at risk for injuries that could affect your bones, boost your intake of calcium and vitamin D with foods such as low-fat milk, yogurt, and low-fat cheese.

## What Not to Eat

Avoid foods that contain glutamate, an excitatory neurotransmitter and amino acid that has been linked to seizure activity. That means avoiding foods that contain monosodium glutamate (MSG), a food additive often used to season Chinese food.

You may also want to avoid alcoholic beverages and foods that contain caffeine. Both substances may worsen seizures.

## Supplements for Epilepsy

Taking a quality multivitamin can help ensure overall health, but in general, you should exercise caution in using supplements if you have epilepsy. Before taking any supplement, discuss it with your physician.

## Stay-Healthy Strategies

- **BE CAUTIOUS WITH EXERCISE.** Regular exercise can help people with epilepsy combat depression, sleep better, and boost energy. But exertion can trigger seizures in some people. Talk with your doctor about the best ways to stay active and choose activities carefully.

- **CONSIDER JOINING A SUPPORT GROUP.** Living with epilepsy can be difficult. Check with the Epilepsy Foundation about support groups or online communities where you can meet others who have this disease.

- **KNOW YOUR MEDS.** There are many drugs used to treat epilepsy, and it isn't always easy to find one that works. Many also cause side effects. When trying a medication, discuss all aspects of it with your doctor.

- **DEVELOP A GOOD RAPPORT WITH YOUR DOCTORS.** Sometimes, treating epilepsy can involve more than one doctor. Make sure you're comfortable with all the people on your medical team. Be honest about your symptoms and side effects, and use your appointment time wisely to gather information.

## When to Call 911

When an epileptic seizure ends within five minutes, you know the cause is epilepsy, and if consciousness returns without incident, there is probably no need to seek further medical care. But some circumstances around an epileptic seizure warrant more medical attention. According to the Epilepsy Foundation, you should call an ambulance if any of the following occurs:

- The seizure has happened in water.

- There's no medical I.D. and no way of knowing whether the seizure is caused by epilepsy.

- The person is pregnant, injured, or diabetic.

- Poisoning, hypoglycemia, high fever, heat exhaustion, or head injury is involved.

- The seizure continues for more than five minutes.

- A second seizure starts shortly after the first has ended.

- Consciousness does not start to return after the shaking has stopped.

# FEVER

MANY PEOPLE—ESPECIALLY PARENTS of small children—react to a fever with alarm, especially when the fever is high. They worry that the fever may affect the brain. But in reality, a fever is a sign that your body is fighting an infection, not a disease itself.

Fevers can occur with numerous bacterial or viral infections, including the flu, a urinary tract infection, or an unidentified virus. A fever is often the first sign that you're ill. But it may also be a reaction to medication or to a vaccine, or the result of being too warm or overdressed.

Most people have a normal temperature that ranges between 97 and 99°F. The average is 98.6°F. But even when you're healthy, your temperature may vary. It's generally lower in the early part of the day and higher in the evening. Your temperature can also go up when you're physically active.

A fever most often occurs as the result of an infection. When a virus or bacteria invades, white blood cells are summoned to defend the body against the offensive microbe. This activity causes the release of chemicals called pyrogens. Pyrogens in turn signal the hypothalamus, the body's thermostat, to crank up the temperature. The higher body temperature kills off the microbes. The extra heat is released when your blood vessels dilate, causing you to sweat.

In most people, a fever by itself is nothing serious and will resolve itself in a few days. In fact, it's normal for toddlers and young children to have fevers of up to 104 degrees for four or five days, as long as they are acting well and drinking plenty of fluids. But if they are listless or inconsolable, they need to see a doctor. You should also call a doctor if your child's fever persists for more than five days or if the temperature spikes to 105 degrees.

A fever in newborns under two months of age, however, is considerably more serious and could signal a viral illness or a severe infection or disease, such as meningitis. If that happens, call your pediatrician immediately.

Although most fevers are not serious, they can be highly uncomfortable. You can alleviate the discomfort with an over-the-counter analgesic such as acetaminophen or ibuprofen. But if the fever is not too bothersome, it might be best to let the fever run its course. Note: Ibuprofen should be used only in infants over six months of age. Anyone taking ibuprofen should do so with food because it can irritate your stomach.

## What It Looks Like

Most people know the fuzzy feeling that accompanies the start of a fever. You may also experience chills, headaches, muscle aches, sweating, and sleepiness. Some people may lose their appetite or experience lethargy.

More severe symptoms that may accompany a fever include severe headaches, skin rash, difficulties breathing, chest pain, persistent vomiting, and confusion. If you have any of these symptoms, you should call your doctor.

## What to Eat

Although the saying claims you should "feed a cold, starve a fever," the truth is you should still eat when your temperature is higher than normal, says Milton Stokes, R.D., a spokesperson for the American Dietetic Association. Eating the right foods will help nourish the immune system, which needs extra support when there's an infection.

Eat foods rich in vitamin C, such as fruits and vegetables, which will strengthen your immune system. Good choices include broccoli, peas, carrots, cauliflower, oranges, grapefruit, strawberries, blueberries, and kiwi. Fruits and veggies will also help ensure you get enough fluids.

Make sure to get plenty of fluids to help you stay hydrated. Try to get at least half of your fluids from water, and get the rest from unsweetened drinks such as vegetable juice, 100 percent fruit juice, herbal teas, broths, or low-fat milk.

Keep in mind that what you eat will also be affected by the presence of other medical problems. For instance, if you have conditions such as vomiting, malnutrition, or loss of appetite, your fluid needs—as well as your energy requirements—could be significantly greater. You may need as much as fifteen cups of fluid a day.

## Fever Q&A

**Q.** What are febrile seizures?

**A.** Some children who have fevers also experience convulsions known as febrile seizures. During a febrile seizure, the child trembles and loses consciousness. Some children may become rigid or develop twitches. The seizure may last only a few seconds or go on for several minutes.

Approximately 4 percent of children younger than age five have febrile seizures. They are rare beyond that age. During a seizure, parents should try to stay as calm as possible and try to prevent the child from getting hurt. Move him away from sharp objects or off a bed. Turn his head to the side so vomit and saliva can drain. If your child has difficulty breathing, turns blue, or suffers several seizures in a row, call 911. In any event, you should talk to your pediatrician. Although febrile seizures can be extremely alarming, most children don't suffer lasting effects.

## What Not to Eat

If you are an adult with a fever, avoid alcoholic beverages, which act as diuretics and may diminish your fluids. And anyone with a fever should also avoid refined sugars, which tend to suppress the immune system. Refined sugars are found in processed foods, desserts, and breads, but also in some fruit juices (ones that are not 100 percent fruit juice).

## Supplements for Fever

Take a quality multivitamin to make sure you're still getting all the essential nutrients you need. You might also consider taking vitamin C, which is an antioxidant that can help strengthen your immune system. Never exceed the upper limit, however, which is 2,000 mg. Too much vitamin C can cause diarrhea and will not provide any added benefit. Another way to get vitamin C is to eat nine to ten servings of fruit each day.

# FIBROMYALGIA

YOU'RE BESIEGED WITH PAIN, exhausted from insomnia, and awaken every morning stiff and uncomfortable. Yet, you look great and your doctors are at a loss as to why you're hurting so much. For approximately 4 percent of the U.S. population, the explanation for this baffling condition is fibromyalgia.

Fibromyalgia is a medical syndrome characterized by widespread pain, sleep disturbance, tender points around the body, and a host of other seemingly unrelated symptoms ranging from irritable bowel syndrome to depression. It is a puzzling condition, one that doctors often have trouble diagnosing and treating. No one knows what truly causes fibromyalgia.

Fibromyalgia is seven times more common in women than men, and it is most likely to occur between the ages of 20 and 55. There also appears to be a genetic tendency toward getting fibromyalgia, and a greater risk for it in people who have a rheumatic illness, such as lupus, rheumatoid arthritis, or scleroderma. In addition, the risk is higher in people who are experiencing severe emotional or physical stress and those who suffer a neck injury (from a car accident, etc.).

To be diagnosed, you must have pain in at least eleven of eighteen tender points and have experienced widespread pain for a span of at least three months.

## 🔎 What It Looks Like

People who have fibromyalgia typically have multiple symptoms, which vary widely from one patient to the next. Almost everyone has widespread pain and fatigue, and most people also have trouble sleeping. Some may have cognitive difficulties such as forgetfulness and trouble concentrating, a problem affectionately called "fibro fog."

Often, fibromyalgia sufferers will also experience other medical problems such as irritable bowel syndrome, restless leg syndrome, headaches, depression, temporomandibular joint disorder (TMJ), and numbness. Others may also have dry eyes and mouth, chronic yeast infections, irritable bladder, and Raynaud's phenomenon, an exaggerated response to cold temperatures that causes fingers to turn white. Women may have painful menstrual periods and vulvodynia, a type of pain in the external female genitalia.

What makes fibromyalgia so frustrating is that most people who have it look perfectly healthy. Even blood tests, X-rays, and magnetic resonance imaging (MRI) reveal no obvious abnormalities. For these reasons, many people are skeptical that fibromyalgia even exists. But in recent years, studies have started to show that levels of certain chemicals and substances occur in abnormal amounts in people with fibromyalgia. Other tests have revealed that the brain activity in people with fibromyalgia shows an exaggerated response in the brain's pain centers.

Most people successfully live with the disease by treating the symptoms. But in some cases, fibromyalgia can be debilitating. At its worst, fibromyalgia has forced some people to give up jobs or abandon hobbies, and it can also affect relationships.

## ¡¶¡ What to Eat

Studies have suggested that eating a vegan diet composed of raw vegetables, nuts, seeds, and grain products can improve the symptoms of fibromyalgia. But most experts agree that there is no single food or diet plan that can relieve fibromyalgia sufferers of their aches and pains or help them achieve a good night's rest. But that doesn't mean you shouldn't strive to eat a healthy, well-balanced diet that helps you maintain your weight and steer clear of disease.

According to Michael McNett, M.D., a family practice physician in Chicago and the co-author of *The Everything Health Guide to Fibromyalgia*, it's important to get a balance of carbohydrates and protein. Your body needs both nutrients to stay well. Fill your plate with nutrient-dense foods such as vegetables, fruits, and whole-grain breads, cereals, and pasta. These foods contain important antioxidants and other disease-fighting substances. To maintain energy levels, be sure to include low-fat sources of protein in your diet, such as fish, lean beef, turkey, and tofu. And make sure to drink plenty of water.

That said, there are certain nutrients that can help relieve your symptoms. According to McNett, people with fibromyalgia should make sure their diets contain vitamins A, C, and B. Vitamin A is an antioxidant that can boost immunity and improve vision. It is found in orange-colored fruits and vegetables such as sweet potatoes, carrots, and apricots. Vitamin C is another immune-boosting antioxidant that is found in citrus fruits and numerous vegetables. B vitamins assist in energy metabolism, brain function, and neurological health. They are found in leafy greens, eggs, fish, milk, and fortified foods, among other sources.

Some minerals are critical as well. Magnesium, for instance, assists in muscle contractions and energy production and is found in nuts, legumes, and whole grains. Calcium, which is involved in bone formation and proper muscle function, occurs in dairy products, leafy greens, and fortified foods. Potassium aids in nerve transmission and muscle function and is found in fruits, vegetables, and chicken.

# What Not to Eat

Reduce your intake of saturated fat and cholesterol, which can promote heart disease and weight gain. Foods high in saturated fat include red meats, whole dairy foods, and butter. Cholesterol is found in seafood, meat, poultry, eggs and dairy foods. Both saturated fat and cholesterol can contribute to high cholesterol.

Avoid processed foods, which are often made with refined sugar and partially hydrogenated oils that contain trans-fatty acids. Like saturated fats and cholesterol, trans-fatty acids have been linked to heart disease.

Cut back on or eliminate alcohol if you're taking medications. Some experts also recommend shunning sugar, artificial sweeteners, preservatives, additives, and caffeine—all substances that can aggravate your fibromyalgia symptoms.

Some people may notice that certain foods can affect their pain. For instance, some people get a headache from eating too much chocolate. Others may experience arthritic pain from eating eggplant. If you have fibromyalgia, it's important to avoid foods that exacerbate your pain. Other foods to avoid include the following:

- **ASPARTAME.** This popular artificial sweetener is commonly marketed as NutraSweet or Equal. Aspartame contains a compound called aspartate. In the body, aspartate is easily converted into a neurotransmitter called NMDA, which stimulates pain fibers.
- **CAFFEINE.** As a stimulant, caffeine can disrupt sleep and worsen fatigue.
- **ALCOHOL.** Drinking large amounts of alcohol will aggravate stress levels and prevent you from dealing effectively with your fibromyalgia.
- **SUGAR.** Too much sugar from refined carbohydrates can worsen stress and cause weight gain. It can also promote yeast overgrowth (*Candida albicans*), which some experts believe is at the root of fibromyalgia.

In addition, avoid eating too many refined carbohydrates when you have carbohydrate cravings, which are common among people with fibromyalgia. Carb cravings are often the result of exhaustion, depression, and low levels of the neurotransmitter serotonin. Too many refined carbs—the kind in cookies, cakes, and white breads—can actually worsen fibromyalgia symptoms, though you may not notice the problem until the next day.

## Do You Need an Elimination Diet?

Because foods can aggravate your fibromyalgia, you might want to try an elimination diet, which involves eating a specific diet (usually one free of foods that tend to exacerbate your condition), and then gradually reintroducing suspect foods to figure out which ones trigger your symptoms. A good place to start is by eliminating the most common allergy triggers, such as milk, wheat, eggs, citrus, and chocolate. To learn more about this diet, consult a nutritionist.

# ✺ Supplements for Fibromyalgia

People who have fibromyalgia might want to consider taking supplements to relieve their symptoms, but not all supplements will help all patients. The supplements you will benefit from depend primarily on your symptoms. Here are some that might be worth a try:

## MAGNESIUM AND MALIC ACID

Combining magnesium with malic acid, a fruit acid found in apples, can stimulate the production of adenosine triphosphate (ATP), an energy source in many body cells. People with fibromyalgia are believed to be deficient in ATP.

## CHLORELLA

Studies show that *Chlorella pyrenoidosa*, a freshwater algae more than two billion years old, may relieve the symptoms of fibromyalgia.

## COENZYME Q10

CoQ10 is produced naturally by the body and used in the production of cellular energy. It also acts as an antioxidant and, in people with fibromyalgia, might help relieve fibro fog.

## GINSENG

Many fibromyalgia sufferers find ginseng helps with mental energy and motivation. *Panax ginseng* has been used for thousands of years in Asia to treat fatigue. But ginseng can be overstimulating and cause high blood pressure and sleep problems in some people.

## SAM-E

SAM-e, or adenosylmethionine, is a natural substance that may relieve pain, fatigue, and depression in people with fibromyalgia. In the body, it helps produce and regulate hormones that affect mood. Research on SAM-e in fibromyalgia patients has been mixed, and any benefit requires very high doses.

## MELATONIN

Melatonin is a naturally occurring hormone involved in regulating sleep-wake cycles. Some experts believe that fibromyalgia sufferers do not produce enough melatonin on their own at night. As a supplement, melatonin can sometimes induce sleep.

## ST. JOHN'S WORT

Although highly regarded in Europe as a treatment for depression, experts in the United States say it is effective only for mild depression. It should never be taken with antidepressants, and it may interact with other medications as well.

## 5-HTP

5-HTP is similar to serotonin, a major neurotransmitter that may occur in lower amounts in people with fibromyalgia. Taking it at bedtime may help promote sleep, and higher doses may relieve depression. But you should never take it if you're on antidepressants.

## ACIDOPHILUS

*Acidophilus* is a bacteria that promotes a healthy digestive tract by inhibiting disease-causing bacteria and fungi. Some people who have irritable bowel associated with their fibromyalgia have noticed that taking *acidophilus* can significantly relieve their symptoms.

Other supplements that might help include feverfew for migraine headaches, valerian for anxiety, enteric-coated peppermint oil for irritable bowel syndrome, and *ginkgo biloba* for memory and brain function.

## 📋 Stay-Healthy Strategies

- **TRY TO EXERCISE,** even for ten minutes a day. Regular physical activity will help you sleep, reduce your stress, and prevent unwanted weight gain.

- **CREATE A HEALTHY SLEEP ROUTINE.** Go to bed and get up at the same time every day. Practice good sleep hygiene by eliminating distractions and keeping the room comfortable and dark or dimly lit.

- **TAME YOUR STRESS.** Learn to change the way you cope with stress by changing the way you perceive events. Eliminate stress wherever possible and incorporate relaxation into your daily routine.

- **CONSERVE YOUR ENERGY.** Save your energy for those tasks that matter most and learn to set aside those that are less important. Get into the habit of saying no to too many demands on your time and energy.

- **LEARN ABOUT THE CONDITION.** Fibromyalgia is a complex illness that varies widely among patients. Knowing as much as you can about how to manage this malady will help you live a better quality of life.

# GALLSTONES

LOCATED ON THE UNDERSIDE OF THE LIVER and on the right side of the abdomen is the pear-shaped gallbladder. This organ is the storehouse for bile, a digestive substance produced in the liver that is secreted into the intestines through the common bile duct. Bile helps the body digest fats. When the liquid stored in the gallbladder hardens into stone-like pieces, you are said to have gallstones.

Bile is made up mostly of cholesterol, water, bile salts, proteins, and bilirubin. Bile salts break up fat, and bilirubin gives bile and stool a yellowish color. When the correct composition of the bile is disrupted, the bile can harden into stones.

There are actually two types of gallstones: cholesterol stones and pigment stones. The more common type is cholesterol stones, which are made up mostly of cholesterol. Pigment stones are small, dark stones made of bilirubin. Gallstones vary in size and can be as small as a grain of sand or as large as a golf ball. Some people have just one gallstone, while others may develop hundreds of tiny stones.

Gallstones are quite common and occur in about one in ten people over the age of 40. They seem to have a genetic basis and are more common in people of Native American and Hispanic heritage.

Gallstones are also more likely in people who take cholesterol-lowering drugs, because the drugs actually increase the amount of cholesterol in bile. People (such as diabetics), who have high triglycerides, a type of fatty acid in the blood, are at greater risk as well. In addition, gallstones are more likely when there is rapid weight loss, which triggers the liver to secrete extra cholesterol into bile, and fasting, which decreases gallbladder activity and causes cholesterol to build up in bile.

Finally, gallstones are more common in women, especially women who take hormone replacement or birth control pills. The added estrogen appears to decrease gallbladder activity and increase cholesterol levels in bile. Cholesterol stones, in particular, are more likely in people who are overweight.

## What They Look Like

Many people have what some experts call "silent stones." The stones do not interfere with the proper functioning of the gallbladder and so they do not need treatment.

But other people may have what is called a gallstone or gallbladder attack. These symptoms occur suddenly and can cause steady pain in the upper abdomen that worsens rapidly and lasts anywhere from 30 minutes to several hours.

Other symptoms include bloating, belching, gas, nausea, vomiting, and indigestion. They may also experience pain in the back between the shoulder blades and pain under the right shoulder. These attacks are more likely to occur after a high-fat meal. Afterward, they may notice a recurring intolerance for fatty foods.

In some people, the stones may block the bile ducts, which interrupts the release of bile. When that occurs, you may develop an inflammation or infection of the gallbladder and bile ducts. These blocked bile ducts may lead to jaundice, which causes the skin or whites of the eyes to turn yellow. The condition may also produce chills and low-grade fever. Some people may also develop pancreatitis, inflammation of the pancreas, if the gallstones block the pancreatic duct.

## What to Eat

The best dietary treatment for gallstones is to eat a high-fiber, low-fat diet, says Joseph Petrosino, a physician's assistant in gastroenterology in Schenectady, New York. Start by eating a lot of fresh fruits and vegetables. Studies have found that a diet high in plant foods may reduce the risk for gallstones. In fact, vegetarians are at significantly lower risk for gallstones than people whose diets include meat. Some of the best choices include apples, oranges, peas, and carrots, which contain pectin, a soluble fiber. Fruits and vegetables are also abundant in disease-fighting antioxidants. Make sure to eat whole grains, too, which are another good source of fiber.

Some experts recommend including olive oil in your diet. Olive oil contains healthy unsaturated fats and may help improve the flow of bile. Some experts say it may even help the passage of gallstones. It's also a good idea to eat flaxseeds, which contain fiber as well as essential fatty acids that can help reduce inflammation.

Try adding soy foods to your diet too. Soy, which is found in tofu, tempeh, edamame, and soy milk, is a healthy protein that may reduce gallstone attacks.

Finally, be sure to drink plenty of water. Water helps improve the consistency of bile and prevents it from being overloaded with cholesterol.

## What Not to Eat

Avoid foods high in saturated fats such as red meat, dairy products, and fried foods. Try to eliminate processed foods made with partially hydrogenated oils, which contain trans-fatty acids. Trans fats are most commonly found in packaged foods such as cookies, crackers, cakes, and snack foods.

Limit your intake of refined carbohydrates and sugars as well. These foods have been linked to a higher incidence of gallstones. The combination of refined carbs and fats reduces the production of bile acids, which makes the bile less soluble.

## Supplements for Gallstones

Start with a quality multivitamin that supplies all the essential nutrients. Always consult a doctor before taking any supplements. Supplements you may want to consider include the following:

## VITAMIN C

This antioxidant vitamin may offer protection against the development of gallstones. One study of 13,000 people found that those with gallbladder disease had less vitamin C in their blood.

## FISH OIL

Fish oil contains essential fatty acids that help reduce inflammation and protect against gallstones. If you're on blood-thinning medications, however, talk to your doctor first. Fish oil can promote bleeding.

## MILK THISTLE

Milk thistle is a plant in the ragweed family that enhances liver function. For gallstones, it may help improve bile flow. But steer clear of it if you have an allergy to ragweed.

## PEPPERMINT OIL

Enteric-coated capsules of peppermint oil may help with the breakdown of gallstones.

## Stay-Healthy Strategies

- **MAINTAIN A HEALTHY WEIGHT.** Being overweight or obese raises your risk for gallstones because it causes increased secretion of cholesterol in the bile.

- **GET PHYSICAL.** Regular exercise will not only help you lose or maintain your weight but also lower your risk for gallstones.

- **BE ON THE LOOKOUT FOR FOOD ALLERGIES.** Foods such as eggs, pork, milk, and citrus foods can sometimes induce a gallbladder attack. To help you pinpoint any offending foods, considering trying an elimination diet (see page 142 for more information).

- **GET PROPERLY DIAGNOSED.** Gallstone symptoms can mimic those associated with irritable bowel syndrome, ulcers, and even heart attack. An ultrasound is considered the most sensitive test for gallstones.

## Surgery for Treatment

Some people with gallstones have no symptoms and require no treatment. But in people who do have symptoms, the most common treatment is a surgical procedure called laparoscopic cholecystectomy.

During this procedure, the surgeon makes several tiny incisions in the abdomen and then inserts surgical instruments and a miniature video camera. The camera provides an enlarged view of the gallbladder and surrounding tissues. The view allows the surgeon to perform the surgery through the incision. The surgery involves separating the gallbladder from the liver, bile ducts, and other structures. The gallbladder is eventually removed through one of the initial incisions.

Recovery from the laparoscopic procedure is relatively quick and may involve as little as just one night in the hospital, plus several days of rest at home. Patients generally have less pain and fewer complications than they did when the only option was doing the procedure by cutting the abdomen.

# GASTROESOPHAGEAL REFLUX DISEASE

ALMOST EVERYONE KNOWS THE BURNING SENSATION that comes from an occasional bout of heartburn. But for some people, heartburn occurs with every meal. These people may suffer from a condition known as gastroesophageal reflux disease, or GERD.

The esophagus is the tube that carries food from the mouth to the stomach. It is separated by the lower esophageal sphincter (LES), a ring of muscle that acts as a valve between the esophagus and stomach. GERD occurs when the LES is weak or overly relaxed and doesn't close properly. As a result, the contents of the stomach leak back into the esophagus, causing reflux. The symptoms are especially common in pregnancy, when the LES becomes extremely relaxed due to high levels of progesterone.

The burning sensation that you feel is the result of the stomach acid touching the lining of the esophagus. You may even taste the acid in the back of your mouth. That is known as acid indigestion.

GERD is a common condition that affects 25 to 35 percent of all people at one time or another. As many as 10 percent of Americans suffer from heartburn every day, and 44 percent have symptoms at least once a month, according to a report in *American Family Physician*.

It's normal to have occasional heartburn, and it certainly doesn't mean that you have GERD. But some people are more likely to develop GERD than others. Elevated hormone levels in pregnancy, for instance, can slow the digestive system, making heartburn and GERD more likely in pregnant women. GERD and heartburn are also more common in people with scleroderma. With scleroderma, the esophagus may not function as well, causing the stomach acid to reflux. But if you start noticing that you have heartburn more than twice a week, you may want to ask your doctor about GERD.

Although GERD is not a life-threatening condition, it can lead to more serious complications, such as Barrett's esophagus. In this condition, the cells lining the esophagus undergo changes that may make you more at risk for esophageal cancer. Fortunately, GERD can be controlled with help from over-the-counter antacid medications, drugs that block the production of stomach acid (known as proton pump inhibitors), or medications that decrease the amount of reflux. In rare cases, surgery may be required.

## What It Looks Like

The primary symptom of GERD is heartburn and acid indigestion, but it is possible to have GERD without heartburn. Some people may have pain in the chest, hoarseness upon waking, or difficulties swallowing food. Sometimes GERD may feel as if you have food stuck in your throat, you are choking, or food is coming back up the throat (regurgitation). GERD may also produce a dry cough, sore throat, and bad breath.

## What to Eat

Focus on eating a diet rich in whole, unprocessed foods, which are less likely to aggravate your symptoms, says Joseph Petrosino, a physician's assistant in gastroenterology in Schenectady, New York. Make sure to eat plenty of healthy whole-grain breads, pasta, and rice, complex carbohydrates that are better able to absorb stomach acids.

The way you eat is important too. Try to eat five or six small meals instead of three large ones. Too much food will trigger the overproduction of stomach acid, causing heartburn and indigestion. Be careful never to overeat, because that aggravates symptoms as well. Don't lie down for two to three hours after you eat so the food has plenty of time to digest.

Make sure to also drink a lot of water. Many beverages can stimulate the production of stomach acid, but water actually helps dilute any excess acid.

## What Not to Eat

A critical part of managing GERD is pinpointing the foods that worsen your symptoms. Start by avoiding foods high in fat such as fried foods, certain fast foods, and red and processed meats. High-fat foods linger in the stomach longer, causing greater secretion of stomach acids.

Many other foods also seem to worsen GERD:

- Citrus foods
- Chocolate
- Caffeinated beverages
- Spicy foods
- Tomato-based foods
- Mint flavorings
- Garlic and onions
- Soda
- Beer and other alcoholic beverages

Not everyone will suffer the same problems with these foods, but it's generally best to limit or eliminate these foods from your diet.

## Supplements for GERD

There are no supplements or herbal remedies used to treat GERD. In fact, the use of supplements in people who have GERD should be done with caution. Some supplements (and medications too) may actually make symptoms worse. These include vitamin C, iron, and potassium. If you take supplements or medications, tell your doctor about them. And if you want to try something, always talk to your doctor first.

## 📋 Stay-Healthy Strategies

- **STOP SMOKING.** Cigarettes contain chemicals that reduce substances that neutralize stomach acids.

- **WATCH YOUR WEIGHT.** Being overweight may increase your risk for GERD and worsen existing symptoms.

- **EXERCISE WITH CAUTION.** Some people develop heartburn when they exercise. Avoid exercising too soon after meals and avoid aggravating foods before a workout. Choose exercises that don't involve a lot of bouncing and bending.

- **RELIEVE STRESS.** Although stress doesn't cause GERD, it can make symptoms worse. Consider taking up meditation, tai chi, or yoga to build more inner calm.

## GERD and Children

It's not uncommon for infants and children to suffer from GERD. Young children have immature digestive tracts. In kids, GERD may cause repeated vomiting, coughing, and respiratory problems.

Simple strategies, like burping your infant more frequently during a feeding, can sometimes help. You might also try keeping him in an upright position for 30 minutes after eating. Older children may want to follow the advice above on avoiding acid-promoting foods.

Talk to your child's doctor if the problem occurs regularly and causes discomfort. The good news is that most children will outgrow GERD.

# GLAUCOMA

TUCKED AWAY IN THE BACK OF YOUR EYE is the optic nerve, a collection of nerve fibers that transmit images to the brain. When the optic nerve is damaged, your vision gradually deteriorates. Damage to the optic nerve is most often the result of a condition called glaucoma.

The healthy functioning of the eye depends in large part on its built-in drainage system. The drains are located on the outer edge of the iris, which is the colored part of the eye that shrinks and grows to let in the proper amount of light. In healthy eyes, there is a steady production of fluid known as aqueous humor. The ongoing production of aqueous humor is balanced out by the proper drainage of this fluid. When drainage doesn't occur properly, the pressure in the eye—known as intraocular pressure—builds up, causing glaucoma.

Glaucoma is actually made up of several different diseases. Most cases are known as open-angle glaucoma, in which the fluid in your eye drains too slowly, causing the fluid to back up and increase pressure within your eye, much like a clogged drain. The process is slow and painless, and by the time it's detected, many people have already experienced some degree of vision loss. No one knows exactly what causes open-angle glaucoma, but advancing age may be one factor.

Another type of glaucoma is angle-closure or closed-angled glaucoma. This form is less common and occurs when the drainage angle canals become blocked. People who develop this type of glaucoma often have a very narrow drainage angle in the eye to begin with. This type of glaucoma is more common among farsighted people, who tend to have smaller eyes that can narrow the angle. The aging process can also cause blockage. As you age, the lens of the eye gets larger, which pushes the iris forward and closes up the space between the iris and the cornea.

Angle-closure glaucoma may progress slowly, but it may also occur suddenly in an acute form. A sudden dilation of the pupils—which can occur when you enter a dark room—may close up the angle and block drainage. Certain medications can cause the pupil dilation that leads to angle-closure glaucoma, including tricyclic antidepressants, antihistamines, and antianxiety drugs. Acute angle-closure glaucoma is a medical emergency that can cause vision loss within hours of its onset. Immediate treatment and laser surgery can help decrease the loss of vision.

In some cases, glaucoma is the result of an eye injury or disease. For example, people who take steroids for longer than six months are at greater risk for glaucoma, as are people who have diabetes and those who are nearsighted. These include asthmatics and people with autoimmune conditions. Some people develop glaucoma because of a structural abnormality of the eye. Less commonly, glaucoma may be the result of eye surgery.

A third form of glaucoma is low-tension or normal-tension glaucoma. In this type of glaucoma, damage occurs to the optic nerve even though intraocular pressure is not every high—it may even be normal. The cause of low-tension glaucoma is a mystery, but some experts think it may be due to an extra-sensitive optic nerve or to a reduction in blood flow caused by a systemic condition such as atherosclerosis, in which the arteries become hardened.

According to the Glaucoma Research Foundation, glaucoma affects about three million people in the United States, though only half know they have it. Glaucoma accounts for 9 to 12 percent of all cases of blindness in the United States and is the leading cause of blindness among African-Americans and elderly Hispanic-Americans.

No one knows why some people develop glaucoma while others do not. But the fact is that everyone is at some risk for this condition. A family history of the disease might make you more vulnerable. You are also at greater risk at a younger age if you are African-American. To better assess your risk, check out www.preventblindness.org/glaucoma.

Although the cause of each form is slightly different, they are all equally stealthy, causing no symptoms until the damage has been done. And in the end, the result is the same: Left untreated, glaucoma can result in vision loss.

Because glaucoma is such a serious and potentially devastating condition, eye exams almost always involve tests to screen for glaucoma. The best way to detect glaucoma is by dilating the pupils. Dilation allows the eye doctor to see the optic nerve inside the eye to look for signs of glaucoma.

Unfortunately, the disease has no cure and damage cannot be reversed. The good news is that if it's caught early, glaucoma can be treated with medications or surgery. For some people, the use of medicated eye drops is enough to reduce the pressure.

## What It Looks Like

Frighteningly enough, glaucoma is often a painless condition with no signs or symptoms. As it progresses, you may start to lose peripheral vision, though you may unknowingly compensate for that loss by turning your head.

If it's an acute attack of angle-closure glaucoma, however, you may experience blurred vision, headaches, eye pain, intermittent colored halos around lights, redness, and nausea. An acute attack of angle-closure glaucoma typically occurs at night in dim lighting, when the eye is most susceptible to rapid dilation. If you suspect you're having an attack, get help immediately. Blindness can occur within hours if you are not properly treated.

## What to Eat

Eating a diet rich in fruits and vegetables may help prevent glaucoma, says Mildred M.G. Olivier, M.D., ophthalmologist and president of the Midwest Glaucoma Center. Recent research looking at food intake in older women found that increased consumption of fruits and vegetables was associated with a lower prevalence of glaucoma.

To reap the benefits of different nutrients, try to eat a variety of fruits and vegetables. Make sure to include leafy greens such as kale, spinach, and collard greens. These foods are rich in lutein and zeaxanthin, two antioxidant carotenoids that have been associated with lowering the risk for macular degeneration, another eye disease. You can also find them in broccoli, celery, green peas, pumpkin, corn, green beans, green peppers, and brussels sprouts. Lutein is found in egg yolks, honeydew, and kiwi as well.

It's also important to eat a diet rich in vitamins C, E, and A, as well as the mineral zinc. These are antioxidants that may help keep eyes healthy. Vitamins C and A are found primarily in fruits and vegetables, while vitamin E occurs mostly in vegetable oils such as soybean, corn, and safflower, as well as nuts and seeds such as sunflower, almonds, and hazelnuts. Vitamin E is also found in wheat germ, and in lesser amounts, in leafy greens.

Zinc, on the other hand, is found in many animal products including beef, seafood, and liver. You can also get zinc from whole-grain foods, wheat germ, and sunflower seeds.

## What Not to Eat

Some studies have suggested that you should limit caffeine. Research has suggested that beverages and foods such as coffee, tea, and chocolate may increase intraocular pressure.

## Supplements for Glaucoma

Take a quality multivitamin to make sure you're getting all the essential nutrients. You may also want to consider taking certain supplements to boost eye health. But always consult your doctor first. Many of these supplements in excess can cause health problems. Supplements you might consider include the following:

### LUTEIN/ZEAXANTHIN

These substances are antioxidant carotenoids that play a vital role in eye health. They may be sold separately or in combination.

### VITAMIN C

Vitamin C is an antioxidant that may help prevent free radical damage to healthy cells.

### VITAMIN A

This fat-soluble vitamin plays an important role in overall eye health. But be careful not to ingest too much, which can cause toxicity.

### BILBERRY

Bilberries grow on low-growing shrubs and are an herbal treatment that may help by strengthening capillaries, tiny blood vessels.

### GINKGO BILOBA

This herbal remedy from China may help relieve the symptoms of glaucoma by improving blood flow to the optic nerve.

### RUTIN

Rutin is a bioflavonoid that may promote healthy blood vessels and help prevent glaucoma.

## Stay-Healthy Strategies

- **GET A DILATED EXAM** for glaucoma every year, even if you have perfect vision. Only careful screening can detect glaucoma before it gets to advanced stages.

- **GET REGULAR AEROBIC EXERCISE.** Physical activity can help reduce intraocular pressure.

- **REDUCE STRESS.** Stress can trigger acute-angle closure glaucoma and worsen other forms of glaucoma. Try meditation or yoga to relieve stress. Find support through a group or by talking to friends or a clergy person.

- **PROTECT YOUR EYES.** Wear sunglasses or a hat whenever you're out in the sun to shield eyes from ultraviolet rays.

### Glaucoma Q&A

**Q.** Can you drive if you have glaucoma?

**A.** It all depends on the severity of your vision loss. As long as you do not have significant visual field loss and your condition is detected early, you can probably still drive, says the National Highway Transportation Safety Board. But if you don't have peripheral vision, you may not see other cars, bicyclists, or pedestrians outside your central vision.

The best thing to do is to ask your doctor to refer you to a specialist (sometimes an occupational therapist) who can check your driving skills.

# GUM DISEASE

MOST PEOPLE DON'T GIVE MUCH THOUGHT to their gums. But this vital structure in your mouth is what holds your teeth in place, allowing you to chew your food. When the gums become infected and inflamed, you develop gum or periodontal disease.

Gum disease is a chronic bacterial infection that affects the gums and bones that support your teeth. It may occur in just one tooth or in several teeth. The condition begins when the bacteria in plaque infiltrate the gums, causing them to become inflamed. Plaque is the sticky, colorless film that forms on teeth and causes cavities.

Periodontal disease actually occurs in several forms. Gingivitis is the mildest form and involves the reddening and swelling of the gums. With gingivitis, the gums bleed easily but there is often little pain or discomfort. The condition can even be reversed with treatment and proper oral hygiene. But left untreated, it can worsen and become periodontitis.

In periodontitis, the plaque spreads and grows below the gum line. Once below the gum line, the bacteria inside the plaque produce toxins that irritate the gums. The toxins, in turn, cause chronic inflammation, which eventually destroys the tissues and bone that support the teeth. The gums separate from the teeth, creating gaps that become infected. Over time, the gaps widen, causing even greater destruction to the gum and bones. Eventually, the teeth loosen and may need to be removed. Treatment for advanced stages of gum disease may involve a combination of surgery, implants, and cosmetic procedures.

Gum disease is a common condition. According to the American Academy of Periodontology, 35.7 million people in the United States have gum disease. The condition affects more than a third of all people over age 30 and more than half of people over age 55.

The root cause of gum disease is plaque, but other factors can raise your risk. A family history of gum disease can significantly increase your risk, as can cigarette smoking. In women, the risk for gum disease is greater during periods of hormonal upheaval, such as pregnancy, puberty, and menopause.

Certain lifestyle factors can also influence your development of gum disease. Being under stress, for instance, can make you more likely to develop gum disease because it lowers your body's resistance to infection. Taking certain medications such as oral contraceptives and antidepressants, having diabetes or heart disease, and clenching or grinding your teeth will increase your risk for gum disease too. And because your body needs vital nutrients to combat any infection, poor nutrition can also make you more vulnerable to gum disease.

## ᵞ|ᵞ What to Eat

Make sure to eat a diet rich in calcium, says Richard Price, D.M.D., a spokesperson for the American Dental Association. One study found that people who ate less than 500 mg of calcium a day were almost twice as likely to have gum disease, especially if they were in their 20s and 30s. Good sources of calcium include low-fat milk and cheese, yogurt, leafy green vegetables, and fortified cereals.

Proper absorption of calcium requires adequate intake of vitamin D, so make sure to get enough of this bone-building vitamin as well. Foods that contain vitamin D include fortified milk and cereal and salmon with bones. You can also get vitamin D by being in the sun, although overexposure could raise your risk for skin cancer and premature aging.

It's also important to get plenty of vitamin C, an antioxidant vitamin that helps fight infection and repair healthy tissues. One study found that patients with gum disease who had reduced levels of vitamin C were able to improve their symptoms after eating two grapefruits a day for two weeks. The change was most pronounced in smokers.

Vitamin C occurs in many fruits and vegetables. It is especially abundant in citrus fruits, broccoli, red bell peppers, strawberries, cantaloupe, and dark leafy greens. To get more vitamin C, aim for a colorful diet.

Make sure to drink plenty of water too. Water helps rinse away bacteria-filled plaque.

## ⊘ What Not to Eat

Avoid eating foods high in saturated fat and trans-fatty acids. These foods promote inflammation and make the body less capable of fending off infection. Foods high in saturated fat include red meat, whole dairy products such as ice cream, fried foods, and greasy foods. Foods that contain trans-fatty acids are usually processed foods made with partially hydrogenated oils. These foods include cookies, crackers, desserts, snack foods, pastries, and margarine.

In addition to being inherently less healthy, high-fat foods promote weight gain, which can lead to obesity and diabetes, two risk factors for gum disease.

Try to limit your consumption of refined carbohydrates and sugar as well. Candy, soda, chewy fruit snacks, and other sweets fill your mouth with cavity-promoting sugar, which adheres to the surface of teeth and causes the formation of plaque. In particular, avoid excessive snacking, which also promotes plaque formation. If you do snack, choose healthier options.

## ⊱ Supplements for Gum Disease

Start by taking a multivitamin that provides all the essential nutrients for overall good health. Other supplements you might consider include the following:

### CALCIUM AND VITAMIN D

Healthy teeth and gums require adequate intake of this bone-building combination. If you don't get enough of these two in your diet, make sure to take a supplement.

## VITAMIN C

Vitamin C is an antioxidant vitamin that helps maintain and repair healthy tissues. It also helps combat infections, including gum disease. A deficiency of vitamin C may contribute to gum disease.

## 📋 Stay-Healthy Strategies

- **PAY ATTENTION TO ANY SYMPTOMS.** If you notice bleeding or irritation in your gums, see a dentist or periodontist right away.

- **QUIT SMOKING.** Cigarette smoking is the single biggest controllable risk factor for gum disease. So do what you can to quit.

- **PRACTICE GOOD ORAL HYGIENE.** Brush your teeth at least twice a day, floss regularly, and see your dentist for a professional cleaning regularly. And look for the American Dental Association's seal of acceptance on the oral care products you use.

- **MANAGE YOUR OTHER MEDICAL CONDITIONS.** Heart disease, diabetes, and osteoporosis all raise your risk for gum disease, so get your gums checked if you have these conditions.

## Could You Have Gum Disease?

According to the American Academy of Periodontology, here are some questions to help you determine whether you have gum disease:

- Do you ever have pain in your mouth?
- Do your gums ever bleed when you brush your teeth or when you eat hard food?
- Have you noticed any spaces developing between your teeth?
- Do your gums ever feel swollen or tender?
- Have you noticed that your gums are receding or your teeth appear longer than before?
- Do you have persistent bad breath?
- Have you noticed pus between your teeth and gums?
- Have you noticed any change in the way your teeth fit together when you bite?
- Do you ever develop sores in your mouth?

If you answered yes to any of these questions, you should see a dentist or periodontist for an evaluation.

# HAIR LOSS

AT ANY GIVEN TIME, 90 PERCENT OF THE HAIR on our head is in a two- to six-year growth phase. The remaining 10 percent is in a two- to three-month resting phase, which is followed by the shedding of that hair. On an ordinary day, we can lose as many as 150 strands of hair.

Such loss is normal, and many of us treat it as a routine occurrence. But in some people, the hair loss may become excessive. You may notice extra strands in the bathroom sink or more hair than usual in your hairbrush. When that occurs, you are said to be experiencing excessive hair loss.

Hair loss, which is technically known as androgenetic alopecia, can occur to anyone at any age, and affects an estimated 30 to 40 percent of all people. In men, the hair loss can lead to male-pattern baldness. The pattern is characterized by a receding hairline and baldness at the top of the head. Women may develop female-pattern baldness, in which the hair loss occurs over the entire top of the scalp.

Hair loss is primarily genetic. The amount you lose, the age at which you start to lose it, and the pattern of your baldness are determined largely by your genes. But some people develop an autoimmune disease called alopecia areata. With this condition, the immune system attacks the hair follicles, causing hair to fall out in patches all over the body, including the eyebrows. The hair in alopecia areata may grow back, but it may also fall out again.

Other causes of hair loss include disease such as diabetes, lupus, and thyroid disease; medications such as chemotherapy and drugs for heart disease; radiation therapy; childbirth; scalp infections; and poor nutrition.

Some people may choose to embrace their hair loss by shaving off the remaining hair. Others may opt to use wigs or have hair transplants. Still others may try to regrow the hair with the use of medications. But once you start taking the medication, you must continue to take it or the hair loss will resume.

## What It Looks Like

Hair loss is just as the term implies—the erosion of hair on the scalp. The result is a thinning of the hair. Men may experience a receding hairline, while women may notice that their entire scalp has become less dense with hair. If alopecia areata is the cause of your hair loss, the hair will fall out in patches.

## ⅼⅼⅼ What to Eat

Eating a healthy, well-balanced diet will provide your body with the nutrients you need to sustain a healthy head of hair, says Christine Gerbstadt, M.D., R.D., a spokesperson for the American Dietetic Association. Start with a diet rich in fruits and vegetables, which may help slow hair loss and strengthen the health of your hair.

Of particular importance are iron and protein, because a deficiency in these nutrients can sometimes lead to hair loss. Iron is an essential mineral found in animal products, which provide what is called heme iron, and plant foods, which contain nonheme iron. Heme iron is generally better absorbed than nonheme iron. Good sources of iron include liver, beef, pork, fish, leafy greens, fortified cereal, beans, and pumpkin seeds. Also, eating nonheme sources of iron with a heme iron can boost absorption of the nonheme iron.

Foods rich in vitamin C enhance absorption of iron too. So it's always a good idea to eat or drink something with a lot of vitamin C when you're eating a food high in iron. For example, if you're eating a sirloin steak, have it with turnip greens or tomatoes on the side. The combination will ensure that you maximize your absorption of the iron. When looking for good sources of vitamin C, choose those foods that are also high in fiber, because too much iron absorption can cause constipation.

Eat foods that contain omega-3 fatty acids. These healthy fats are found in cold-water fish such as tuna, salmon, and mackerel, as well as in flaxseed and walnuts. These fats help keep hair healthy and can prevent dry, brittle hair.

Make sure to also eat enough protein, which contains the amino acids that can help strengthen hair. Healthy sources of protein include chicken, turkey, fish, and eggs.

Finally, eat foods rich in biotin, a B vitamin essential for healthy hair. Biotin is found in brewer's yeast, bulgur wheat, lentils, sunflower seeds, soybeans, and walnuts.

## ⊘ What Not to Eat

Stay away from very low-calorie liquid diets. These types of weight loss plans can result in hair loss as well as other health problems such as fatigue, nausea, and diarrhea.

Do not eat raw egg whites. Raw egg whites contain a substance that binds biotin and prevents it from being properly absorbed.

Also, make sure your hair loss isn't the result of celiac disease, a condition in which the body cannot tolerate gluten, a protein that is found in wheat, rye, and barley. Research has found that people with alopecia areata sometimes also had celiac disease.

## ⁀⁀ Supplements for Hair Loss

Healthy hair benefits from regular intake of all the essential vitamins and minerals, so take a quality multivitamin to start. You might also consider taking other supplements, but always consult a physician first. Supplements to consider include the following:

### BIOTIN

This B vitamin is known to strengthen hair and may help prevent hair loss.

### INOSITOL

Inositol is another B vitamin that has been linked to hair health.

### IRON

Taking iron can help prevent hair loss. But always take iron under a doctor's supervision. Too much iron can cause iron overload and damage to the organs.

### VITAMIN C

Vitamin C is an antioxidant that boosts overall health and immunity. It aids with the absorption of iron, which is essential to hair health.

### SAW PALMETTO

Saw palmetto is an herbal remedy commonly used to treat prostate enlargement. Some experts believe it may help stimulate hair growth, especially in men.

## Stay-Healthy Strategies

- **TREAT YOUR HAIR KINDLY.** Avoid the overuse of chemicals and blow dryers. Comb wet hair with a wide-toothed comb. Don't style it with tight hair fasteners or rollers.

- **REDUCE STRESS.** Too much stress can spur hair loss, so look for ways to buffer yourself against anxiety and stress.

- **EXERCISE REGULARLY.** Physical activity enhances circulation throughout the body, even the scalp. So make a point to exercise.

- **CONSIDER TREATMENT.** Medications can slow or prevent hair loss. Minoxidil (Rogaine) is available for men and women and is sold over-the-counter. Finasteride (Propecia) is prescribed for men only and is available with a doctor's prescription.

### Your Hair During Pregnancy

One of the most profound changes during pregnancy occurs in your hair. While you're pregnant, you may notice that your hair is thicker and fuller. Other women may notice that their hair is dull and lifeless. These changes are attributed to the extra hormones surging through your body, which is causing hair to grow faster and shed more slowly.

After pregnancy, however, your hair may undergo a period of rapid loss. This increase in hair loss is simply a sign that your hormone levels are returning to normal.

# HALITOSIS

YOU'RE STANDING BESIDE SOMEONE when you suddenly catch a whiff of bad breath. Maybe it's the smell of garlic from last night's dinner. Or maybe it's the aroma of stale cigarettes. Maybe it just smells plain bad. In some people, bad breath is a persistent problem that doesn't go away even with careful attention to oral hygiene.

Bad breath is called halitosis. Many people have bad breath for extrinsic reasons (i.e., they eat odorous foods that tend to linger). Usually, the odor dissipates after a few hours or, in some cases, a couple of days.

In cases of persistent bad breath, the person may have a buildup of anaerobic bacteria in the back of his or her mouth. No one knows exactly why some people have an excess of these bacteria, but in some cases it's caused by chronic post-nasal drip or from taking medications that dry out the mouth. According to Richard Price, D.M.D., a spokesperson for the American Dental Association (ADA), there are about 400 medications that can cause a reduction in saliva flow. The drier the mouth, the worse the breath.

In other people, bad breath may be caused by an underlying health problem, such as diabetes, gum disease, or a poor diet. All these health problems can be reflected in your breath.

Whatever the cause may be, bad breath is a source of embarrassment. Some people with bad breath don't even know they have it. But if you are aware, you should consult your doctor or dentist about it. A conversation about your lifestyle, diet, and health can help pinpoint the cause so you can figure out the best way to treat it.

## What It Looks Like

Most people have bad breath when they awaken in the morning. Long hours without any fluids dries out the mouth, causing morning breath. After breakfast and a good brushing, however, the breath is usually clean.

Unless you have an underlying illness or suffer from intrinsic bad breath, most people do not have bad breath unless they eat strong-smelling foods. The severity of the odor will vary depending on the individual.

## What to Eat

Make sure you're eating enough fruits and vegetables, which can help eliminate any underlying infections at the root of poor health and are less likely to cause bad breath, Peterson says. A crunchy fruit such as an apple or pear is naturally good for bad breath because it lubricates the mouth and stimulates saliva flow. You should also make sure your diet is composed mostly of whole, unprocessed foods, which is easier on the digestive tract.

Consider eating yogurt, if you don't already. Yogurt contains *acidophilus*, a healthy bacteria that can improve digestive health. A healthy digestive tract can help eliminate some of the problems with bad breath.

Finally, drink water—lots of it. Keeping the mouth moist can help flush out the anaerobic bacteria that are at the root of your bad breath. Another good drink is green tea, which contains polyphenols that can help eliminate bacteria.

## What Not to Eat

Avoid garlic and onions, which tend to produce noxious odors for several hours. Other potent-smelling foods include tuna fish, salami, beer, wine, coffee, and spicy foods.

Also, try not to eat foods with a tendency to stick to your teeth or get caught in between teeth. The stickiness will stimulate the production of plaque, which, in turn, will lead to a buildup of bacteria. These foods include caramel-type candies, sugary gum, fruit snacks, and hard candies.

In addition, steer clear of foods that are slow to digest. These foods are typically high in fat and include red meat, fried food, and processed foods. Because they tend to linger in your body longer, they are more likely to cause halitosis.

## Stay-Healthy Strategies

- **BRUSH TWICE A DAY** with fluoride toothpaste to remove food and plaque. Make sure to brush your tongue too. Floss once a day to remove food particles from between teeth.

- **SCRAPE THE TONGUE.** Consider purchasing a tongue scraper that will remove the bacteria from the mouth. Go as far back into the throat you can and give it a good scrape.

- **QUIT SMOKING.** Stale cigarettes are a major culprit behind bad breath—and a cause of many illnesses. Do what you can to quit.

- **GET CHECKED BY YOUR DENTIST FIRST.** If severe bad breath continues, it may be an indication of a more serious underlying illness, such as a respiratory infection or diabetes. Talk to your primary care doctor if you can't resolve halitosis.

- **RESIST THE URGE TO SUCK ON MINTS ALL DAY.** Mints are a temporary solution and, in the end, stimulate acid production in the mouth that will increase your risk for cavities.

- **CONSIDER DOING A DETOX DIET,** as described on page 87. Sometimes, bad breath is the result of a build up of toxins in your diet, and doing a detox diet may help eliminate these substances that are the underlying cause of your bad breath.

# The Worst Remedies for Bad Breath

In 2002, the American Academy of Periodontology asked its members for the most ineffective home remedies and practices that their patients have used to tackle bad breath. Among them are the following:

**1. Excessive use of mouthwash.** Too much mouthwash produces stinky tissue that is worse than what your breath is already like.

**2. Breath mints.** A sweet-smelling mouth doesn't mean a healthy mouth. Long-lasting sugar candies subject teeth to acid attacks, increasing your risk for cavities.

**3. Chewing gum.** True, chewing gum can increase your flow of saliva, but it's only a cover-up for the odors underneath.

**4. Mint chew tobacco.** Smokeless tobacco causes gums to recede, increases the chance of losing the bone and fibers that hold your teeth in place, and causes oral cancer.

**5. Products sold on infomercials.** Only use items that have the American Dental Association's Seal of Approval. Unapproved items could do more harm than good.

**6. Vodka martinis or sour mash whiskey.** Alcohol may worsen the problem by making your mouth dry and eliminating the saliva you need to remove oral bacteria.

**7. Brushing with household cleansers.** Many chemicals used for household cleaning are poisonous and should not be consumed.

**8. Intestinal cleansing methods.** Bad breath does not originate from the stomach, so resist the use of products that are intended to clean out your intestines.

**9. Rinsing with kerosene.** Talk about setting your mouth on fire!

# HANGOVER

LAST NIGHT'S PARTY WAS CERTAINLY FUN, but this morning you awaken with a miserable hangover. Your head is pounding, your stomach is queasy, and your mouth feels as parched as sandpaper.

Hangovers are the result of drinking too much alcohol. Alcohol contains ethanol, which causes dehydration, dry mouth, and fatigue. Alcohol also takes a toll on the stomach lining, which causes nausea and, in some cases, vomiting. During the breakdown of ethanol, toxic substances are produced. Some of these substances impair the liver's ability to supply glucose to the brain, which, in turn, causes tiredness, moodiness, and reduced concentration.

Certain alcoholic beverages also contain congeners, which are produced during fermentation and distillation. Congeners are present in distilled or fermented drinks such as wine, rum, vodka, and gin. They also have a toxic effect on the body.

The best way to avoid a hangover is to drink in moderation and to drink on a full stomach (or at least with some food in your system) because food slows the absorption of alcohol. It's also wise to drink slowly. A lot of alcohol consumed over a short period of time will cause drunkenness more rapidly and put you at greater risk for a hangover in the morning. While drinking, make sure to consume a lot of water, which will help you stay hydrated.

## What It Looks Like

Hangovers can vary depending on how much alcohol was consumed. Mild hangovers may involve some dry mouth and headache. More severe hangovers may cause nausea, vomiting, and extreme fatigue. Regardless of severity, however, a hangover hurts.

## What to Eat

The best cure for a hangover is time, but drinking a lot of water can help prevent dehydration, says Milton Stokes, R.D., a spokesperson for the American Dietetic Association (ADA).

If you wake up feeling nauseated or you're vomiting, don't rush to eat. When you do eat, try eating a bland diet with foods such as crackers or dry toast, applesauce, bananas, and tea.

## 🚫 What Not to Eat

If your hangover is severe, you probably won't want to eat, which is perfectly okay. But when you do eat, try to avoid high-fat, high-sugar foods, which are void of nutrients, are heavier on the stomach, and can make you feel worse after eating.

## 💊 Supplements for Hangovers

There are no supplements that can effectively cure a hangover.

## 📋 Stay-Healthy Strategies

- **LIMIT YOUR INTAKE.** It isn't always easy, but the best way to manage hangovers is to prevent them in the first place.

- **ALWAYS EAT BEFORE YOU DRINK ALCOHOL.** A full stomach slows the absorption of alcohol.

- **GET PLENTY OF R&R.** Don't overdo it on the day you have a hangover. Make sure to rest and relax.

- **FOLLOW UP EACH ALCOHOLIC DRINK WITH A GLASS OF WATER.** This strategy will help you stay hydrated.

## What's Moderation, Anyway?

Experts agree that the only way to drink healthfully is to drink in moderation. But what exactly is moderation? According to the American Dietetic Association, moderation for women means drinking no more than one drink a day; for men, it means no more than two. One drink is the equivalent of twelve ounces of beer, five ounces of wine, or one and a half ounces of 80-proof distilled spirits. Each serving contains 14 grams of pure ethanol.

# HEADACHES AND MIGRAINES

NEARLY EVERYONE KNOWS THE AGGRAVATING PAIN and tension that comes from having a headache. They can strike when you're stressed out, tired, or hungry. Some women get them when they have their periods. Men and women get headaches with fevers, sinus infections, or a multitude of other conditions. In any case, headaches are highly common.

According to the American Council on Headache Education, 90 percent of men and 95 percent of women experienced a headache in the past year. While the occasional headache is normal, however, chronic headaches can be disruptive and interfere with daily activities.

Most people suffer from tension headaches, which afflict approximately 78 percent of all adults. These headaches are generally the result of tight muscles, or tension, in the neck or shoulders. A smaller number of people suffer from cluster headaches, severe recurring headaches that affect about one million people in the United States.

Many people suffer from a type of headache known as a migraine. Approximately thirty million people in the United States experience migraines, the vast majority of them women. Migraine headaches are a specific type of headache in which there is intense pain, usually on one side of the head, which worsens with ordinary activities.

A lot of women develop migraines during their periods, a condition known as menstrual migraines. This type of migraine can last longer and recur more often than regular migraine headaches. Other women may have menstrual-related migraines, which can occur any time of the month. Experts suspect that the drop in estrogen levels during menstruation is the cause of menstrual migraines. These migraines can be brought on the by the use of hormonal contraceptives, which affect estrogen levels as well.

Many other factors can trigger a headache as well. Foods, smells, and even the weather can lead to headache pain. Strong emotions such as stress, depression, anxiety, disappointment, and frustration also can cause headaches. Some people get headaches from spending too much time in front of a computer, sleeping in an awkward position, or drinking too much caffeine.

Most headaches are treated with an over-the-counter (OTC) analgesic. People who have migraines may require prescription medications. But keep in mind that overusing OTC remedies can cause a rebound effect that only triggers more headaches.

## 🔎 What They Look Like

The intensity of a headache or migraine varies depending on the cause of the headache and your tolerance for pain. In general, a tension headache might feel like a band tightening around your neck or head. You may feel a pressing sensation on both sides of your head, and it may move into your temples, the back of your head, and/or your neck. But performing routine activities generally doesn't worsen the pain, nor do you experience sensitivity to light or noise.

Cluster headache pain is severe and tends to occur on just one side of the head. Cluster headaches may last for several days and then disappear, only to return later on. This type of headache is more common in men.

Migraine headaches make you sensitive to light and noise. In the early and later phases of a migraine attack, some people also experience muscle tenderness, fatigue, and mood changes. You may also feel nauseated and even vomit. The pain of a migraine is usually severe, but it may also be moderate. Migraines can last four to seventy-two hours or more.

Some migraine sufferers experience what experts call an aura, during which they often see zigzag lines, shimmering lights, or bright flashes of lights. An aura may also be accompanied by numbness and tingling in the arm. People with auras often need to lie down in a dark place until the aura passes.

## 🍴 What to Eat

Eat a healthy, well-balanced diet that includes fruits, vegetables, and whole grains, says Marielle Kabbouche, M.D., a neurologist at Cincinnati Children's Hospital Medical Center. Make sure to eat regularly and to avoid skipping meals, including breakfast. Include dark green vegetables in your meals. Green vegetables such as broccoli, spinach, and kale contain riboflavin, a B vitamin that helps prevent migraines. It is also found in yogurt, eggs, and low-fat milk.

Include foods rich in magnesium in your diet too. Some migraine sufferers may actually be deficient in this mineral, which helps relax the blood vessels and preserve proper cell function throughout the body. Good sources of magnesium include wheat germ, nuts (almond and cashews are especially high in magnesium), whole grains, tofu, soybeans, and many vegetables.

Make sure to drink plenty of water to help stay hydrated. Proper hydration can keep headache pain at bay and prevent migraines.

# What Not to Eat

Avoid any food that you think might set off a headache. But keep in mind that not everyone experiences headaches from the same foods. The most common offenders are foods and beverages that contain caffeine, such as coffee and tea, and tyramine, a substance found in red wine and aged cheeses.

Before you ban these foods from your diet, try an elimination diet. Give up potential offenders for seven to ten days and then gradually reintroduce them back into your routine. Eliminate those that cause headache pain.

It might also help to keep a headache diary so you can record the circumstances that surrounded the pain, including foods you ate, your mood, how well you slept the night before, and even the weather conditions. After a while, you should be able to identify a pattern and pinpoint the offending foods and situations.

# Supplements for Headaches and Migraines

Taking a quality multivitamin can ensure that you get all the vital nutrients you need. In addition, you might want to consider taking certain supplements, including the following:

### RIBOFLAVIN
Riboflavin, or vitamin B2, has been used to prevent migraines in both children and adults.

## Mind Over Matter

Some experts recommend biofeedback for the treatment of frequent and debilitating migraines. Biofeedback involves first measuring physiological function and then training the patient's mind to respond in a way that relieves the pain. It's been used for numerous health problems, such as temporomandibular joint (TMJ), stress, and fibromyalgia. Biofeedback can also lessen stress and help relax tight muscles, which may be contributing to headaches.

During a biofeedback session, you are attached to an electronic monitor that measures bodily functions such as your brain waves, skin temperature, and blood pressure. While you're hooked up, you will do relaxation techniques that alter these functions. You will see changes in body functions on the monitor and learn how you feel when your blood pressure slows, your body temperature goes up, and your brain waves calm down.

With practice, biofeedback will empower you to control your migraine pain. For more information, and to find a qualified biofeedback counselor in your area, check out the Biofeedback Certification Institute of America (www.bcia.org).

## COENZYME Q10

CoQ10 is an enzyme naturally produced in the body and essential to the production of energy in mitochondria, the energy-producing part of all body cells. Although it's still being investigated as a remedy for migraines, a deficiency of CoQ10 may trigger migraines.

## MAGNESIUM

This major mineral may help reduce migraines, especially in women who get them before their menstrual periods.

## Stay-Healthy Strategies

- **GET YOUR SLEEP.** Adequate rest is essential to preventing headaches, especially in people who have migraines. So make sleep a priority every night.

- **CONSIDER RELAXATION EXERCISES.** Meditation, deep breathing, prayer, yoga, and other forms of relaxation can help buffer you from the stress that often triggers headaches.

- **MAKE IT A POINT TO EXERCISE.** Regular physical activity can relieve stress, boost mood, improve sleep, and even reduce migraine headaches. Try to do something active every single day.

- **WATCH YOUR POSTURE.** Poor posture can sometimes lead to headaches, so make sure you're standing and sitting tall.

### TIP

*Consider doing a short detox diet. A detoxification diet eliminates all the toxins in your body and gives you a chance to cleanse your system of substances, including those that may be causing headaches. Among the symptoms a detoxification diet can relieve are headaches—though you may experience some headaches if you're a regular caffeine drinker. Check out page 87 for more information on doing a detox diet.*

# HEARTBURN

*See Gastroesophageal Reflux Disease on page 148.*

# HEART DISEASE

HEART ATTACK. CORONARY ARTERY DISEASE. Heart failure. All these medical conditions belong to a category of illnesses known as heart disease. The various forms of heart disease affect approximately seventy million Americans, according to the Centers for Disease Control and Prevention (CDC).

Heart disease refers to several different and distinct conditions, all affecting the body's network of blood vessels and/or heart. It occurs when the vessels or heart are damaged and unable to perform the vital task of pumping blood to all the organs of the body. The following are some forms of heart disease:

- **CORONARY ARTERY DISEASE (CAD).** CAD occurs when blood flow to the arteries leading to the heart becomes obstructed. Most often, the cause of the obstruction is atherosclerosis, a hardening of the arteries caused by the buildup of plaque. CAD refers to those conditions that affect only the arteries. When CAD leads to other complications such as angina (chest pain) or heart attack, you are said to have coronary heart disease.

- **CARDIOMYOPATHY.** When the heart itself becomes diseased, you are said to have cardiomyopathy. The heart may be weakened by a loss of muscle, dilated or enlarged, or thickened. In some people, the heart may become enlarged without an identifiable cause.

- **HEART FAILURE.** Once known as congestive heart failure, heart failure occurs when your heart can't pump enough blood to the rest of the body. Because of the heart's reduction in pumping power, the rest of the body is deprived of oxygen. Some people may develop heart failure as the result of another heart condition such as CAD.

- **HEART ATTACK.** Also known as myocardial infarction, a heart attack occurs when the blood supply to the myocardium, the muscular wall of the heart that pumps blood out of the heart, is severely reduced or completely stopped. If the obstruction lasts more than a few minutes, the heart may experience irreparable damage or the person may die. Prompt treatment, in some cases, can be lifesaving.

- **STROKE.** A stroke happens when a vessel supplying blood to the brain bursts or develops a blockage such as a clot, depriving the brain of much-needed oxygen and nutrients. A stroke can cause life-altering changes in a person's senses, motor skills, and mobility. Some people become paralyzed, while others may die. (See the Stroke chapter on page 301.)

There are many other illnesses that can also affect the blood vessels and heart. High cholesterol, high blood pressure, and even varicose veins are all considered types of heart disease. So is vasculitis, inflammation of the blood vessels, and peripheral arterial disease.

These days, we hear a great deal about heart disease and its dubious distinction as the nation's number-one killer. Together with stroke, heart disease accounts for 40 percent of all deaths in the United States, according to the CDC. In fact, one American will die of heart disease every 34 seconds.

The good news is you can actually prevent many forms of heart disease. The key is practicing good lifestyle strategies that include regular exercise, a healthy diet, not smoking, and maintaining your weight. These efforts can go a long way toward preventing disease.

## What It Looks Like

The signs and symptoms of heart disease will vary greatly depending on the type of illness you have. High blood pressure, for example, often produces no signs and symptoms at all. The only way to know you have it is to have regular blood pressure checks. Atherosclerosis is also a silent disease that produces no symptoms.

Cardiomyopathy, on the other hand, may cause shortness of breath, dizziness, and chest pain, while heart failure often results in fatigue, swelling, and shortness of breath.

Most heart attacks produce distinct symptoms, too, though they don't always resemble the ones we see in the movies. During a heart attack, many people feel chest discomfort as well as pain or discomfort in one or both arms, the back, neck, jaw, or stomach. Some people may experi-

ence shortness of breath, cold sweat, lightheadedness, or nausea.

Symptoms of a stroke often come on suddenly. Some people may feel numbness or weakness on one side of the body, in the face, arm, or leg. They may also experience confusion and have trouble hearing or comprehending speech. Other symptoms include difficulties walking

### Fast Facts on Heart Disease

Here are some facts about heart disease from the Centers for Disease Control and Prevention:

- About 90 percent of middle-aged Americans will develop high blood pressure at some point in their lives.

- Approximately 70 percent of people with high blood pressure do not have it under control.

- More than 106 million people were diagnosed with higher than normal cholesterol levels in 2002.

- Reducing systolic blood pressure by just 12 to 13 mmHg—the top number in a reading—over four years results in a 21 percent reduction in coronary heart disease and 25 percent reduction in total heart disease deaths.

- A 10 percent decrease in total cholesterol reduces the incidence of heart attack and stroke by almost 30 percent.

and a sudden lack of coordination, headaches, or troubles with vision.

## ⫶|⫶ What to Eat

People who have heart disease or who are at risk for heart disease should focus on eating a diet that lowers risk factors such as high cholesterol, diabetes, and high blood pressure, says Marie Savard, M.D., author of *The Body Shape Solution for Weight Loss and Wellness.*

It's also important to follow an eating plan that helps you lose weight and trims inches from your waist. Studies show that waist circumference may be a more accurate predictor of heart disease risk than even body mass index (BMI), which is a measure of your weight in relation to height. A study in *The Lancet* in November 2005 found that waist-to-hip ratio was closely associated with risk for heart attack—the higher the ratio, the greater the risk. Meanwhile, BMI was only modestly associated with heart attack risk. Others vulnerable to heart disease include people who have a family history of heart disease and who are overweight, inactive, or smokers.

Any heart-healthy diet should include fish, which contains omega-3 fatty acids that may lower your risk for heart disease. Healthy fish include salmon, tuna, and mackerel. Omega-3s are also found in walnuts, flaxseed, and fortified foods such as peanut butter and breakfast cereal.

A heart-healthy diet must also incorporate a lot of fruits and vegetables—try to eat a colorful array that supplies your body with a variety of phytonutrients and antioxidant vitamins that can help prevent disease. Eating fruits and veggies will help ensure you get adequate fiber as well. Soluble fiber, the kind that dissolves in water, is especially critical because it will help slow down digestion and keep blood sugar in check. It will also help lower LDL cholesterol (the bad, or "lousy," cholesterol), triglycerides, and high blood pressure, while raising levels of HDL (the good, or "healthy," cholesterol).

Both soluble and insoluble fiber can help minimize weight gain by making you feel full. Sources of soluble fiber include oats, kidney beans, peas, flaxseed, apples, oranges, and carrots. Insoluble fiber is found in whole-wheat foods, cauliflower, beans, spinach, peas, and apples. As you see, some foods supply both.

Other good sources of fiber include whole grains, such as brown rice, bulgur wheat, and quinoa. You should also include legumes such as chickpeas, kidney beans, pinto beans, and black beans, which are a healthy source of protein as well. Other good protein sources include chicken, fish, and soybean products. Soy foods come in many forms, including tempeh, tofu, edamame, soy milk, and soy burgers.

In addition, try to get your fat primarily from monounsaturated fats, which are healthier and less damaging to arteries than saturated fats. Good sources of monounsaturated fats include avocados, almonds, and pecans. Monounsaturated fats are also found in olive or canola oil.

Finally, consider using margarine-like spreads made of soybean extract (such as Benecol and Take Control), which contain plant stanols that have been found to lower cholesterol.

# What Not to Eat

Avoid foods high in saturated fats, which occur primarily in animal products such as red meat, dairy products, and butter. You should also steer clear of foods that contain trans-fatty acids, which are often found in packaged foods such as candy bars, cookies, muffins, and crackers—the kinds commonly found in vending machines. The tip-off on trans-fatty acids is the presence of anything partially hydrogenated in the ingredient list.

In addition, try to restrict or eliminate foods high in sugar, which can elevate insulin levels and cause an increase in cholesterol, triglycerides, and blood pressure.

People who already have high blood pressure should avoid high-sodium foods such as canned soups, packaged meals, and deli meals. Also stay away from processed meats such as hot dogs, pastrami, and bologna; fried foods of any variety; and foods made with white flour.

# Supplements for Heart Disease

Consider taking a quality multivitamin, which supplies the basic nutrients you need for good health, especially on days when you don't eat as well. You might also consider taking the following:

## FISH OIL

Studies show that omega-3 fatty acids are beneficial to the prevention of heart disease, so you may consider taking a fish oil supplement. If you're on blood-thinning medication, talk to your doctor first, because fish oil may increase your risk for bleeding.

## CERTAIN B VITAMINS

Taking folic acid and vitamins B6 and B12 may help reduce levels of homocysteine, a substance that has been implicated in the development of heart disease.

## MAGNESIUM

Some people may consider taking magnesium, a mineral that may help lower blood pressure, relax blood vessels, and promote healthy contractions of the heart.

## PSYLLIUM

Psyllium is a seed husk and a soluble fiber that can help with bowel regularity and lowering cholesterol. Talk to your doctor first before taking psyllium, especially if you have food allergies, because some people react to psyllium.

## ASPIRIN

Research has shown that one baby aspirin a day can prevent a heart attack in men and stroke in women. Talk to your doctor before starting on aspirin, which can cause a number of side effects including stomach irritation and bleeding.

# 📋 Stay-Healthy Strategies

- **QUIT SMOKING.** Cigarette smoking is a major risk factor for heart disease. Make a serious effort to quit.

- **MAKE EXERCISE A PRIORITY.** Do whatever you can to move, because regular physical activity can lower your risk for heart disease and improve overall health.

- **LOWER STRESS.** Take up meditation, guided imagery, or another form of relaxation. Learn to avoid stressful situations, and take the ones you can't dodge in stride.

- **GET TREATMENT FOR DEPRESSION.** People who have depression are at higher risk for heart disease. If you suspect you may have it, seek medical treatment.

## Get Moving

A key component to heart disease prevention is exercise. Here's how to make sure you move:

- Build it into your day. Park far way from the entrance, take the stairs, and do errands on foot.

- Enlist a buddy to exercise with you.

- Write it on your schedule like any other appointment.

- Do it first. A morning routine will ensure you get your activity for the day before other commitments get in the way.

# HEPATITIS

CONSIDER ALL THAT THE LIVER DOES, and it's easy to see why an unhealthy liver causes serious health problems. The liver is a storehouse for iron, the production center of essential digestive juices, and the detox center for toxins including alcohol and drugs. It also holds a high concentration of glycogen, the stored form of energy in the body.

Hepatitis is an inflammation of the liver that can sometimes result in liver damage. The condition is most commonly caused by one of three hepatitis viruses—A, B, or C—though it's also possible to get hepatitis from drinking too much alcohol or using illicit drugs. In some cases the condition is acute, or short-term, but in others, hepatitis may be chronic.

Hepatitis is spread through the sharing of unsterilized needles and syringes with infected people and through the use of personal care items that are tainted with contaminated blood. Having sex with infected persons can spread the disease, too, but it is rare. Babies can contract the disease in utero if their mothers have it.

The most common cause of the illness is the hepatitis C virus. Unlike hepatitis A and B, there is no vaccine for hepatitis C. In recent decades, the incidence of hepatitis C has declined. In the 1980s there were an average of 240,000 new infections each year, according to the Centers for Disease Control and Prevention (CDC). By 2004, that number had dropped to an average of about 26,000. Experts believe the decrease is due in large part to the screening of blood donors (prior to 1992, unscreened blood was used for blood transfusions). In all, there are about 4.1 million Americans who are infected by hepatitis C.

A similar decline has occurred with hepatitis B, thanks to routine vaccinations, which started in 1982. According to the CDC, the number of new infections has fallen from about 260,000 in the 1980s to about 60,000 in 2004. There are currently 1.25 million people in the United States infected with hepatitis B. Hepatitis B is the deadliest of the three viruses, with about 15 to 25 percent of infected persons dying of chronic liver disease.

Hepatitis A, on the other hand, is an acute infection transmitted through contact with others who have an infection. It is usually transmitted by putting something in the mouth that has been contaminated by the feces of an infected person. In some parts of the world, hepatitis A is quite common. Travelers to those areas are advised to get vaccines beforehand.

Once you've had hepatitis A, you will not contract it again. However, about 15 percent of people who get infected will experience a relapse or a prolonged case of the illness that lasts six to nine months. The arrival of a vaccine in the late 1990s has reduced the incidence of new infections.

## 🔍 What It Looks Like

Many times, people with hepatitis will have no signs or symptoms at all. Those who do may notice a yellowish hue in their skin or in the whites of their eyes, which is a sign of jaundice, meaning that there is too much bilirubin circulating in their blood. Bilirubin is a substance normally produced by the breakdown of red blood cells and then processed by the liver. Hepatitis can interfere with that process.

Hepatitis may also cause fatigue, loss of appetite, abdominal pain, and nausea. Hepatitis C may cause the urine to darken, while hepatitis B may cause joint pain. Hepatitis A, which is more likely to cause signs and symptoms, especially in adults, may cause fever and diarrhea.

## 🍴 What to Eat

Eating a healthy, well-balanced diet that prevents excess weight gain or loss is essential for someone with hepatitis, says Milton Stokes, R.D., a spokesperson for the American Dietetic Association. Start by eating a lot of fruits and vegetables, whole grains, low-fat dairy products, and nutrient-dense proteins. The antioxidants in fruits and vegetables will help prevent damage to body cells. Fruits and veggies are also naturally low in calories and high in fiber, which will help prevent weight gain.

When choosing breads, cereals, and pastas, look for foods that are whole grain. Check the ingredient list for words such as "whole wheat," "oatmeal," or "whole-grain corn." These are whole-grain foods containing fiber and nutrients that are lacking in refined grains such as white bread. For protein, try eating low-fat dairy products and nutrient-rich sources such as fish, dried beans, soy, eggs, and nuts. And don't overlook lean red meat. When buying red meat, look for cuts with "loin" in the title, such as sirloin, which tend to have less fat.

People with hepatitis are at risk for malnutrition, especially if they have other infections as well. The condition can sometimes lead to anorexia, loss of taste, early satiety, nausea, and vomiting. Separately or combined, these conditions can wreak havoc on your nutritional status if they're not kept in check. In fact, some people with hepatitis need as many as 3,000 calories a day and double the amount of protein of an average healthy person to sustain their body weight. Whether you're trying to prevent weight loss or gain, proper management of body weight is important for anyone who has hepatitis.

Regular meals and snacks are also vital to sustaining your energy levels. Eating regularly is very important if you're being treataed for hepatitis C, which can sometimes cause nausea.

Be sure to drink plenty of fluids, too, especially if you have other conditions such as vomiting or diarrhea.

## 🚫 What Not to Eat

Limit your intake of high-fat foods. Fat is high in calories and can cause unwanted weight gain. Beware of saturated fats in red meat, whole dairy products, and butter, as well as trans-fatty acids found in fried foods and processed foods such as cookies, cakes, and crackers.

Avoid eating too much sugar. Foods high in sugar are generally lower in nutrients and can promote weight gain. You should also try to reduce your intake of salt, which is found primarily in canned and processed foods. If you prefer canned foods—and many canned beans are perfectly healthy—drain the foods and rinse them in a strainer. This simple technique will eliminate as much as 40 percent of the sodium.

Finally—and perhaps most important—do not drink alcohol. Alcohol is a toxin that stresses the liver. Drinking too much can lead to cirrhosis, liver disease, and even liver cancer. If you already have a drinking problem and develop hepatitis, get counseling to overcome the alcoholism. And if you don't drink, don't start now. Alcohol is too serious a toxin to be ingested by someone whose liver is compromised by hepatitis.

## ⚇ Supplements for Hepatitis

When it comes to hepatitis, excess amounts of certain vitamins can tax the liver. At the same time, your body needs essential vitamins and minerals.

Strike a balance by taking a high-quality multivitamin to ensure you get all the essential nutrients, especially if your appetite is suppressed. But be careful of the vitamin you choose; some people with hepatitis C have elevated levels of iron, which can damage organs. Look for a multivitamin that does not have iron.

Also, be careful about taking too much vitamin C, A, or D. Excess vitamin C promotes the absorption of iron, while too much A and D is toxic to the liver.

Before taking any supplements or herbal remedies, talk to your doctor first. Some supplements you might consider include the following:

### MILK THISTLE
Milk thistle has been used for centuries for the treatment of liver disease. Studies on this plant have been mixed, but the National Center for Complementary and Alternative Medicine is currently doing a clinical trial on milk thistle's potential in treating hepatitis C. People allergic to ragweed, however, should avoid milk thistle, which belongs to the same plant family.

### LICORICE ROOT
The active component in licorice root is glycyrrhizin. Studies of licorice root have found that it shows potential for reducing long-term complications from hepatitis C. Again, people with hepatitis C should not take licorice without first talking to their doctors.

### GINSENG
Ginseng is an herb that's been used for centuries in Asia to stimulate the immune system. Animal studies have shown some benefits for the liver.

### SCHISANDRA
Schisandra is a plant used in Chinese medicine. Some small studies have suggested that it may have some protective effects on the liver.

## Stay-Healthy Strategies

- **WATCH YOUR WEIGHT.** Too many pounds can cause fatty deposits in the liver and make it harder to treat hepatitis. But being too thin can deprive your body of the energy it needs to stay well. Aim to be at a healthy weight.

- **BE WARY OF HEALTH CLAIMS.** It's easy to fall prey to ads promising better health when you have a chronic illness, but remember, some supplements—such as chaparral, skullcap, and pennyroyal—are toxic to the liver. Two good sources to check are www.quackwatch.com and www.nutrition.gov. Remember: If a supplement or diet remedy sounds too good to be true, it probably is.

- **STEER CLEAR OF ENVIRONMENTAL POLLUTANTS.** Fumes and the toxins from these chemicals are also processed in the liver.

- **TAKE PREVENTIVE MEASURES** to protect yourself from contracting hepatitis. Always wash your hands before handling food. Get vaccinated before traveling to high-risk areas. Avoid sharing needles or personal care items. And practice safe sex.

---

## Are You at Risk for Hepatitis C?

It's frightening but true: Most of the 4.1 million Americans with hepatitis C don't even know they have it. That's why some experts recommend that you be tested, regardless of whether you have signs or symptoms.

According to the Hepatitis Foundation International, those who are most at risk include the following:

- Intravenous drug users—current and in the recent past

- People who have multiple sex partners or partners with other sexually transmitted diseases

- People who have tattoos done without sterilized equipment

- Anyone who had a blood transfusion before 1992

- Anyone who received clotting factors before 1987

- Hemodialysis patients

# HERPES

HERPES IS GENERALLY CONSIDERED a genital infection, though a different virus from the same family also causes cold sores. The herpes simplex virus-2 is the culprit behind the genital form of herpes, while HSV-1 is the virus that causes cold sores on the lips.

Most people get genital herpes by having sex with someone who has the virus. The virus can also be transmitted by having oral sex or close skin-to-skin contact with an infected person. Genital herpes is the most common sexually transmitted infection in the United States. According to the Centers for Disease Control and Prevention, one out of five American teenagers and adults is infected with HSV-2. The condition is more common among women than men. In fact, one out of four women in the United States is infected with HSV-2. Since the late 1970s, the number of people with genital herpes has increased 30 percent nationwide, with the largest increase among teens and young adults.

Although there is no cure for genital herpes, there are antiviral medicines that treat the symptoms and can help prevent future outbreaks. Taking these medications can also decrease the risk of passing herpes on to other sexual partners. These drugs include acyclovir (Zovirax), famciclovir (Famvir), and valacyclovir (Valtrex).

## 🔎 What It Looks Like

Oftentimes, genital herpes presents no symptoms. But in people who do have signs and symptoms, genital sores usually occur within two weeks after the initial infection. During this time, urination may be painful and the sores may feel itchy or painful. Within two to four weeks, the sores will heal. But once you are infected, you will always have the virus and may experience recurrent sores.

In some people, the first episode may involve flu-like symptoms such as fever and swollen glands. You may also experience a second cycle of sores. Many people who develop sores will go through four or five outbreaks in the first year. After that, the number of outbreaks will diminish. But some people with HSV-2 will never have any sores.

In some cases, genital herpes sores can be quite painful. In people who have suppressed immune systems, the sores can be severe. When the sores recur, the first signs are often tingling and itching.

Fortunately, herpes is not a life-threatening disease, though some experts believe it may play a role in the spread of HIV, the virus that causes AIDS. People who have active herpes sores may be more susceptible to HIV infection, and those who are already infected with HIV may spread both infections more easily.

Psychologically, having herpes can be extremely distressing. Many people may feel tainted and undesirable. Others may question the fidelity of their partners.

Pregnant women may worry about transmitting herpes to their unborn babies. For pregnant women, the key to keeping your baby healthy is to tell your doctor you have herpes or that you had sex with someone who has herpes. If the infection is active at the time of delivery, the baby may need to be delivered by cesarean section.

## 🍽 What to Eat

Boost your immunity by eating a lot of fresh, unprocessed foods such as fruits, vegetables, and whole grain foods, says Fred Pescatore, M.D., a New York City physician who uses nutrition to treat patients and the author of *The Hamptons Diet Cookbook*.

Make sure to eat foods that are rich in L-lysine, an amino acid that may block the activity of the herpes virus. L-lysine occurs in beans, fish, red meat, and dairy products.

## 🚫 What Not to Eat

Stay away from foods that contain arginine, an amino acid that helps promotes the replication of the herpes virus. These foods include peanuts, almonds, raisins, nuts, and seeds, as well as anything with chocolate.

Avoid drinking caffeine or alcohol, which, in excess, can weaken immunity by interfering with sleep. Pass up processed foods, which may also weaken the immune system. Some experts also believe that highly acidic foods may aggravate the infection, so avoid grapefruit, oranges, and tomatoes during an outbreak.

## 💊 Supplements for Herpes

Take a high-quality multivitamin to ensure overall health and well-being. You might also consider taking the following:

### L-LYSINE

L-lysine has long been regarded as a treatment for herpes infections. It works by inhibiting replication of the herpes virus.

### ZINC

Some studies have suggested that zinc may help reduce the duration and severity of a herpes outbreak. You might also ask your doctor about topical creams that contain zinc.

### NATURAL ANTIVIRAL REMEDIES

Certain plants contain substances with antiviral properties. These herbal remedies may help reduce the incidence of genital sores and prevent their recurrence. Among them are the following:

- Olive leaf extract or oil. The oil and extract from the olive tree contains phytochemicals that help fight disease.

- Oregano oil. This oil derived from oregano, a Mediterranean plant, is a potent germ fighter.

- Lemon Balm. This herb contains terpenes and tannins, substances in plants that may have antiviral properties.

- Lauric acid. This fatty acid occurs naturally in human milk and coconut milk and is available in a supplement called monolaurin.

## Stay-Healthy Strategies

- **MINIMIZE STRESS.** Stress can trigger a recurrence of the infection.

- **STAY HEALTHY THE BEST YOU CAN.** Even illnesses such as the common cold can compromise your immune system, so do your best to stay well.

- **USE CONDOMS WHENEVER YOU HAVE SEX.** Condoms can help prevent the spread of herpes, especially if you aren't sure whether you're infected.

- **CONSIDER JOINING A SUPPORT GROUP.** Having herpes can cause a lot of stress and problems, especially when it comes to forming close, intimate relationships. Talking to others in the same predicament can help make it a little easier.

---

### Prevent the Spread

A key problem with herpes occurs when someone doesn't know he has the infection and passes it on to others. But if you know you have herpes, you should take actions to reduce your risk of spreading the disease. Here's how:

- Avoid touching the infected area during an outbreak and wash your hands after contact with the area.

- Do not have sexual contact (vaginal, oral, or anal) from the time the symptoms first appear until symptoms are completely gone.

# HIGH BLOOD PRESSURE

BLOOD COURSING THROUGH OUR VESSELS exerts a certain amount of pressure on the artery walls, a measure we know as blood pressure. It's lowest when you sleep and rises when you get up. Blood pressure also goes up during exercise and in times of stress, excitement, and fear. But high blood pressure can occur in even the calmest people.

In healthy people, blood pressure is no more than 120/80 mmHg. The top number of a blood pressure reading—the higher number—is systolic pressure, which occurs when the heart beats and pumps the blood. When the heart rests between beats, the pressure falls—even as the blood continues to travel through the blood vessels—producing the bottom number, which is called diastolic pressure.

Nearly a third of all American adults have high blood pressure, or hypertension, a condition characterized by a blood pressure reading of 140/90 mmHg. Having high blood pressure means your heart is working harder than it should to get blood through your vessels. The extra exertion eventually takes a toll. People with untreated high blood pressure may suffer a heart attack, stroke, or kidney failure. Unfortunately, the lack of symptoms means some people have no idea they have hypertension.

In an effort to prevent high blood pressure, some doctors are now diagnosing patients with prehypertension, in which systolic blood pressure is between 120 and 139 and diastolic pressure is between 80 and 89. At this stage, lifestyle changes can help lower blood pressure and may prevent full-blown hypertension.

Once you are diagnosed with high blood pressure, it usually doesn't go away, though you may have a brief return to normalcy. Eventually, you may need medications to keep it normal. It also sets the stage and raises your risk for other cardiovascular problems such as heart disease, diabetes, and insulin resistance. Fortunately high blood pressure can be treated and controlled. A healthy lifestyle that includes a nutritious diet and exercise is one way you can manage high blood pressure.

## ⚲ What It Looks Like

High blood pressure presents no symptoms, which is why it's often called a "silent killer." The key to catching it is knowing the risk factors for it. People who are at risk for high blood pressure include adults over the age of 35, African-Americans, and people who are overweight or obese. It is also more likely to occur in people who are heavy drinkers and in women who take oral contraceptives. In addition, people who have diabetes, gout, or kidney disease are at greater risk. But these are only risk factors. High blood pressure also occurs in thin people from a Caucasian background who do not have preexisting diseases. The only way to know for sure is to have your blood pressure taken regularly.

## 🍴 What to Eat

People who have high blood pressure should strive for a heart-healthy diet that helps to maintain weight and trim inches off your waist, says Marie Savard, M.D., author of *The Body Shape Solution for Weight Loss and Wellness*. Studies show that waist circumference may be a more accurate predictor of heart disease and high blood pressure risk than even body mass index (BMI), which is a measure of your weight in relation to height.

Any heart-healthy diet should include several fruits and vegetables each day, which will fortify your body with disease-fighting phytonutrients and antioxidant vitamins. Eating fruits and veggies will help ensure you get fiber as well. Soluble fiber, the kind that dissolves in water, is especially critical because it will help slow down digestion and can help lower blood pressure.

Both soluble and insoluble fiber can help with weight loss or maintenance by making you feel full. Good sources of fiber include oats, kidney beans, peas, cauliflower, flaxseed, apples, oranges, and carrots.

Another good source of fiber is whole grains such as brown rice, bulgur wheat, and quinoa. Other high-fiber foods include legumes such as chickpeas, kidney beans, pinto beans, and black beans, which are healthy sources of protein as well.

When it comes to protein, look for lean varieties. Good proteins include chicken, fish, and soy products such as tempeh, tofu, edamame, soy milk, and soy burgers. Fish has the added bonus of omega-3 fatty acids, which may lower your risk for heart disease. Healthy fish include salmon, tuna, and mackerel. Omega-3s are also found in walnuts, flaxseed, and fortified foods including peanut butter and breakfast cereal.

You should also try to eat low-fat dairy foods such as yogurt, skim milk, and cheese. These foods supply magnesium, calcium, and protein. Research has shown that the combination of fruits and vegetables with low-fat dairy foods helps lower blood pressure.

In addition, try to get your fat primarily from monounsaturated fats, which are healthier. Good sources of monounsaturated fats are found in avocados, almonds, pecans, and other nuts, as well as in olive or canola oil.

# 🍴 What Not to Eat

For people with high blood pressure, one of the worst dietary villains is salt. Studies by scientists at the National Heart, Lung, and Blood Institute (NHLBI) found that eating a low-sodium diet (1,500 mg compared with 3,300 mg in a typical American diet) significantly lowered blood pressure. Be on the lookout for high-salt foods such as canned soups, packaged meals, and processed meats including hot dogs, pastrami, and bologna. Beware of condiments and convenience foods that are often high in sodium.

Avoid foods high in saturated fats, too, which are found mostly in red meat, dairy products, and butter. You should also steer clear of foods that contain trans-fatty acids, which are often found in packaged foods such as candy bars, cookies, muffins, and crackers—foods commonly found in vending machines. Check the ingredient list for anything "partially hydrogenated," which means the product contains trans-fatty acids. Both saturated fats and trans fats damage arteries and are high in calories.

Try to cut back or eliminate foods high in sugar and white flour. These foods are high in calories and supply few nutrients. They can also raise your cholesterol, triglycerides, and blood pressure.

Finally, drink alcohol in moderation, if at all. Alcohol can raise blood pressure and is high in empty calories—energy without the presence of healthy nutrients.

# 💊 Supplements for High Blood Pressure

Start with a quality multivitamin, which supplies the basic nutrients you need for good health. Other supplements you might consider taking include the following:

### FISH OIL
Studies show that omega-3 fatty acids are beneficial to the prevention of heart disease, so you may consider taking a fish oil supplement. If you're on blood-thinning medication, talk to your doctor first since fish oil may increase your risk for bleeding.

### CERTAIN B VITAMINS
Taking folic acid and vitamins B6 and B12 may help reduce levels of homocysteine, a substance that has been implicated in the development of heart disease.

### CALCIUM AND VITAMIN D
Some studies have suggested that the bone-building mineral calcium can help lower blood pressure. But you also need vitamin D in order to make sure the calcium gets absorbed. Many seniors are deficient in vitamin D because their skin can no longer make it from sunlight.

### MAGNESIUM
Some people may consider taking magnesium, a mineral that may help lower blood pressure, relax blood vessels, and promote healthy contractions of the heart.

## PSYLLIUM

Psyllium is a seed husk and soluble fiber that can help promote bowel regularity and lower cholesterol. Talk to your doctor first before taking psyllium, especially if you have food allergies, because some people react to psyllium.

## ASPIRIN

High blood pressure raises your risk for heart disease. Research has shown that one baby aspirin a day can prevent a heart attack in men stroke in women. But talk to your doctor before starting on aspirin, which can cause a number of side effects including stomach irritation and bleeding. Your doctor may delay starting aspirin until your blood pressure is under control.

## Stay-Healthy Strategies

- **WATCH YOUR WEIGHT.** Being overweight has a direct link to high blood pressure, so do what you can to lower and maintain it.

- **LEARN TO SPEAK UP IN RESTAURANTS.** When choosing an entrée, ask that foods be prepared without salt and that condiments be placed on the side.

- **GET ACTIVE.** Regular exercise helps lower blood pressure. Do whatever you can to move your body.

- **MONITOR YOUR BLOOD PRESSURE.** Consider purchasing a home device so you can track your blood pressure regularly and gauge your efforts to control it.

- **TAKE YOUR MEDICATIONS EVERY DAY.** Make it a habit by taking your pill at the same time. Post reminder notes if necessary.

## What's DASH?

Back in 1997, the National Heart, Lung and Blood Institute of the National Institutes of Health (NHLBI) released a study called "Dietary Approaches to Stop Hypertension" (DASH). The study looked at the effect of different eating patterns on blood pressure in more than 450 adults. It compared a typical American diet with two modified diets: one high in fruits and vegetables, and a combination version that was high in fruits and vegetables and included low-fat dairy, which became known as the DASH eating plan. Of the three diets, the combination diet resulted in the greatest drop in blood pressure.

A subsequent study looked at the effect of sodium restriction on 412 adults who ate either a typical diet or the DASH diet. The results showed that the biggest reductions in blood pressure occurred in people who ate the DASH diet *and* consumed the least amount of sodium.

The bottom line: A diet rich in fruits, vegetables, and low-fat dairy and low in sodium is the best choice for people with hypertension.

Check out the NHLBI Web site at www.nhlbi.nih.gov/health/public/heart/hbp/dash/ for information on DASH and sample menus.

# HYPERTHYROIDISM

EVERYONE NEEDS THYROID HORMONE to survive, but people who have hyperthyroidism are getting more thyroid hormone than they need. With hyperthyrodism, your metabolism speeds up considerably, and you feel anxious, nervous, and unsettled. Your heart beats rapidly and you can't get to sleep at night. You may be losing weight despite an increase in appetite.

Hyperthyroidism is much less common than hypothyroidism, which occurs when you don't have enough thyroid hormone. According to the American Association of Clinical Endocrinologists, hyperthyroidism affects about 1 percent of the U.S. population, most of them women. The condition can occur for various reasons, but the most common cause is Graves' disease, an autoimmune condition in which autoantibodies attack the thyroid gland, causing it to release too much thyroid hormone.

Other conditions that may cause hyperthyrodism include the following:

- Toxic multinodular goiter, in which an enlarged thyroid develops nodules that make their own thyroid hormone.

- Plummer's disease, in which a single toxic nodule is producing excess thyroid hormone.

- Subacute (painful) or silent (nonpainful) thyroiditis, an inflammation or enlargement of the thyroid gland.

- Postpartum thyroiditis, which occurs shortly after giving birth.

Some people become hyperthyroid from eating too much iodine, the mineral the thyroid uses to produce thyroid hormone. Hyperthyroidism may also occur in people who take certain medications such as Cordarone, which is used to treat abnormal heart rhythms. In addition, hyperthyroidism may occur in people being treated for hypothyroidism when the dose of thyroid hormone replacement is too high.

## 🔍 What It Looks Like

Too much thyroid hormone can cause myriad symptoms, including a very rapid heartbeat. In some cases, it can be as fast as 100 beats per minute. Some people also become extremely nervous and irritable. They may experience ravenous hunger, even as they lose weight. The revved up metabolism often causes exhaustion and fatigue.

If hyperthyroidism becomes severe, they may develop a wide-eyed, startled look. In people with Graves' disease, an eye condition known as exophthalmos, or thyroid eye disease, may result. The condition is characterized by a distinct bulging of the eyeball. In addition, hyperthyroidism may cause the following:

- Enlarged thyroid
- Diarrhea
- Profuse sweating
- Thin skin
- Hair loss
- Light, infrequent menstrual periods

Left untreated, hyperthyroidism can lead to heart failure, abnormal heart rhythms, and osteoporosis. The condition steps up the production of osteoclasts, substances that naturally break down bone, but does not affect the production of osteoblasts, substances that counter osteoclasts by building bone. Taming the conditions of hyperthyroidism requires antithyroid medications, radioactive iodine treatments, or surgery to remove all or part of the thyroid gland. Some people may be given beta blockers to lower blood pressure, slow a rapid heartbeat, and reduce tremors. Eating the right foods can help relieve some of the symptoms and improve a person's overall health.

### Diarrhea: An Uncomfortable Symptom

Some people with hyperthyroidism will develop diarrhea when their digestive systems speed up. If you do have diarrhea, try eating a bland diet that includes bananas, applesauce, plain toast, and broth. Avoid high-fiber foods which may worsen it. And make sure you get plenty of fluids to prevent dehydration.

## ⑪ What to Eat

According to Theodore C. Friedman, M.D., Ph.D., co-author of *The Everything Health Guide to Thyroid Disease*, anyone with a thyroid condition needs to eat a healthy diet that sustains the immune system, especially if Graves' disease is at the root of your hyperthyroidism. That means eating a diet comprising plenty of fresh fruits and vegetables, lean protein, and complex carbohydrates.

Pay special attention to your fruit and veggie choices. Some of these are known as goitrogens, substances that promote the formation of goiters by inhibiting the production of thyroid hormone. In people with hyperthyroidism, goitrogens may help reduce the amount of thyroid hormone. Good vegetables to eat include brussels sprouts, cabbage, corn, cauliflower, kale, and rutabagas. Good fruits include peaches, pears, and strawberries.

You also need to eat foods rich in calcium, the bone-building mineral. Good sources of calcium include milk, yogurt, and cheese. Opt for the low-fat varieties to keep weight gain to a minimum. You can also find calcium in leafy greens, fortified orange juice, tofu, and sardines with edible bones.

In addition to calcium, you need to make sure you get enough vitamin D, which ensures absorption of calcium. Vitamin D can be found in some of the same foods as calcium, such as milk, cheese, and sardines. It's also found in fortified breakfast cereals and eggs. Although your body can make vitamin D after exposure to sunlight, you should guard against too much sun exposure because it raises your risk for skin cancer.

## ⊘ What Not to Eat

If hyperthyroidism already has you anxious and jittery, it's important to give up caffeinated foods and beverages such as coffee, tea, and cola. Caffeine is also found in chocolate, energy drinks, diet aids, cold remedies, and certain menstrual pain relievers. Even without a thyroid problem, caffeine can cause insomnia, anxiety, and heart palpitations.

That's because caffeine is a stimulant that boosts the body's production of adrenaline, one of the fight-or-flight hormones. Although the adrenaline initially gives you an energy boost, it subsequently causes a crash that can trigger carb cravings and overeating. Caffeine also causes blood pressure to increase temporarily and urination to become more frequent, which can boost your excretion of calcium.

If hyperthyroidism has you concerned about bone health, you should also restrict or eliminate alcohol. Too much alcohol reduces bone density and can affect your balance and coordination, putting you at increased risk for falls and hip fractures. Alcohol is also high in empty calories–seven calories per gram.

Be wary of eating too much iodine as well. Excess iodine in someone with hyperthyroidism can worsen the symptoms. Iodine is found in high-sodium foods such as canned soups, prepackaged foods, and snack foods.

## Supplements for Hyperthyroidism

Some people with hyperthyroidism may require supplements to enhance their health. A quality multivitamin, for instance, can help meet your body's revved-up metabolic needs. In addition, you may consider the following:

### CALCIUM

People with hyperthyroidism are at risk for bone loss. Choose a supplement with the right amount of elemental calcium in it. To maximize absorption, take calcium with food or orange juice. Also, if you take more than 750 mg of calcium per day, split the dosage between morning and bedtime because your body can only absorb so much calcium at one time.

### VITAMIN C

Because your body is under stress, you may need vitamin C to keep your immune system strong.

## Stay-Healthy Strategies

- **GET A THOROUGH MEDICAL EXAM** and treatment for hyperthyroidism. Do not attempt to self-treat this condition.

- **GIVE THE MEDICATIONS TIME TO WORK.** Antithyroid drugs often take a while to kick in, and you may need to adjust the dosage to your particular condition.

- **TRY STRESS-MANAGEMENT TECHNIQUES.** Because you are already in a hyper-stressed state, try to avoid stressful situations and practice relaxation techniques such as meditation.

- **PRACTICE GOOD SLEEP HYGIENE.** Sleep may not come easily to people with hyperthyroidism, but laying the foundation for good sleep can help, especially once the condition is effectively under control.

# HYPOTHYROIDISM

FATIGUE. WEIGHT GAIN. DEPRESSION. For some people, this constellation of symptoms traces its cause to a small but powerful gland located near the base of your neck called the thyroid gland. This small butterfly-shaped gland produces thyroid hormone, which regulates everything from your weight to your mood. When the thyroid gland becomes underactive, you don't produce enough thyroid hormone, causing a condition called hypothyroidism. As a result, all your bodily functions will slow down.

According to the American Association of Clinical Endocrinologists, hypothyroidism affects about 10 percent of all women and 3 percent of men in the U. S. Hypothyroidism is also more common with advancing age. By age 60, 17 percent of all women and 9 percent of men will have an underactive thyroid. Studies suggest that approximately thirteen million Americans are living undiagnosed.

Several factors can reduce the thyroid's production of thyroid hormone, including age. Worldwide, it's most often caused by a lack of iodine. But here in the United States, where our diets have been fortified with iodized salt since the 1920s, the most common cause is an autoimmune disorder called Hashimoto's thyroiditis, in which the body attacks its own healthy thyroid tissues and destroy the gland's ability to produce thyroid hormone.

Some people develop hypothyroidism as a result of other medical conditions or from medications they take. For instance, people who have been treated with radioactive iodine to treat hyperthyroidism often develop hypothyroidism. People who take medications such as lithium, prednisone, and propranolol are also at higher risk for hypothyroidism. In addition, anyone who has had her thyroid removed or undergone radiation to the neck or upper chest is at greater risk for developing an underactive thyroid.

## 🔍 What It Looks Like

Hypothyroidism is tricky to detect because it frequently resembles other health conditions and lifestyle factors. Symptoms like fatigue, weight gain, body aches, and depression are easily blamed on a busy schedule or advancing age. In women, they may be dismissed as evidence of menopause. But for millions of people—especially women—your thyroid may be the culprit.

When you first start developing hypothyroidism, you may have no symptoms at all. But over time, your body functions will start to slow down and you will start to notice signs and symptoms that something isn't right. Although you may not have all of these symptoms, here are some common ones:

- Unexplained weight gain
- Difficulties concentrating and remembering
- Depression
- Dry skin, hair, and nails
- Frequent constipation
- Heavier, more frequent periods
- Difficulties getting pregnant
- Swollen thyroid gland called goiter
- Increase in blood pressure
- Intolerance of the cold
- Muscle aches
- Low libido
- Frequent headaches
- Worsening of allergies and PMS
- Slow healing of infections, cuts, and bruises
- Anemia, or low red blood cell count
- High cholesterol

Hyperthyroidism is detected with a simple blood test for the thyroid-stimulating hormone (TSH)–high TSH levels mean the pituitary is signaling the thyroid to make more thyroid hormone, in an effort to stimulate the gland–this indicates an underactive thyroid. Hypothyroidism is easily treated with thyroid hormone replacement.

## ¶¶¶ What to Eat

Having hypothyroidism means your energy levels and propensity for weight gain are already compromised by your thyroid problems. That's why it's important for you to maximize your nutrition. Healthy eating is also important because you're at greater risk for high cholesterol and high blood pressure, which puts you at risk for serious diseases such as heart disease and diabetes.

According to Theodore C. Friedman, M.D., Ph.D., co-author of *The Everything Health Guide to Thyroid Disease*, you should eat a moderate amount of complex carbs, which will help keep cholesterol levels down and minimize weight gain. Limit simple carbs to fruits and vegetables, which supply healthy nutrients such as vitamins A and C.

It's also important to choose your proteins wisely. Stick with lean proteins such as chicken, fish, and turkey. Protein helps you feel full and can prevent unwanted weight gain by taming your appetite.

Be sure to include some healthy fats in your diet. Although high in calories, fats are essential to the brain and nervous system. The best type of fat you can eat is the monounsaturated variety found in avocados and olive oil. Another healthy type of fat is the omega-3 fatty acids found in fish. These polyunsaturated fats have been touted as healthful for blood flow, brain function, and the reduction of inflammation.

If you have hypothyroidism and are battling weight gain, it's important to eat a lot of fiber. Fiber is a component of complex carbohydrates and can be either soluble–it dissolves in water–or insoluble. Soluble fibers reduce the time it takes to empty the stomach and lower cholesterol levels. Good sources include dried peas and beans, apples, and oats. Insoluble fibers–known as roughage—cannot dissolve in water but absorb water. They add bulk to the stool and help move food through the digestive tract, thereby preventing constipation, a common problem for people with hypothyroidism.

High-fiber foods also help promote weight loss by displacing unhealthy foods with healthy ones. In addition, fiber can help relieve constipation and reduce cholesterol by binding bile acids, which are rich in cholesterol.

If you do increase your intake of fiber, make sure to keep tabs on your thyroid function with routine tests. A diet rich in fiber may decrease the amount of thyroid medication that your body absorbs.

## 🚫 What Not to Eat

Because a key goal is minimizing weight gain, it's important to reduce your intake of refined carbs such as cakes, cookies, juices, and most snack foods—foods with no nutrients and plenty of empty calories.

Limit the amount of saturated fats in your diet. These are the unhealthy fats that clog arteries and raise the risk for heart disease. These fats are solid at room temperature and are found in meat, whole dairy foods, butter, and palm and coconut oils.

Also, steer clear of foods with trans-fatty acids. These fats are produced when oils are hydrogenated to make them solid at room temperature. They're commonly found in processed foods such as breakfast cereals, frozen pancakes, potato chips, crackers, and cookies. They're also found in margarine and shortening.

In addition, limit your intake of iodine, a mineral found in iodized salt, plants and animals found in saltwater (such as seafood, seaweed, and kelp), milk, meat, spinach, and eggs. While people with healthy thyroids usually can get away with eating more iodine, those with hypothyroidism should be wary of eating too much iodine, which can inhibit the thyroid's production of thyroid hormone.

Watch your intake of soy, a bean found in foods such as tofu, tempeh, soy milk, soy sauce, and miso, a soybean paste. The bean is also used to make soy burgers, soy shakes, and soy cereals. Too much soy can further aggravate a thyroid problem because isoflavones found in soy can increase your thyroid-stimulating hormone (TSH) levels, which in turn can cause an increase in thyroid hormone requirements. Soy can also inhibit absorption of thyroid medications. So if you do eat soy, wait at least four hours after taking your thyroid medication to do so.

Finally, limit caffeine, which is found in coffee, tea, soft drinks, and chocolate. It is also found in energy drinks, diet aids, cold remedies, and certain menstrual pain relievers. Caffeine can trigger carb cravings and overeating. It also causes a temporary rise in blood pressure and more frequent urination, which can increase your excretion of calcium. In excess, caffeine can cause insomnia, anxiety, and heart palpitations. The lack of quality sleep can also stimulate your appetite, which could cause weight gain.

Finally, limit your intake of foods called goitrogens, which can enlarge the thyroid. Goitrogens include cruciferous vegetables such as broccoli, cauliflower, brussels sprouts, and cabbage. Other foods such as spinach, strawberries, radishes, peaches, millet, soy products, corn, sweet potatoes, carrots, peanuts, and walnuts are also considered goitrogens. Eat these foods in moderation and at a relatively constant amount from one day to the next.

## 🫙 Supplements for Hypothyroidism

Consider taking a quality multivitamin for overall health. Two other supplements you might consider taking include the following:

### SELENIUM

People with hypothyroidism who take levothyroxine may want to take selenium, which aids in the conversion of thyroid hormone into its active form. Selenium supplements also have been shown to improve autoimmune thyroiditis.

### IRON

Iron is needed to help convert the inactive form of thyroid hormone into the active form. So if you have hypothyroidism, consider testing your ferritin levels. Ferritin is a protein that stores iron in the liver. Low ferritin levels will reveal a drop in your iron stores and may indicate a need for iron supplements. But do not take iron with your thyroid medication. Take your thyroid medication first and take the iron at least four hours later. Taken together, iron can inhibit absorption of the thyroid medication.

## 📋 Stay-Healthy Strategies

- **READ UP ON HYPOTHYROIDISM.** The more you know about managing this lifelong condition, the better you'll be at keeping symptoms and problems at bay.

- **LISTEN TO YOUR BODY.** Hypothyroidism can fluctuate in severity. Learn to identify symptoms that show you need to change the dose of your medications.

- **MAKE EXERCISE A PRIORITY.** Regular exercise will promote sound sleep and help prevent weight gain.

- **PRACTICE MINDFUL EATING.** Eat slowly and deliberately and avoid eating on the run or while doing other tasks. Putting the focus on enjoying your meals will help you naturally achieve a healthy weight.

### Listen to Your Body

Being on thyroid hormone replacement doesn't mean the end of managing your condition. It's still important to pay close attention to how you feel. Excess fatigue, mild depression, or inexplicable weight gain may signal that your thyroid hormone levels are off and that you may need to talk to your doctor about changing the dosage of your medication.

Any time you don't feel right, call your doctor. Describe your situa-tion and ask for the soonest possible appointment.

# INDIGESTION

ALMOST EVERYONE SUFFERS from an occasional bout of indigestion: the wrong mix of foods, too much stress, eating on the run. All these factors can lead to indigestion. But unless you experience additional symptoms with it, it's rarely a serious problem.

Indigestion can strike for any of a number of reasons. Maybe you ate a food that irritates your stomach. Or maybe you ate too fast or too much. Sometimes indigestion is the result of eating foods that are too fatty, spicy, or greasy. Drinking too much alcohol or caffeine can also bring on indigestion. Some people get indigestion when they're feeling nervous or anxious.

People who are prone to indigestion may suffer from a condition called hydrochloric acid (HCL) deficiency. HCL is a stomach acid needed for proper digestion. Levels of HCL can diminish with age. To find out whether you are deficient in HCL, talk to your physician.

## 🔎 What It Looks Like

Indigestion can cause a variety of symptoms and may be mild or severe. Sufferers may notice pain in the upper part of the torso as well as nausea, bloating, or burping. In some cases, it may be accompanied by heartburn, which causes a burning sensation in the throat. Most cases of indigestion go away within hours, but some cases require medical attention.

If your symptoms persist for more than a few days, your symptoms change, or you develop severe abdominal pain, call your doctor. You should also seek medical attention if you vomit, experience inexplicable weight loss, develop yellow jaundice, or pass blood in the stool.

Sometimes, a heart attack is mistaken for indigestion. Call 911 immediately if you develop jaw pain, chest pain, back pain, profuse sweating, anxiety, or a feeling of impending doom. These are symptoms of a heart attack.

## 🍴 What to Eat

To help improve digestion, try eating yogurt that contains the live culture *acidophilus*, says Christine Gerbstadt, M.D., R.D., a spokesperson for the American Dietetic Association. It's also important to eat a diet rich in fruits and vegetables, which are high in fiber and can naturally help prevent indigestion. But choose your fruits and veggies carefully. Some vegetables, such as beans, cabbage, and broccoli, are more likely to cause gas.

The way you eat plays a significant role in the development of indigestion. Chew your food carefully and avoid eating too fast or too much. Try eating small, more frequent meals and eating in a leisurely fashion. Also, make sure to drink plenty of water, which can lessen the symptoms of indigestion.

If you are suffering from heartburn along with indigestion, see the chapter on Gastroesophageal Reflux Disease on page 148 for more information.

## What Not to Eat

Avoid foods that irritate the digestive tract, such as spicy foods, greasy foods, and refined carbohydrates, such as white sugar and white flour. Limit your intake of alcohol and caffeine, substances that can aggravate and cause indigestion.

Look for food sensitivities in your diet by keeping a food diary that lists the foods you eat and any symptoms you experience. A food diary kept for a couple weeks can help pinpoint foods that may be triggering your indigestion.

## Acupuncture for Tummy Troubles

Acupuncture is a traditional Chinese medicine that originated in China more than 3,000 years ago and has been used for ages to relieve pain, including gastrointestinal discomfort. A recent study at the Duke University Medical Center has found that acupuncture may help relieve all sorts of stomach problems including indigestion, gastroesophageal reflux disease, and irritable bowel syndrome.

The premise of acupuncture is based on the notion that the body has patterns of energy flow that are essential for good health. When that energy—or qi (pronounced chi), as the Chinese call it—is disrupted, a person's health falters. Acupuncture helps to restore that flow with the insertion of tiny needles along meridian lines on the body, which correspond to various organs.

If you do decide to try acupuncture, find a licensed therapist. Discuss your plans with your doctor to make sure you're healthy enough. Be honest with the acupuncturist about your health; tell him about your conditions and any medications you take. If your acupuncturist recommends herbal supplements, talk to your doctor before taking them.

## ✂ Supplements for Indigestion

Take a quality multivitamin to make sure you get all the essential nutrients if you're prone to indigestion, which can result in poor absorption of nutrients. Other supplements you might consider include the following:

### BETAINE HCL
Betaine HCL is a supplement form of hydrochloric acid that may aid in digestion if you are deficient in HCL.

### VITAMIN B6
This vitamin, also called pyridoxine, is essential for the production of HCL.

### PROBIOTICS
Taking healthy bacteria such as *Lactobacillus acidophilus* can help enhance the digestive process.

### GINGER
The root of this pungent spice can help relieve symptoms of indigestion.

## ▯ Stay-Healthy Strategies

- **DINE WITH LEISURE.** Avoid eating on the go or while you're rushing about. Make time for your meals and try to really enjoy them.

- **DON'T CHEW GUM.** Chewing gum can cause you to swallow excess amounts of air.

- **RELIEVE STRESS.** When you're in a state of stress, anything you eat can result in indigestion. So look for ways to manage stress in your life, such as changing your thoughts about stressful events and taking up an exercise such as yoga or mediation.

- **MOVE AFTER A MEAL.** A short bout of exercise such as a walk can help with the digestive process and prevent indigestion.

- **DON'T WEAR TIGHT CLOTHES.** Garments that are too restrictive may make you more vulnerable to indigestion.

# INFLAMMATORY BOWEL DISEASE

*See Crohn's Disease on page 104 and Ulcerative Colitis on page 307.*

# INFLUENZA

FEVER. ACHES. CHILLS. For some people, these symptoms add up to a nasty virus. But for others, it may be the flu, a highly contagious respiratory illness caused by influenza viruses.

Every year, 5 to 20 percent of the U.S. population comes down with the flu, according to the Centers for Disease Control and Prevention. More than 200,000 people are hospitalized, and about 36,000 people die of the flu. The timing of flu season varies each year and can start as early as October and end as late as May.

Influenza spreads the same way the cold does, in droplets caused by coughing and sneezing. You can also catch it by having close contact with someone who is infected or by touching something that a sick person has touched, then touching your mouth, eyes, or nose. Unfortunately, you can infect other people even before you know you're sick and for as long as five days while you're actually sick.

The severity of the flu varies widely. Some people may experience mild cases that go away after a short time, while others may wind up with complications such as pneumonia. The elderly, young children, and those who have preexisting health conditions are generally at higher risk for complications.

For these high-risk populations, getting a vaccine each fall is the best way to prevent the flu. The flu shot contains an inactivated vaccine—a dead version of the virus—while the nasal-spray flu vaccine is made with live, weakened flu viruses that do not cause the flu. The flu shot is intended for people over six months of age. The nasal vaccine is approved for use in healthy people between the ages of five and forty-nine who are not pregnant. The vaccines work by stimulating the development of antibodies that guard against influenza viruses. It's best to get vaccinated in October or November.

Anyone who wants to lower the risk for contracting the flu should get vaccinated, as should those at high risk for complications. Visit www.cdc.gov/flu/keyfacts.htm for a specific list of high-risk populations who should get the vaccine.

## ⌕ What It Looks Like

The flu is a respiratory illness that in mild cases may resemble a bad cold. Common symptoms include fever, headaches, extreme fatigue, muscle aches, sore throat, dry cough, and a stuffy and runny nose. Children may also suffer from nausea, vomiting, stomach pain, and diarrhea.

Some people, especially those age sixty-five or older, may develop complications from the flu such as bacterial pneumonia and dehydration. Those who have chronic medical conditions such as heart failure, diabetes, or asthma may notice a worsening of those symptoms. And children may develop sinus problems and ear infections.

It isn't always easy to determine whether you have the flu or another respiratory infection. Sometimes seeing a doctor is the only way to know for sure. Although there are antiviral medications that can help treat the flu, the best treatment is getting plenty of rest and drinking lots of fluids. Analgesics such as acetaminophen or ibuprofen can help reduce fever and body aches but will not shorten the duration of the flu.

## ⫴ What to Eat

Chicken soup may be one of the best nutritional remedies for someone battling the flu, says Fred Pescatore, M.D., a physician in New York City and the author of *The Hamptons Diet Cookbook*. Chicken soup has been used since the twelfth century as a way to relieve upper respiratory ailments.

It's also essential to drink plenty of fluids, preferably water, hot tea, or broths. Staying hydrated will prevent the mucus from becoming too thick and worsening congestion.

To strengthen immunity, eat foods that are light but rich in immune-strengthening vitamin C, such as fruit or steamed vegetables. Good sources of vitamin C include oranges, grapefruit, kiwi, and papaya. In addition, try to eat foods that contain selenium and zinc, minerals that are also antioxidants. Good sources of both include chicken, eggs, and whole grains.

## ⊘ What Not to Eat

Limit your intake of sugar, even the natural kinds such as honey and maple syrup, which can strain your immune system. Watch out for sugary fruit juices. If you do drink them, dilute them with water so you reduce the sugar. Steer clear of dairy products, which in some people can increase the production of mucus. You should also avoid drinks that can cause dehydration, including alcohol and caffeinated beverages.

## ⚕ Supplements for the Flu

Make sure to take a quality multivitamin. You may also want to consider taking certain supplements, such as the following:

### VITAMIN C

Boost your intake of vitamin C, a potent antioxidant that can help strengthen your immunity.

### ZINC

Zinc is an antioxidant mineral that may help lessen your symptoms. The best way to use zinc, Pescatore says, is to apply it topically to the mucous membrane of the nose. Simply taking a zinc supplement will not do anything.

### ECHINACEA

Echinacea enhances the immune system and may help shorten the duration of the flu and lessen its symptoms.

## AHCC

Active hexose correlated compound is a Japanese medicinal mushroom extract that may strengthen the immune system and decrease the duration of colds and flus.

## ELDERBERRY

The extract of this berry is an antiviral agent that may help to reduce coughing and promote healing.

## OSCILLOCOCCINUM

Oscillococcinum is a homeopathic remedy for treating the flu. Taken at the first signs, it may help shorten the flu's duration.

## Stay-Healthy Strategies

- **MAKE PREVENTION THE GOAL.** During flu season, do your best to stay well. Sleep well, eat a diet rich in fruits and vegetables, and exercise.

- **STAY HOME IF YOU DO GET SICK.** Going to work or school will only spread the flu to others.

- **GET YOUR REST.** The best thing you can do when you have the flu is take it easy. Otherwise, you put yourself at risk for other complications such as pneumonia.

- **MINIMIZE STRESS.** Too much stress puts you at risk for illness, so do what you can to relax during flu season.

### Who Should *Not* Be Vaccinated

Every fall, we hear a great deal about the flu vaccine and the need for some people to get it. While the flu vaccine is helpful for some people, there are others who should not be vaccinated. According to the Centers for Disease Control and Prevention, these populations include the following:

- People who have a severe allergy to chicken eggs.
- People who have had a severe reaction to an influenza vaccination in the past.
- People who previously developed Guillain-Barré syndrome within six weeks of getting a flu shot.
- Children younger than 6 months of age.

In addition, people who have a fever as the result of illness should postpone vaccinations until their symptoms lessen. If you have any questions about whether to get the flu vaccine, consult your health care provider.

# INSOMNIA

ALMOST EVERYONE HAS EXPERIENCED sleeplessness before: You lie in bed tossing and turning, waiting for sweet slumber to set in. Or perhaps you're the type who falls asleep fast only to awaken in the middle of the night. In either case, you spend the next day feeling very tired.

The inability to get to sleep is called insomnia. If you suffer from insomnia, you're in good company. According to the National Sleep Foundation (NSF), 58 percent of all adults in the United States experience insomnia at least a few nights a week. People who can't maintain sleep or awaken too early every morning are also suffering from insomnia. The end result is always the same: You go through your days feeling tired and miserable.

Insomnia can be a condition on its own, or it can be a symptom of another health problem such as depression, fibromyalgia, or hyperthyroidism. Difficulties sleeping are more prevalent among the elderly and in women but can affect anyone at any age. Women may be more prone to it during hormonal shifts that occur during menstruation, menopause, or pregnancy. People who are obese are also more likely to experience bouts of insomnia.

In addition, sleep conditions such as restless legs syndrome (RLS) and sleep apnea can lead to insomnia. RLS is a condition in which you feel an overwhelming urge to move your legs. Sleep apnea is a dangerous condition that occurs when your airways close repeatedly during sleep and disrupt breathing.

Some people are lucky enough that they never have troubles getting enough sleep. But according to a 2005 poll by the NSF, insomnia is exceedingly common. The poll found that 86 percent of adults have daytime sleepiness at least three times a week.

## 🔍 What It Looks Like

The severity of insomnia varies and can fluctuate. Some people may have short-term insomnia, which lasts as little as one night or as long as a few weeks. Others may have intermittent insomnia, which is short-term and occurs sporadically. Still others may have chronic insomnia, which is defined as sleep difficulties at least three nights a week for a month or more.

While difficulty falling asleep, difficulty staying asleep, or waking too early are the most obvious signs of insomnia, you may also notice other signs and symptoms, such as feeling unrefreshed after a night's sleep, daytime sleepiness, trouble concentrating, and irritability.

Insufficient or poor sleep isn't just tiring, though. It can actually cause several health problems such as high blood pressure, diabetes, and weight gain. So don't ignore insomnia or any other sleep problem. Talk to your doctor about your insomnia and make an effort to improve sleep.

## ¶¶ What to Eat

Focus on eating foods that contain tryptophan, an amino acid that gets converted into serotonin and melatonin in the body, says Marilyn Tanner, R.D., a spokesperson for the American Dietetic Association. These substances are natural sedatives. Good sources of tryptophan include turkey, tuna, chicken, milk, eggs, and almonds.

The way you eat can affect your sleep too. Make sure you're getting enough food so you aren't kept awake by hunger. By the same token, make sure you're not overeating or eating too late. Either way, your stomach may be keeping you up.

## What Not to Eat

Eliminate all caffeine from your diet. According to the NSF, people who consume four or more caffeinated beverages a day are more likely to have difficulty falling asleep and to wake up unrefreshed. Caffeine is found in coffee, tea, sodas, chocolate, and certain medications. It's also found in coffee ice cream, chocolate chips, and

energy drinks. The effects of caffeine can linger in your body for several hours, so it's best to avoid any foods or beverages with caffeine if you're susceptible to insomnia.

Avoid foods that contain tyramine, a compound derived from tyrosine, an amino acid. Tyramine is a brain stimulant that can aggravate insomnia. Foods that contain tyramine include chocolate, bacon, cheese, sauerkraut, tomatoes, wine, ham, and soy, including soy milk.

In addition, cut alcohol from your diet. Many people think of alcohol as a sedative, but it actually causes more frequent awakenings and less restful sleep. It also contains tyramine.

Finally, don't load up on fluids or heavy foods before bedtime. Too many fluids may have you running to the bathroom frequently, and heavy foods such as high-fat or spicy foods tend to cause indigestion.

## ⁜ Supplements for Insomnia

Some supplements may help induce sleep in people who are having trouble nodding off. Others may help relieve the stress that is keeping you awake. Before taking anything, talk to your doctor. Supplements to consider include the following:

### MELATONIN

Melatonin is a hormone naturally produced by the body that helps regulate the sleep-wake cycle. It can help induce sleep and promote a deeper sleep.

## VALERIAN

Extracts of the root of this pungent vine help alleviate anxiety and relax muscle tension so you're better prepared for sleep.

## CHAMOMILE

Chamomile is a flowering plant native to Europe and now grown in North America. Drinking chamomile tea can have a tranquilizing effect that promotes relaxation and sleep.

## PASSIONFLOWER

This perennial vine is available as an herbal tea and can relieve insomnia.

## 📋 Stay-Healthy Strategies

- **KEEP A REGULAR SCHEDULE.** Wake up and go to sleep at the same time every day, even on weekends. Resist the urge to sleep in on weekends. A strict schedule will keep your body on a consistent sleep-wake cycle.

- **RELAX BEFORE BED.** Doing something that relaxes you before you get into bed will help prepare you for sleep. Avoid activities that will rouse you, such as paying bills or exercising. Instead, try taking a bath, listening to music, or reading a book.

- **CREATE A SLEEP-FRIENDLY BEDROOM.** Keep it cool, quiet, and dark. Minimize noise or try using fans or humidifiers that create white noise. Sleep on a comfortable mattress.

- **USE YOUR BEDROOM ONLY FOR SLEEP.** Don't work or watch TV in your bedroom. Limiting activities will help you associate the room with sleep.

- **EXERCISE REGULARLY.** Getting daily exercise will help you sleep better. Ideally, you should do it in the later afternoon and at least three hours before bedtime.

---

## National Sleep Foundation Poll Says Many Don't Sleep Well

In 2005, a poll by the National Sleep Foundation showed that many Americans are sleep deprived. Respondents revealed that at least a few nights a week the following occurs:

- 54 percent experience at least one symptom of insomnia
- 38 percent wake up feeling unrefreshed
- 32 percent wake often during the night
- 21 percent awaken too early and can't get back to sleep, or they aren't able to fall asleep

Among those who can't fall asleep, almost 25 percent said it takes them at least 30 minutes to doze off. Most of the people having trouble are women, and most tend to sleep alone.

# INSULIN RESISTANCE

WHENEVER YOU EAT, FOOD BREAKS DOWN into simple sugar, also called glucose, which supplies your body cells with the energy they need to function. But in order for the cells to use glucose, you need insulin, a hormone produced in the pancreas. In some people, their body cells become resistant to the effects of insulin, causing a condition known as insulin resistance or metabolic syndrome.

Many people who have insulin resistance also develop prediabetes, which occurs when blood glucose levels are higher than normal but not high enough to be classified as diabetic.

Unfortunately, for many people the end result is diabetes, a metabolic disease in which the body cells no longer respond to insulin. Diabetes is a serious medical condition that puts you at risk for numerous problems including heart disease, blindness, and kidney failure.

It's difficult to know exactly how many people have insulin resistance, but estimates suggest it affects 20 to 25 percent of the population. The risk for insulin resistance is partly inherited and can increase with age. It may also be brought on by the use of certain medications such as Prednisone, a steroid. But one of the biggest risk factors for insulin resistance is weight gain. A poor diet and a lack of exercise greatly increase your risk for becoming insulin resistant.

The good news is that the condition can be reversed. Losing weight and exercising regularly can help you avoid diabetes. In fact, a study known as the Diabetes Prevention Program found that making lifestyle changes could lower the risk for diabetes by 58 percent. The regimen helped bring study subjects' blood glucose levels back to normal.

## What It Looks Like

One of the primary reasons for insulin resistance is extra body fat, especially if the weight is concentrated around your waist. Being overweight or obese significantly raises your risk for becoming insulin resistant. That's because the extra weight interferes with the body's ability to use insulin. The problem is compounded if you do not exercise regularly, because activity helps the body use insulin.

How do you know if you have insulin resistance? According to the National Institutes of Health, you are said to have insulin resistance if you have any of these conditions:

- Excess weight around the waist. In men, that's a waist measuring more than 40 inches; in women, it's more than 35 inches.

- High triglyceride levels (150 mg/dL or higher)

- Low levels of HDL, or "good," cholesterol (below 40 mg/dL for men and below 50 mg/dL for women)

- High blood pressure (130/85 mmHg or higher)

- High fasting blood glucose levels (110 mg/dL or higher)

If you have any of these conditions, consider making lifestyle changes that will help you lose weight. Improving your diet and getting regular exercise will go a long way toward preventing the development of diabetes, heart disease, and other life-threatening illnesses.

## 🍴 What to Eat

According to Lynn Sutton, R.D., C.D.E., a registered dietitian in Albany, New York, who specializes in treating people with insulin resistance and diabetes, people with insulin resistance should eat a high-fiber diet rich in a variety of fresh fruits and veggies as well as whole-grain foods such as brown rice, oatmeal, and whole-wheat bread. Instead of the recommended 25 grams of fiber, people with insulin resistance should aim for 35 grams a day.

Although humans cannot digest fiber, fiber has many benefits for people with insulin resistance. Soluble fiber, the kind that dissolves in water, is especially critical because it holds water, which helps slow down digestion. In turn, the release of glucose into the bloodstream is slowed, and blood sugar levels are less likely to spike. It

also helps lower LDL cholesterol, triglycerides, and high blood pressure, while raising levels of HDL cholesterol. Good sources of soluble fiber include oats, kidney beans, peas, flaxseed, apples, oranges, and carrots.

Insoluble fiber is beneficial, too, because it helps prevent constipation by moving waste more quickly through the colon. Good sources of insoluble fiber include whole-wheat foods, cauliflower, beans, spinach, peas, and apples. As you can see, some foods supply both. Both types of fiber can help minimize weight gain by making you feel full.

Other good sources of fiber include whole grains such as brown rice, bulgur wheat, and quinoa. You should also include legumes such as chickpeas, kidney beans, pinto beans, and black beans into your diet. When choosing whole-wheat breads, look for those that contain at least two grams of fiber in a serving.

For protein, focus most on lean meats and fish that are grilled, baked, or broiled. Fish contain omega-3 fatty acids, a healthy type of polyunsaturated fat that can help lower cholesterol, triglycerides, and blood pressure. You can also get omega-3s in flaxseed and walnuts.

Other good sources of protein include seeds, legumes, and soy foods, which contain beneficial plant sterols and stanols. Soy foods come in many forms, including tempeh, tofu, edamame, soy milk, and soy burgers.

For fat—yes, your diet should still contain some fat—eat foods that contain monounsaturated and polyunsaturated fats, which can help lower cholesterol. Good sources of monounsaturated fats include olive oil, canola oil, walnuts, avocado, and peanuts. Polyunsaturated fats can be found in safflower, sesame, corn, and sunflower-seed oils as well as nuts and seeds.

Also, consider using margarine-like spreads made of soybean extract (such as Benecol and Take Control), which contain plant stanols that have been found to lower cholesterol.

It's also important to eat a well-balanced mix of all the macronutrients at each meal. Eating com-plex carbs with lean proteins and healthy fats at each meal will help slow digestion, slow the rise of blood glucose, and help you feel full longer.

Pay special attention to portion sizes and calo-ries, too, when you eat. Because losing weight is important for people with insulin resistance, you should try to make sure you aren't overeating.

## What Not to Eat

For people with insulin resistance, it's important to reduce fat intake and lower calories in an effort to lose weight and shrink the waist. To do that, avoid foods high in saturated fats, which occur in animal products such as red meat, whole dairy products, and butter. You should also stay away from foods with trans-fatty acids, which are often found in packaged foods such as candy bars, cookies, muffins, and crackers. Be on the lookout for anything on the ingredient list that is partially hydrogenated.

Try to cut out fried foods, too, such as french fries, doughnuts, and fried chicken, which are high in fat and calories.

In addition, restrict or eliminate refined foods, which are typically high in sugar and can elevate insulin levels and cause an increase in choles-terol, triglycerides, and blood pressure. That means avoiding white bread, rolls, muffins, and bagels as well as candy bars, desserts, and sugary beverages such as soda. It also means substitut-ing whole dairy foods with low-fat versions.

People who already have high blood pressure should avoid high-sodium foods such as potato chips, processed meats, and canned soups.

### Is Stress Making You Fat?

Taming stress can often help reduce your food intake. Why? Stressful events—or the perception that something is stress-ful—trigger the release of life-saving hor-mones such as cortisol and adrenaline, which are essential when you need to fight or flee from a real threat. These hor-mones tell you to stock up on your energy stores (by eating) so you have the strength to escape a threat.

But in the absence of a real threat, the hormones are still there, telling you to replenish your energy stores. In particular, you may find yourself craving sweets and unhealthy carbs, which provide quick bursts of energy—but also a lot of empty calories.

If you think stress is making you fat, take steps to control it. Learn a relaxation method or try to avoid stressful situa-tions. Develop a strategy for confronting stress that doesn't involve eating, such as taking a walk or writing in a journal.

## 🍬 Supplements for Insulin Resistance

Beyond taking a quality multivitamin, which supplies the basic nutrients you need for good health, also consider taking the following:

### NIACIN

As a B vitamin, niacin occurs in wheat and rice bran and in Brewer's yeast. It is also found in whole grains, legumes, fish, and peanuts. Some studies have found that niacin can help lower total cholesterol and LDL while increasing HDL.

### GARLIC

As a supplement, this pungent spice may help lower cholesterol and triglycerides. If you want to try garlic supplements, make sure to choose one that has allicin, the most bioavailable form of garlic.

### PSYLLIUM

Psyllium is a seed husk and a soluble fiber that can help with bowel regularity and lowering cholesterol. Talk to your doctor first before taking psyllium, especially if you have food allergies, because some people react to psyllium.

### COENZYME Q10

Your body naturally produces CoQ10, a substance involved in energy production. It's found in every plant and animal cell. As a supplement, it may help lower blood pressure, blood glucose, and body weight.

## 📋 Stay-Healthy Strategies

- **MASTER THE ART OF READING NUTRITION LABELS.** You can find information from the American Dietetic Association (www.eatright.org) or from the U.S. Food and Drug Administration's Center for Food Safety and Applied Nutrition (www.cfsan.fda.gov).

- **EXERCISE!** Do whatever you can to move your body. Whether it's gardening, housework, or climbing stairs, it's important to do something active every day. Take a walk during lunch, join a gym, or take up a childhood sport you once enjoyed.

- **GO HIGH-FIBER SLOWLY.** If you're not accustomed to eating a lot of fiber, introduce it gradually. Your stomach needs time to adjust, and doing it quickly can cause gas, diarrhea, and bloating. Be sure to also drink more water as you increase your fiber intake.

- **EAT ONLY WHEN YOU'RE HUNGRY.** Avoid eating when you're stressed, bored, or angry. Learn to look for cues that you're truly hungry.

# IRRITABLE BOWEL SYNDROME

EVERYONE EXPERIENCES OCCASIONAL bouts of stomach distress. A low-fiber diet may cause constipation. Too much spicy food can set off stomach pain. And sometimes we just experience the need to go to the bathroom frequently.

But in some people, these symptoms persist and become disruptive, causing a chronic condition known as irritable bowel syndrome (IBS). IBS is a functional disorder of the gastrointestinal (GI) tract that causes abdominal pain and diarrhea or constipation in its sufferers.

In IBS, the nerves and muscles in the large intestine may contract too much or be overly sensitive to certain stimuli such as foods or stress. Some people experience symptoms after eating a large meal or taking certain medications. Women may experience it when they menstruate. In any case, IBS results in excessive contractions that cause the stool to pass too quickly or slowly through the intestines. The end result is diarrhea or constipation, or difficulty having a bowel movement even when the urge is there.

IBS affects as many as 20 percent of all adults in the United States, most of them women. The cause of the condition remains a mystery, but experts do know it involves a malfunction of the large intestine.

Treating IBS means treating the symptoms. Some people use laxatives to relieve constipation, while those with loose stools may require antidiarrheal medications. But be careful to use laxatives only for the short term because they can be habit-forming.

In some cases, if your symptoms are severe and you don't respond to dietary changes and stress management, your doctor may prescribe tegaserod (Zelnorm), the only medication specifically approved for IBS.

## 🔎 What It Looks Like

The signs and symptoms of IBS vary greatly. Almost everyone with IBS has abdominal pain and abnormalities with their bowel movements. In addition, there may be bloating, cramping, gas, and nausea. Some people also experience weight loss, headache, fatigue, difficulties concentrating, anxiety, and depression. The condition can last for many years with symptoms that fluctuate.

For sufferers, IBS can be extremely disruptive. The unpredictability and discomfort make it difficult to travel, work, or socialize with friends.

Some people are embarrassed by the condition. Even ordering a meal in a restaurant can become a challenge.

But as annoying and painful as IBS can be, the condition does not cause permanent damage to the intestines. It is not contagious and does not lead to serious disease such as cancer.

However, don't just assume you have IBS if you have these symptoms. These can also be symptoms of other intestinal diseases. Be sure to get checked out by an intestinal specialist, known as a gastroenterologist.

## An Antidepressant for IBS?

The brain isn't the only organ that houses neurotransmitters such as serotonin. The intestines do too. IBS is thought to be a disruption of serotonin signals between the gut and the brain. Antidepressants work by restoring balance to serotonin levels in the intestines as well as the brain.

## ⑪ What to Eat

A healthy diet for IBS involves eating more high-fiber foods such as fruits, veggies, flaxseed, and whole-grain foods such as brown rice and whole-wheat pasta and breads, says Jeannie Moloo, R.D., a nutritionist in Sacramento, California, and the co-author of *The No-Salt, Lowest Sodium* cookbook series. Experts recommend getting 20 to 35 grams of fiber in your diet each day, but those with IBS may fare better if they try eating slightly more.

Fiber works by absorbing water and preventing diarrhea. It also stimulates the large intestine to work faster to eliminate waste, which prevents constipation. In addition, fiber speeds up transit time—the time it takes for food to move through the digestive tract—which encourages the intestine to function more normally.

When selecting the best high-fiber foods to eat, make sure to choose those that don't trigger your IBS symptoms, which will vary from one person to the next. Consult with a registered dietitian, if necessary, to work out a tailor-made eating plan.

The way you eat can help too. Try eating smaller, more frequent meals if you're susceptible to IBS after a large meal. Chew slowly to avoid swallowing excess air, which can cause gas. Make sure to also drink a lot of water. The extra fluids will help you prevent constipation.

## ⊘⑪ What Not to Eat

Avoid any food that seems to trigger your IBS symptoms. To find out which foods are problematic, keep a food diary and record any symptoms you experience after eating a certain food.

Reduce or eliminate high-fat foods such as fried foods, red meats, cured meats, and heavy desserts. Fat stimulates the bowels. You should also cut out all sugars, including sugar alcohols such as xylitol and sorbitol, because sugar can trigger IBS symptoms. In addition, avoid dairy products such as cheese or ice cream, which can also stimulate the bowels.

Other foods and drinks to eliminate include anything that contains caffeine or carbonation. These foods and beverages tend to aggravate the

GI tract. If you're sensitive to the gas-producing effects of vegetables such as broccoli, cabbage, and eans, eliminate those foods from your diet too.

## ♻ Supplements for IBS

Take a multivitamin to ensure you get the essential nutrients. Other supplements you might consider include the following:

### PSYLLIUM

Psyllium is a seed husk and soluble fiber that can help stabilize any bowel irregularities. Talk to your doctor first before taking psyllium, especially if you have food allergies, because some people react to psyllium.

### PEPPERMINT OIL

Try taking enteric-coated peppermint oil, which is a muscle relaxant that can sometimes help calm spasms in the GI tract.

### PROBIOTICS

Probiotics can help restore healthy bacteria such as *Lactobacillus acidophilus* to the GI tract. If IBS is causing diarrhea, you may be losing healthy bacteria essential for healthy digestion.

## Consider the Specific Carbohydrate Diet

People who suffer from irritable bowel syndrome (IBS) may benefit from the Specific Carbohydrate (SC) Diet. The SC Diet involves eating few or no carbohydrates and instead focuses on eating foods that contain monosaccharides, specific carbohydrates that are rapidly absorbed.

The SC Diet is based on the premise that sicknesses such as IBS, Crohn's disease, and ulcerative colitis and are caused by an imbalance of intestinal flora. The diet permits most fresh, raw, or frozen vegetables; legumes; unprocessed meats; natural cheeses low in lactose; homemade yogurt; most fruits; and select oils including olive, coconut, soybean, and corn.

But it prohibits many other foods including all sugars except honey; all starchy foods such as bread, potatoes, yams and pasta; all milk products except homemade yogurt; and all grains and canned vegetables. It also bans canola oil, mayonnaise, ice cream, candy, chocolate, and all products that contain baking powder.

The diet is intended to restore balance to your digestive tract and tame the bacterial overgrowth that is making you sick. Over time, the diet is believed to heal the gut, which will in turn relieve your symptoms. For more information, see page 75 and check out www.scdiet.org and www.breakingtheviciouscycle.org.

# 🗒 Stay-Healthy Strategies

- **TAKE STEPS TO ALLEVIATE STRESS.** Stress is the most common trigger of IBS. Do what you can to minimize it. Learn to say no to unnecessary obligations. Adopt a new perspective. Consider trying meditation, biofeedback, or hypnosis.

- **GET EVALUATED FOR LACTOSE INTOLERANCE.** Some people cannot tolerate this sugar, which is found in dairy products. A food diary may help you to determine whether you have this problem.

- **SEEK MEDICAL HELP.** Some people may suspect they have IBS but are too embarrassed to take their concerns to a doctor. But these symptoms may or may not be IBS and warrant medical attention regardless.

- **FIND SUPPORT.** It isn't easy to live with IBS. Consider joining a support group with other sufferers to help you cope. If you'd rather do it online, check out www.ibsgroup.org, which is also a source of information about IBS.

## A More Nourishing Alternative

Some experts believe that lacto-fermented foods eaten every day can help enhance bowel function. These foods work by neutralizing unhealthy chemicals found in modern foods and produced by grains and beans, while increasing the microorganisms that enhance digestion. They may be especially beneficial to people who suffer from irritable bowel syndrome (IBS), says Sally Fallon, author of *Nourishing Traditions* and president of the Weston A. Price Foundation, an organization that works to restore nutrient-dense foods to the human diet.

But be picky about the lacto-fermented foods you choose. Stick with foods that have not been heated, so that the live microorganisms are preserved. If you want to eat grains and legumes, soak them in a warm acidic medium such as warm water with a little lemon juice, vinegar, or homemade whey or yogurt before cooking, which will neutralize many components that are hard to digest and ease IBS symptoms.

Other good foods that relieve symptoms of IBS include broth made from animal bones and healthy fats such as coconut oil and organic cultured butter.

# KIDNEY STONES

KIDNEY STONES ARE HARD MASSES formed from substances and minerals in the urine that accumulate on the inner surface of the kidneys. Some crystals remain small and pass through the urinary tract without a problem. But others may become larger, and their passage causes tremendous pain.

The majority of kidney stones are made up of calcium and oxalate, substances that occur naturally in foods and drinks you consume. A less common type of kidney stones is struvite stones, which are the result of chronic urinary tract infections that cause a buildup of ammonia. Struvite stones are generally more common in women. Uric acid stones are rare and often the result of a high-protein diet, a genetic predisposition, or chemotherapy treatment. Even less common are cystine stones, which occur in people with an inherited disorder that causes them to excrete excessive amounts of certain amino acids.

According to the National Institutes of Health, the incidence of kidney stones has risen steadily for the past 30 years. Kidney stones are more common in men than women. They're also more prevalent in Caucasians than in African-Americans. Kidney stones are especially common in men between their 40s and 70s. Women are more likely to get them in their 50s. Having a kidney stone puts you at greater risk for more stones in the future.

If stones are small and cause no symptoms, you may not ever know they're there unless you have an X-ray for other reasons during a health exam. But usually pain or blood in the urine will send you to your doctor who can do X-rays and blood and urine tests that can help confirm a kidney stone.

Treatment for kidney stones may be as simple as drinking large amounts of water or as complicated as surgery to remove the bothersome stone.

## What It Looks Like

Not everyone who has kidney stones will experience symptoms. For these people, the stones are small and pass easily through the urinary tract without causing any problems.

But when you do have symptoms, they can be rather dramatic. Pain is typically the first symptom, and it can be excruciating. The pain is usually felt in the middle of your back, on either the right or left side, and extends around the front to the pelvic area. The pain may also spread to your groin. Some people suffer nausea and vomiting.

If you can't pass the stone, the pain continues as the ureters—the tubes in the urinary tract—try to squeeze the stone and push it through the bladder. This may cause blood in the urine. While the stone travels down the ureters toward the bladder, you may notice a more frequent urge to urinate and a burning sensation when you do go.

In some cases, a kidney stone can cause an infection, which brings on fever and chills. If this happens, call your doctor immediately.

## ∦ What to Eat

Make sure to drink a large amount of fluids, which can help prevent the formation of kidney stones, says Jacob Teitelbaum, M.D., author of *Pain Free 1-2-3*. According to the National Kidney Foundation, you should drink at least three to four quarts of fluid a day and even more in hotter weather to make up for fluids lost to sweating. Drinking fluids will help dilute your urine, which in turn lowers the risk for stone formation. Try to drink mostly water.

Eating calcium is also important for combating kidney stones. Although experts used to discourage calcium consumption, they've now learned that calcium may help prevent kidney stones by binding to oxalates in the intestine and reducing the amount that gets absorbed. In a study look-ing at diet and the incidence of kidney stones over time in men, the benefits of calcium were most notable in men under the age of 60. But calcium had no impact on men older than 60. Similar benefits have also been found in women.

It's important to eat foods rich in magnesium too. Magnesium has been associated with a lower risk for kidney stones. Good sources of magnesium include avocados, spinach, peanut butter, pecans, and quinoa.

Another important mineral is potassium, which is involved in regulating fluids and minerals in body cells. Good sources of potassium include bananas, haddock, tomatoes, turkey, milk, and potatoes.

## ⊘ What Not to Eat

People prone to kidney stones may need to avoid foods rich in oxalates. Foods high in oxalates include the following:

- Almonds
- Beets
- Chocolate
- Coffee
- Cola
- Rhubarb
- Spinach
- Tea
- Wheat bran

Some foods contain moderate amounts of oxalates and should be eaten in small quantities. These include berries, sweet potatoes, oranges, nuts, and tomatoes.

Avoid eating too much salt. Salt promotes the excretion of calcium, so that more of it winds up in the urine. Reducing the amount of animal protein can help as well. Too much protein, such as beef, chicken, pork, fish, and eggs, can increase kidney stone formation in some people. One study in men found that protein had a great impact on kidney stone formation in men with a body mass index below 25.

Some experts also recommend limiting your intake of some sources of vitamin C, which may be linked to a higher incidence of kidney stones. But many foods rich in vitamin C also contain potassium, a mineral that seems to counterbalance the negative effects of vitamin C.

Finally, reduce your intake of caffeine and alcohol. Both substances act as diuretics that deplete fluids.

## ⚕ Supplements for Kidney Stones

Consult a health care professional before determining which supplements to take. Some supplements, such as vitamin C, vitamin D, and fish oils, may raise your risk for kidney stones. On the other hand, the following supplements may help lower your risk for kidney stones:

### MAGNESIUM

Taken as a supplement, this major mineral may help lower the incidence of kidney stones.

### VITAMIN B6

Pyridoxine may help decrease the production of oxalate, especially when it is combined with magnesium.

## 📋 Stay-Healthy Strategies

- **WATCH YOUR WEIGHT.** Studies have linked being overweight or obese to a higher incidence of kidney stones.

- **CONSULT A REGISTERED DIETITIAN (R.D.) FOR SPECIFICS.** Not everyone responds the same way to every food. For a custom plan, talk to an R.D. about specific foods to eat and avoid.

- **STRAIN YOUR URINE IF YOU SUSPECT A KIDNEY STONE.** A strainer will help you retrieve the stone so you can take it to your doctor for evaluation. Knowing the type of stone you have will help you make the right dietary changes. For example, cutting back on meat will not necessarily help prevent a calcium oxalate stone from forming.

### Little-Known Facts about Kidney Stones

- Astronauts are more vulnerable to kidney stones due to an increase in the amount of calcium in their blood. The elevated levels of blood calcium are the result of a loss in bone density from being in zero gravity.

- The famous Greek philosopher Epicurus is said to have died from a kidney stone blockage that lasted two weeks.

- Science fiction writer Isaac Asimov suffered from kidney stones and was treated with morphine to relieve the pain.

# LACTOSE INTOLERANCE

GOT MILK? NOT EVERYONE DOES. People with an intolerance for lactose, a sugar in milk, can't properly digest it. If they do drink too much, they'll experience uncomfortable symptoms.

Inside the digestive tract, most people have an enzyme called lactase that breaks down lactose into glucose and galactose. These simple sugars are absorbed into the bloodstream for use as energy in body cells. People who have lactose intolerance don't have enough lactase, making them incapable of digesting significant amounts of lactose, the major sugar found in milk and milk products.

Left undigested, the lactose is then fermented by healthy bacteria that live in the intestinal tract. It is this fermentation process that causes the bloating, cramping, nausea, gas, and diarrhea that most people associate with lactose intolerance.

Lactose intolerance is a common condition that affects about thirty million people in the United States, according to the American Dietetic Association. It tends to develop gradually after the age of two, as the body begins to produce less lactase. Although it can affect anyone, it is more common among Asian-, African-, and Native Americans. The condition is less prevalent among Caucasians, especially those whose ancestors come from northern or western Europe. Lactose intolerance can also emerge in advancing age as the body produces less lactase.

But other factors also influence lactase production. Some people have a reduction in lactase as the result of taking certain medications. Having certain intestinal diseases or conditions such as celiac disease or Crohn's disease can also cause a decrease in lactase that results in lactose intolerance.

Keep in mind that lactose intolerance is not the same thing as an allergy to cow's milk, though the symptoms are similar. An allergy is a malfunction of the immune system, not the digestive tract. People who have a milk allergy are having an allergic reaction, often to casein, a protein in the milk. If you have a milk allergy, you must avoid all dairy products.

But people who have lactose intolerance may still be able to digest small amounts of milk because the condition can range from mild to severe. Your symptoms may also vary depending on the quantity of dairy products you consume and whether you eat or drink them with other foods.

## 🔍 What It Looks Like

If you're lactose intolerant, you'll start to notice discomfort anywhere from a few minutes to several hours after you've consumed a dairy product. But not everyone who is deficient in lactase has these symptoms. It also depends on how much milk you drink, the amount of lactose you can tolerate, your age, and your digestion rate.

## 🍴 What to Eat

Try drinking lactose-reduced milk and eating lactose-reduced foods, says Susan Krantz, M.A., R.D., assistant director of clinical nutrition services at Shore Memorial Hospital in Somers Point, New Jersey. The milk contains all of the nutrients found in regular milk but is free of the lactose that can produce bothersome symptoms.

Eat yogurt. The kind that contains live cultures, which helps to breakdown the lactose, can help reduce your symptoms of lactose intolerance. Another good option is kefir, a fermented milk product that can improve lactose digestion and boost calcium intake. Like yogurt, kefir contains active bacteria cultures that help break down the lactose in the beverage.

If you'd like to still eat dairy products, try consuming a little at a time. Gradually increase your intake over a few weeks so you can build up your tolerance.

You'll also find that certain types of dairy foods contain less lactose than others. Aged cheeses such as cheddar and Swiss have little or no lactose. There are also variations in the types of milk. Whole milk may be better tolerated than skim milk because the higher fat content can slow digestion; however, remember the trade-off is that the fat is saturated, which is not good for your heart.

To ensure you still get enough calcium in your diet, eat and drink calcium-fortified foods such as soy milk, orange juice, and breakfast cereals. You can also get calcium from leafy green vegetables, sardines, salmon with bones, almonds, brewer's yeast, and broccoli. Another good source is tofu, but check the label to make sure it is processed with calcium sulfate.

Make sure you also eat foods that contain vitamin D. Some good sources of vitamin D in the diet are milk, cheese, eggs, salmon, mackerel, tuna, and fortified cereals. You can also get vitamin D from sunshine. Ultraviolet rays from the sun can initiate vitamin D production in your skin.

# ⊘ What Not to Eat

Which foods you should avoid depends primarily on how much lactose you can tolerate. It also depends on your age. Babies and young children who are lactose-intolerant for instance, should not consume any formulas or food that contains lactose. But most older children and adults do not have to avoid lactose completely. Remember, you can become more tolerant of lactose by having smaller amounts of it at a time.

Milk and other dairy products are the only natural sources of lactose, but keep in mind that lactose is often added to prepared foods. Those who suffer from a low tolerance of lactose should know that lactose may be found in bread, baked goods, processed breakfast cereals, and many instant foods, such as soup. Lactose is also found in the following foods:

- Pancake mixes
- Luncheon meats
- Margarine
- Whipped cream
- Candies
- Salad dressings
- Powdered meal-replacements

You should also learn to read food labels, which can help identify less obvious sources of lactose. Look for tip-off ingredients such as whey, curds, milk by-products, dry milk solids, and nonfat dry milk powder, which are all indicators of lactose.

Finally, be wary of medications. According to the National Institutes of Health, lactose is used in more than 20 percent of prescription drugs and about 6 percent of over-the-counter medicines. Lactose is found in many types of oral contraceptives, as well as in antacids. The good news is that the amount found in these products is usually only problematic for people with severe lactose intolerance.

## 🫛 Supplements for Lactose Intolerance

People with lactose intolerance may benefit from taking a lactase enzyme. Taking a tablet with the first bite of a dairy product can help you break down the lactose. Other supplements to consider include the following:

### PROBIOTICS

Some people may benefit from the use of probiotics (healthy bacteria such as *Lactobacillus*). Probiotics are available as supplements in capsule, tablet, and powdered form.

### CALCIUM

If you're not eating enough foods rich in bone-building calcium, consider taking a supplement. Remember to break up your calcium intake throughout the day because you can't absorb more than 500 to 600 milligrams at one time. Check with your health care provider to see how much you may need.

### VITAMIN D

Proper absorption of calcium requires vitamin D. If you are not spending much time in the sun (without sunscreen) and don't get enough vitamin D in your food, you probably should take a supplement. But don't take too much; Vitamin D is a fat-soluble vitamin that is stored by the body. Again, check with your health care provider to see how much you should take.

## 📋 Stay-Healthy Strategies

- **CONSULT WITH A REGISTERED DIETITIAN.** She can help you determine whether you're getting enough calcium and identify foods that may be aggravating your intolerance.

- **EAT A LACTOSE-CONTAINING FOOD** paired with a food that doesn't contain lactose.

- **TRACK YOUR FOOD AND SYMPTOMS.** If you think you suffer from lactose intolerance, try keeping a food diary to track the dairy foods you eat, when you eat them, and how you feel afterward.

- **GET TESTED.** Talk to your doctor if you suspect lactose intolerance. Your doctor can perform breath tests (the hydrogen breath test is most commonly used), blood tests, and stool tests (for infants and young children) that will definitively identify lactose intolerance.

# LUPUS

A LOW-GRADE FEVER. FATIGUE. ACHY JOINTS. For some people, these symptoms add up to lupus, a baffling and chronic disease that is often tough to diagnose.

Lupus is an autoimmune disorder that occurs when the body's immune system attacks its own cells and tissues. With an autoimmune illness, the body cannot distinguish between foreign substances and its own healthy cells and tissues. As a result, it attacks healthy tissue. In lupus, the attack is waged against the body's connective tissue, which includes bone, blood, ligaments, cartilage, and tendons. Experts estimate there are 500,000 to 1.5 million Americans who have been diagnosed with lupus.

No one knows what causes the immune system to go awry. Only about 10 percent of people who have lupus have a parent or sibling with the illness, and only about 5 percent of children born to parents with lupus eventually develop it. Because the genetic link is relatively weak, experts believe the environment plays a role in the onset of lupus. Possible environmental triggers include infections, stress, antibiotics, ultraviolet light, and hormones.

Lupus can strike at any age. Although the condition occurs in both men and women, women are ten to fifteen times more likely to get it, which leads some experts to suspect that hormones play a role. It is also more common in ethnic women than it is in Caucasian women.

Once it's diagnosed, lupus often involves treatment with multiple medications. The goal is to prevent flares, treat them appropriately when they occur, and minimize damage to body organs. Treatment often involves a cocktail of medications that may include nonsteroidal anti-inflammatory drugs, antimalarial drugs, corticosteroids, and immune suppressants. Just as the disease will change over time, so too will the treatments.

## What It Looks Like

Getting a diagnosis for lupus can be difficult. Many symptoms of the disease are vague and resemble those of other medical conditions. To make it more difficult, there are actually three different kinds of lupus:

- **SYSTEMIC LUPUS ERYTHEMATOSUS (SLE)** is the most serious form of the disease, and it can affect almost any organ or system in the body. It is a chronic inflammatory condition that alternates between flares and periods of remission. Almost everyone with SLE will experience joint and/or muscle pain brought on by inflammation or arthritis. Many will also suffer fatigue, rashes, anemia, and sensitivity to light. Some develop a butterfly-shaped rash across the cheeks and nose. In addition, symptoms may include: Raynaud's phenomenon (a vascular disorder in which the blood vessels constrict abnormally in response to cold temperatures, changes in temperature, or stress), hair loss, and problems with the kidneys.
- **DISCOID LUPUS** is a less serious form that is confined to the skin. It typically causes a rash on the face, neck, and scalp. About 10 percent of cases will develop into SLE.
- **DRUG-INDUCED LUPUS** is just as the name implies, a form of lupus that results from taking certain medications. Drugs that can provoke a bout of lupus include hydralazine, which is used for hypertension, and procainamide, which is used to treat irregular heart rhythms. This condition is extremely rare and occurs only in about 4 percent of people who take these drugs. Once the drug is discontinued, it typically goes away.

In order to be diagnosed with lupus, you must have four of the following eleven symptoms:

- Arthritis pain in two or more joints
- Rash over the cheeks
- Red raised patches on the skin
- Sensitivity to sunlight, resulting in rash or increase in rash
- Ulcers in the mouth or nose
- Excess protein or other abnormalities in the urine
- Inflammation of the lining of the heart or lungs
- Seizures or psychosis
- Low red or white blood cell count
- Positive antinuclear antibodies in the blood
- Positive auto-antibody tests

Many of these symptoms may occur at varying times. Some may come and go or simply change. As a result, getting a diagnosis of lupus can sometimes take months, or even years.

## What to Eat

Eating a healthy, well-balanced diet is essential to anyone suffering from a chronic disease like lupus, says Elizabeth Lipski, Ph.D., C.C.N., author of *Digestive Wellness*. Focus on getting a lot of whole foods, specifically fruits and vegetables, seeds, nuts, and whole grains, in your diet. Plant-based foods are less inflammatory and supply important disease-fighting antioxidants.

Boost your consumption of foods rich in omega-3 fatty acids. These healthy fats are found in cold-water fish such as salmon, mackerel, halibut, and tuna as well as flaxseed and walnuts. The omega-3 fatty acids can help reduce inflammation, which can lessen pain.

Make sure to get plenty of calcium, too, especially if you're taking steroids. Long-term use of steroids can affect bone health and put you at risk for osteoporosis.

## 🚫 What Not to Eat

Be wary of eating foods high in saturated fat and trans-fatty acids. Foods high in fat, which include fried foods and greasy foods, provoke inflammation, which will worsen your symptoms. High-fat foods also put you at risk for weight gain. People who take steroids are already at greater risk for weight gain because these medications stimulate the appetite.

Avoid eating alfalfa sprouts, which have been linked to a worsening of lupus symptoms. They contain an amino acid called L-canavanine that is believed to provoke an autoimmune response.

## 💊 Supplements for Lupus

Start by taking a quality multivitamin that ensures you get all the essential nutrients. According to Lipski, many of the same supplements for arthritis may also benefit people with lupus. But always consult your physician first. Supplements to consider include the following:

### FISH AND FLAXSEED OIL

These oils contain omega-3 fatty acids, which may help reduce the symptoms of lupus. But beware of taking too much, because fish oil has a blood-thinning effect that can cause excess bleeding.

### DHEA

Dehydroepiandrosterone (DHEA) is a naturally occurring hormone that may help relieve symptoms of lupus. In one study, low doses of DHEA boosted mental well-being and libido. But avoid taking high doses, which can cause unwanted hair growth.

### CALCIUM AND VITAMIN D

People with lupus who take steroids are at risk for osteoporosis. Taking a calcium supplement that contains vitamin D can help counter that effect.

## Stay-Healthy Strategies

- **LIMIT SUN EXPOSURE.** Lupus causes photosensitivity, so too much sun can result in a rash and trigger flares. If you're going to be outdoors for more than five minutes, wear sunscreen and a hat. Wear long sleeves and pants whenever possible.

- **EXERCISE REGULARLY.** Low-impact workouts like walking and swimming can help keep muscles strong. People with lupus are at greater risk for heart disease and diabetes, a risk that can be lowered with regular exercise.

- **PACE YOURSELF.** Lupus causes fatigue, so learn to control your activity levels and to rest when your body demands it. Doing too much can trigger a flare.

- **FIND A DOCTOR YOU LIKE.** A good relationship with your physician is vital to the management of a disease like lupus because doctor visits are frequent. Find one you trust and who is willing to work with you.

### Can Women with Lupus Have Children?

Young women make up the bulk of people with lupus, and many wonder if they can safely get pregnant. The good news is, yes, they can become pregnant and deliver healthy babies. According to the Lupus Foundation, more than 50 percent of all lupus pregnancies are completely normal. About 25 percent result in premature deliveries. Less than 20 percent result in miscarriage or stillbirths.

But it isn't always easy to be pregnant with lupus. All pregnancies should be considered high risk, and patients should always work closely with their OB/GYNs to ensure good health.

Delivery of the baby should be done at a hospital that has access to care for premature newborns. Also, moms with lupus should not attempt a natural delivery because complications may arise and require treatment.

# LYME DISEASE

LYME DISEASE IS A RELATIVELY RECENT PHENOMENON, and has emerged in the past few decades as a serious warm weather health hazard in some parts of the country. The story of Lyme disease began in the mid-1970s in Lyme, Connecticut, where a group of children developed what experts first thought was an outbreak of juvenile arthritis. But the cause of their arthritis was eventually traced to a bacterium called *Borrelia burgdorferi*, and doctors named the condition Lyme disease.

Lyme disease is transmitted by deer ticks that become infected by feeding on small rodents. When an infected tick bites a human or animal, it can pass along the bacterium, which then travels into the bloodstream and causes a constellation of symptoms. Untreated, some of these symptoms can be quite severe. Within days or weeks, the infected person may develop a circular rash that resembles a bull's eye around the site of the bite and evolves into a flu-like illness.

According to the Centers for Disease Control and Prevention, the incidence of Lyme disease has climbed steadily. In 1991, there were fewer than 10,000 cases of Lyme reported, while in 2004 there were 19,804 cases. The incidence was especially high in the Northeast, in states such as New Jersey, New York, Connecticut, and Massachusetts.

Lyme disease can potentially affect anyone who lives, works, or spends time outdoors in areas where deer live. The best way to prevent Lyme disease is to avoid the areas where deer live, such as overgrown fields or dense woods, or to check your body for small ticks after visiting these areas. Ticks usually lurk within three feet of the ground, and often on foliage such as leaves, plant stems, and blades of grass. But they can also be found in well-kept lawns and gardens.

Caught early, the disease almost always can be effectively treated with antibiotics, which may be given for as long as four weeks. People who develop arthritis may need a second course of treatment.

## 🔍 What It Looks Like

Days or weeks may pass before you notice that you've been infected. To make it more difficult, the symptoms may be vague and resemble other conditions. In 80 to 90 percent of cases, Lyme disease starts as an expanding rash that usually radiates from the site of the tick bite. On some people, the rash may resemble a bull's eye. But in people with dark complexions, the rash may look more like a bruise. Others may never see a rash at all.

About the same time, you may start to experience flu-like symptoms such as joint pain, fever, chills, and fatigue. These symptoms are usually mild and may even disappear, only to recur later.

Over time, the symptoms may become more severe. You may experience a stiff neck, facial paralysis, severe fatigue, numbness, and tingling. Weeks or months later, you may develop severe headaches, painful arthritis, swelling of the joints, cardiac abnormalities, and neurological problems characterized by memory loss, disorientation, and confusion.

Determining whether you actually have Lyme disease is usually a two-step process. The first test is usually an enzyme-linked immunoassay (ELISA) test. The ELISA test can detect elevated blood levels of antibodies produced in response to the *Borrelia burgdorferi* bacterium. The ELISA test is most effective if it's done at least four weeks after a tick bite.

The problem with the ELISA test is that even people who do not have Lyme disease may still test positive, and many with Lyme will test negative. That's why a positive or negative ELISA test needs to be confirmed by the Western blot test. The Western blot test can pick up more specific Lyme antibodies in the blood. While no test is currently considered 100 percent accurate, the combination of the ELISA and Western blot is for now the best diagnostic tool for detecting Lyme disease.

If Lyme disease goes undetected, the symptoms can become more severe. Patients may develop painful arthritis, cardiac abnormalities, and dementia.

## 🍴 What to Eat

A healthy diet is essential to support the immune system when you're infected with Lyme disease, says Jacob Teitelbaum, M.D., author of *Pain Free 1-2-3*. Eating a lot of vegetables and one or two fruits a day is especially important, because these foods are rich in antioxidants that can help strengthen the immune system.

But specific nutritional recommendations will vary depending on your symptoms. Those who are experiencing a lot of pain should eat cold-water fish such as tuna, salmon, and mackerel. These fish contain omega-3 fatty acids, which can help reduce inflammation. Certain fruits, such as cherries and pineapple, may also help lessen inflammation.

People with Lyme disease who suffer from low blood pressure may benefit from increasing their intake of salt and drinking more water. If you have low adrenal function—you become extremely irritable when you're hungry—try eating more high-protein foods such as chicken, fish, turkey, and legumes, which will help maintain a stable blood sugar level.

## 🚫 What Not to Eat

Avoid eating a lot of saturated fats, which can promote inflammation and worsen pain. Saturated fat is found primarily in red meats, whole milk, and butter. It's also essential to avoid sugar, which acts as an inflammatory as well.

Reduce your intake of alcohol and caffeine too. Both alcohol and caffeine are diuretics, which can cause dehydration that results in excess fatigue.

## 💊 Supplements for Lyme disease

Take a high-quality vitamin powder, which will contain all the essential nutrients for good health. A powder is better than a tablet because it's more apt to cover any deficiency without the need for taking too many pills. Other supplements that might help include the following:

### FISH OIL

Taking fish oil can help lessen inflammation in people with a lot of pain. But if you're taking a blood-thinning agent such as warfarin (Coumadin), talk to your doctor first, because fish oil could cause excess bleeding.

### D-RIBOSE

This naturally occurring sugar is involved in enhancing the production of energy in body cells and can also decrease pain.

### L-THEANINE

This compound is found in a green tea called Suntheanine. It can help relieve stress and induce a higher quality of sleep.

### WILD LETTUCE

Wild lettuce is an herbal remedy derived from the *Lactuca virosa* plant that promotes sleep.

### HOPS

Hops, which is derived from the *Humulus lupulus* plant, contains substances that relieve anxiety, insomnia, and stress. It is the same substance used to flavor beer.

### VALERIAN

This pungent herb can help relieve anxiety, ease pain, and promote sleep.

### PASSIONFLOWER

Passionflower can help relieve anxiety and reduce insomnia.

### MELATONIN

Melatonin is a hormone naturally produced by the body that helps regulate the sleep-wake cycle. It can help induce sleep and promote a deeper sleep.

### BOSWELLIA

If you're suffering from pain, consider taking this herbal remedy to relieve swelling.

### WILLOW BARK

Willow bark is a natural analgesic and can help with pain relief. Aspirin is derived from compounds found in willow trees.

## Watch Out for Ticks

The best way to prevent Lyme disease is to steer clear of the ticks that cause it. Ticks are arachnids and belong to the same family as spiders and scorpions. Like tiny vampires, they feed off mammals by embedding their mouths into the host's skin and sucking the blood. Ticks cause at least nine different known diseases in humans in the United States, including Rocky Mountain spotted fever, babesiosis, and ehrlichiosis.

To avoid ticks, do your best to stay out of areas where they thrive. If you must go outside, wear long sleeves and pants and tuck pants into your socks or boot tops. Use an insect repellent that contains DEET or permethrin, a chemical that kills ticks on contact.

Once you go back indoors, check for deer ticks. If you do see a tick, remove it by its head with tweezers, firmly and steadily without twisting.

But don't assume you're infected if you find a tick. Not all ticks are infected with Lyme, and transmission of the disease doesn't usually begin until 36 to 48 hours after they've been attached. That's why it's critical to scan your body after an outing in tick-infested areas. To be sure, contact your physician who can do an exam to look for symptoms and perform blood tests.

# MACULAR DEGENERATION

INSIDE THE EYES, IN THE CENTER OF THE RETINA, is a tiny area called the macula. The macula is the eye's most highly developed area of vision. It allows us to see the fine details of patterns on a vase, the sparkles in a rock, and the spectrum of colors. When the macula deteriorates, it is known as macular degeneration.

Macular degeneration is a progressive eye condition that affects approximately fifteen million Americans. Some people may have the "wet" form, in which abnormal blood vessels start to grow under the macula. The new blood vessels are fragile and may leak blood and fluid, causing the macula to become raised.

Others may have the "dry" form, in which the light-sensitive cells of the macula gradually break down. In either case, macular degeneration gradually erodes your vision until all that is left is your peripheral vision and the ability to see dim images and black holes at the center of your sight. Eventually, looking straight ahead for everyday tasks such as reading, driving, and identifying people becomes impossible. Skills required for daily living may become significantly impaired.

Macular degeneration is the leading cause of vision loss and legal blindness in adults over age 60. According to the Macular Degeneration Partnership, the condition affects an estimated 14 to 24 percent of Americans aged 65 to 74, and 35 percent of all people over age 75.

These days, with the aging of the Baby Boomers, the most common form is age-related macular degeneration. But age is only one risk factor. Cigarette smoking, obesity, and a family history for the condition also raise your risk.

As of now, there is no cure for macular degeneration. Treatment depends on the type of disease you have and how far along it is. If detected early, you can delay the intermediate form of the disease from becoming the advanced form.

## What It Looks Like

Macular degeneration usually develops slowly and has few symptoms. It typically starts in one eye and goes unnoticed while the other eye compensates. Eventually, when the disease affects both eyes, the signs and symptoms may become more apparent.

The signs and symptoms of macular degeneration vary, depending on the type of disease you have. People who have the dry form of the disease may notice the following symptoms:

- The need for more lighting when reading or working
- Greater difficulty seeing in low lighting
- Blurring of printed words
- Dullness of colors
- Trouble recognizing faces
- Increasing haziness in overall vision
- Blurred or dark spot in center of visual field
- A need to scan your eyes around an object to get a fuller image

With wet macular degeneration, the following symptoms may progress rapidly:

- Distortions such as straight lines that look wavy or close-up objects looking farther away
- Decrease or loss of central vision
- Blurry spot in center of vision

## ¶¶¶ What to Eat

A healthy diet can play a significant role in the prevention or delaying of macular degeneration, says Milton Stokes, R.D., a spokesperson for the American Dietetic Association. Make sure to eat a diet rich in the antioxidant vitamins A, E, and C, as well as foods that contain the carotenoids lutein and zeaxanthin.

Vitamin A is found in red, orange, and yellow foods such as sweet potatoes, mangoes, cantaloupe, apricots, and carrots, as well as dark leafy greens such as kale and spinach. It's also abundant in beef liver and found in smaller quantities in eggs, fish oil, and fortified milk.

Vitamin E occurs in vegetable oils such as soybean, cottonseed, and safflower; nuts (almonds are a good source); wheat germ; peanut butter; and dark leafy greens.

Vitamin C is prevalent in citrus fruits, red bell pepper, tomato, strawberries, orange juice, and grapefruit. For lutein and zeaxanthin, eat dark leafy greens of any variety as well as peas, broccoli, and pumpkin. Lutein actually accumulates in the center of the retina and is part of the macula.

Other healthy foods include lean red meat, eggs, and seafood. These foods contain the antioxidant minerals zinc and selenium, which are also helpful for guarding against macular degeneration. Make sure to also eat cold-water fish such as tuna, salmon, and mackerel, which contain omega-3 fatty acids that may lower the risk for macular degeneration.

## 🚫 What Not to Eat

Steer clear of foods high in fat, especially saturated fats and trans-fatty acids. Too much fat causes oxidation that leads to cell damage. In particular, limit your intake of red meat, whole dairy products such as ice cream and cheese, and desserts such as cakes and cookies.

# 💊 Supplements for Macular Degeneration

In 2001, the Age-Related Eye Disease Study found that high doses of certain supplements may help slow the progression of macular degeneration. But any supplements taken for this condition should be done with the guidance of your physician. Supplements used in the study include the folowing:

### BETA CAROTENE

Beta carotene is a type of carotenoid, the colorful family of antioxidants found in many fruits and vegetables. Certain forms, including beta carotene, can be converted into active vitamin A, which has been linked to combating several diseases, including macular degeneration. But make sure to talk to your doctor about taking beta carotene. High doses may increase the risk for lung cancer in current and former smokers.

### VITAMIN C

This antioxidant vitamin helps combat infection, strengthens immunity, and may guard against further vision loss.

### VITAMIN E

Vitamin E is another antioxidant that may help slow the progression of the disease. Exercise caution with vitamin E if you are on anticoagulant therapy, such as warfarin (Coumadin) or aspirin. Vitamin E is a blood thinner that can cause bleeding problems resulting in hemorrhaging.

### ZINC

Zinc is an essential mineral that is also involved in healthy cell production, tissue growth and repair, and the metabolism of foods. But don't use zinc for extended periods. Chronic use of zinc could lead to copper deficiency, impaired immune function, and a possible disruption in iron absorption.

### COPPER

This trace mineral was included in the formulation used in the study because high levels of zinc can cause copper deficiency. Copper is essential for the manufacture of hemoglobin, the function of enzymes, and the production of energy.

The following are supplements not used in the study that you might also consider:

### LUTEIN/ZEAXANTHIN

These substances are antioxidant carotenoids that play a vital role in eye health. They may be sold separately or in combination.

### BILBERRY

Bilberries grow on low-growing shrubs and are an herbal treatment that may help by strengthening capillaries, tiny blood vessels. Bilberries have a blood-thinning effect, so talk to your pharmacist or doctor first if you are taking anticoagulants. Too much bilberry may cause digestive upset.

# Stay-Healthy Strategies

- **QUIT SMOKING.** Cigarette smoking boosts your risk for macular degeneration.

- **GET REGULAR EYE EXAMS.** Early detection is the key to preventing serious vision loss.

- **WEAR SHADES.** Sunglasses can help block out ultraviolet light. Look for eyewear that filters out both UVA and UVB rays.

- **STAY ACTIVE.** Regular exercise improves blood flow and can help guard against macular degeneration. It will also help prevent excess weight, which can raise your risk too.

## Boost Your Vision

It's frustrating when your vision starts to erode. But there are steps you can take to aid your sight, says the Macular Degeneration Partnership. Here are a few tips from the organization:

- Improve the lighting in your home. This might mean getting brighter lights or looking for lights that reduce glare.

- Read books published in large print.

- Use a hand-held magnifying glass to enlarge words.

- Write in large letters with a broad felt-tip pen on white paper.

# MENOPAUSE

MENOPAUSE IS NOT A DISEASE OR A MEDICAL CONDITION. Instead, it's a natural biological process, a life change that heralds the end of a woman's reproductive years. Some women sail through these years with relative ease and few symptoms except the absence of regular menstrual periods. But for others, menopause is an incredibly difficult time, fraught with numerous physical symptoms, including the infamous hot flashes.

Although your menstrual period doesn't often stop completely until you're in your early 50s, the process of menopause actually begins in your late 30s and 40s, when periods start to become increasingly irregular. This irregularity is caused by a natural decline in the body's production of estrogen and progesterone, two vital hormones involved in menstruation and reproduction. Eventually, when you don't have a period for twelve consecutive months, you are said to have reached menopause. Most women will experience menopause between the ages of 45 and 55.

For years, women relied on hormone replacement therapy (HRT) to treat the symptoms of menopause. Many experts believed that HRT shielded women from the increased risk for heart disease that occurred with menopause. But the Women's Health Initiative in 2002 concluded that HRT—either a combination of oral estrogen and progestin or oral estrogen only—actually put women at greater risk for heart attacks, breast cancer, and stroke. HRT is now prescribed primarily for women with severe hot flashes and vaginal dryness. Other doctors may prescribe non-oral forms of estrogen for menopause-related problems.

For some women, medications are unnecessary. Simple lifestyle changes such as exercise, relaxation, and nutrition may be all it takes to make menopause an easier passage.

## What It Looks Like

Every woman will experience menopause differently, but the most common symptoms include the following:

- Spotting between periods
- Mood swings and irritability
- Muscle aches and pains
- Hot flashes in which you feel warm in the chest and face, especially at night
- Weight gain, especially in the abdomen area
- Memory and concentration problems
- Dryness in the vagina
- Low libido

It isn't always easy to separate these symptoms from other health problems that also occur in middle age. Some of these resemble hypothyroidism, especially weight gain and memory and concentration problems. Others such as hot flashes and muscle aches and pains may suggest hyperthyroidism. Mood swings and irritability may also be signs of depression.

If you do experience these symptoms, it's important to have a thyroid test. While it's true that you may be experiencing menopause, you may also be dealing with a simultaneous thyroid disorder. Women who have a thyroid disease during menopause are at greater risk for heart disease than those without thyroid disease. They're also at increased risk for osteoporosis. That's why a thyroid test is always critical if you're experiencing these symptoms.

## 🍴 What to Eat

For menopausal women suffering from hot flashes, one of the best foods you can eat is soy, according to Mary Jane Minkin, M.D., co-author of *A Woman's Guide to Menopause and Perimenopause* and clinical professor of obstetrics and gynecology at Yale University School of Medicine. Soy products contain substances called isoflavones, plant estrogens that act as natural estrogens.

But choose your soy foods wisely. "The soy that comes in the plastic containers with water around it doesn't really contain [many] isoflavones." Minkin says. Better options are tempeh, edamame, soy nuts, and soy milk.

Another good food is flaxseed, which is abundant in a plant estrogen called lignan. Flaxseed also contains omega-3 fatty acids, which can help lower your risk for heart disease and prevent vaginal dryness during menopause. Other good sources of omega-3 fatty acids are cold-water fish such as salmon, trout, and mackerel.

Make sure to also eat foods rich in calcium and vitamin D, the nutritional duo that can help stave off osteoporosis. Postmenopausal women are at greater risk for low bone density, so foods rich in these nutrients can help strengthen bone. Good choices include low-fat or skim milk, yogurt, cheese, and fortified orange juice.

Finally, eat a lot of fruits and vegetables. These foods are generally high in fiber and rich in

## Make It More Positive

Many women have a tendency to view menopause as a negative transition. But there are ways to make it a more positive experience, in spite of the uncomfortable symptoms and mood swings. Here are some suggestions from the North American Menopause Society:

- Start a gratitude journal. Every night, write three things you're thankful for.
- Find ways to laugh more.
- Make time for relaxation exercises.
- Connect with friends regularly.
- Live in the moment.

Combining all these practices on a regular basis can help make the passage a more joyful experience.

nutrients that can help prevent disease. They will also help prevent unwanted weight gain.

## 🚫 What Not to Eat

Avoid spicy foods, which can set off hot flashes in women who are susceptible. You should also eliminate foods that are thermally hot, such as hot soup, which can trigger hot flashes as well. In addition, steer clear of alcoholic beverages, which not only cause hot flashes but can disrupt much-needed sleep during this time.

Reduce your intake of foods high in saturated fat as well. These foods are more likely to promote weight gain and raise your risk for heart disease. Foods rich in saturated fat include red meat, butter, and whole dairy products. Red meat is also rich in animal proteins, which can cause depletion of bone.

## 💊 Supplements for Menopause

Take a quality multivitamin to make sure you get all the essential nutrients. You might also consider taking the following:

### BLACK COHOSH
Products that contain this herbal remedy may help reduce the hot flashes associated with menopause, especially in the short-term. It is derived from a plant in North America.

### CALCIUM
A supplement of this mineral will help you sustain stronger bones as the body naturally starts to break down more bone than it builds.

### VITAMIN D
Vitamin D, known as the sunshine vitamin, is essential for the proper absorption of calcium and, therefore, bone health.

## 📋 Stay-Healthy Strategies

- **GET YOUR EXERCISE.** Regular exercise can help improve your symptoms, especially insomnia.

- **TREAT VAGINAL DRYNESS.** It is not only uncomfortable but can cause low libido. There are several over-the-counter and prescription remedies that can help.

- **BE WARY OF IRON SUPPLEMENTS.** After menopause, women start to store iron more efficiently, so it's highly unusual for post-menopausal women to have an iron deficiency. Taking too much iron may put you at risk for iron overload, which in extreme cases could damage vital organs.

- **PRACTICE GOOD SLEEP HABITS.** It isn't always easy to get a good night's rest, but good habits can help. So keep the room dark, limit the bedroom to sleep and sex, and go to bed and get up at the same times every day.

# METABOLIC SYNDROME

*See Insulin Resistance on page 203.*

# MONONUCLEOSIS

MONONUCLEOSIS IS OFTEN CALLED THE KISSING DISEASE, thanks to its mode of transmission, which is saliva. But you don't necessarily have to kiss someone to come down with mono. Sharing a straw with an infected person or using the same eating utensil can also lead to mono.

Most cases of mono are caused by infection with the Epstein-Barr virus (EBV), a member of the herpes virus family. Another culprit is the cytomegalovirus, a common virus also in the herpes family. Not everyone who is exposed to these viruses comes down with mono, even if they become infected. Some people may carry the virus their entire life and never have any sign of illness.

Mono is most common among teenagers and young adults who overexert themselves. When people at this age are infected, mono occurs in 35 to 50 percent of the cases, according to the Centers for Disease Control and Prevention (CDC). But most people are infected by the time they're 35 to 40 years old. According to the CDC, as many as 95 percent of adults between these ages have been infected with EBV.

Like many common viral illnesses, there is no cure for mononucleosis except plenty of rest and fluids. Even if you do nothing, the illness will go away on its own after three to four weeks. Over-the-counter analgesics can help relieve fever, headaches, and sore muscles, and warm drinks can help with a sore throat. But the most important thing to do is to listen to your body and get your rest.

## What It Looks Like

The symptoms of mono don't appear right away. They usually emerge about four to seven weeks after you've been infected. Symptoms of mono resemble most other viral illnesses and include the following:

- Fatigue
- Fever
- Sore throat
- Loss of appetite
- Headaches
- Skin rash
- Abdominal pain
- Swollen glands
- Enlarged liver and spleen

Not everyone who has mono will have all these symptoms. The combination of symptoms varies, as does the severity. Some people may have no symptoms at all.

It isn't always easy to figure out whether you have mono. Many other ailments are similar, and it requires a blood test by a doctor to make an official diagnosis.

Although rare, the main concern with mono is that it could cause the spleen to rupture. The spleen is an organ that helps the body filter blood, and it becomes enlarged when you have mono. If your spleen ruptures, you may experience pain in the upper left part of your abdomen, lightheadedness, a rapid heartbeat, and difficulties breathing.

In the month or so after the illness goes away, it's best to avoid contact sports because the spleen may still be vulnerable.

## ¶¶ What to Eat

Battling mono requires a strong immune system, so load up on foods rich in vitamin C, zinc, and folic acid, says Jacob Teitelbaum, M.D., author of *Pain Free 1-2-3*. Good sources of vitamin C include brightly colored fruits and vegetables such as broccoli, red bell peppers, tomatoes, strawberries, blueberries, grapefruit, and oranges.

Zinc is a major mineral found in meats, seafood, and whole grains. It's also found in wheat germ, sunflower seeds, eggs, milk, and fermented soybean paste.

Folic acid is a B vitamin that may be low in people who have viral illnesses. Folic acid helps boost immunity and is found in spinach, navy beans, orange juice, fortified breakfast cereals, and wheat germ.

Also, pay attention to how your body feels when you eat while you're sick. You may have a low appetite initially, in which case you might want to eat lighter foods such as steamed vegetables or chicken soup. As you heal and become stronger, you may want to eat more protein.

## Ⓜ What Not to Eat

Avoid foods that contain sugar, which may suppress the immune system for several hours at a time, Teitelbaum says. That means restricting most baked goods as well as fruit juices, soda, and many packaged foods. You should also minimize your intake of foods high in saturated fats, which also weaken immunity. Saturated fat is found in red meats, whole dairy foods, and fried foods.

Do not drink caffeine or alcohol, which can disrupt your body's need for sleep. In excess, alcohol and caffeine can also weaken immunity.

## ⚕ Supplements for Mono

Ensure overall health by taking a quality multivitamin. Other supplements you might consider taking include the following:

### VITAMIN C
This antioxidant vitamin strengthens immunity and helps defeat the viruses behind mono.

### ZINC
Zinc is an antioxidant mineral that helps combat viral infections.

## LIPOIC ACID

Lipoic acid is a substance naturally manufactured by the body. It acts as an antioxidant and can help reduce any inflammation in the liver.

## 📋 Stay-Healthy Strategies

- **STOP THE SPREAD.** If you have mono, take steps to prevent others from getting sick. Cover your mouth and nose when you sneeze or cough. Don't share drinks or food. Wash your hands frequently.

- **CURTAIL YOUR ACTIVITIES.** Whether you're busy at school, in college, or on your first job, resist the urge to overdo it. Make rest your priority.

- **GET DIAGNOSED.** If you suspect mono, see your doctor. She can do tests to figure out the cause of your symptoms.

- **DO NOT GIVE ASPIRIN TO CHILDREN WITH MONO.** Aspirin puts children at risk for Reye's syndrome, a potentially fatal disease that occurs in children afflicted with viral illness.

### Epstein-Barr

Mononucleosis isn't the only disease linked to the Epstein-Barr virus (EBV). The virus, which was discovered in 1964 by Michael Epstein and Yvonne Barr, has also been implicated in many other illnesses including chronic fatigue syndrome, non-Hodgkin's lymphoma, and Alice in Wonderland syndrome, a neurological condition in which objects are viewed as being much smaller than they are. Some experts have also linked EBV to multiple sclerosis.

# MOTION SICKNESS

FOR SOMEONE WHO SUFFERS FROM MOTION SICKNESS, a simple car ride can be torture, a luxury cruise an impossibility. But motion sickness can also occur on a train, an airplane, or even an amusement park ride.

Motion sickness occurs when the movement you're undergoing does not correspond with the cues your brain is receiving. Sensory receptors in the skin and muscles, visual cues received in the eyes, and the fluid shifting in the inner ear send different and conflicting information to the brain, causing you to feel dizzy. For instance, if you're standing inside the cabin of a boat, your eyes tell you that you are standing still. But your inner ears and sensory receptors will sense that you are actually moving.

When you suffer from motion sickness, your sense of balance is disturbed. The condition is common when airplanes encounter turbulence, boats get caught in rocky waves, and cars meander along winding or bumpy roads. Some people also seem more naturally prone to motion sickness than others.

The best way to cope with motion sickness is to try and prevent it in the first place. You might also consider taking an over-the-counter remedy that can help lessen or prevent motion sickness. But keep in mind that these medications may cause drowsiness. If necessary, talk to your doctor about the possibility of a prescription remedy such as scopolamine.

## What It Looks Like

Motion sickness typically causes dizziness, nausea, and fatigue. If it's severe enough, you may even vomit. Some people also develop a cold sweat and feelings of anxiety.

For most people, the symptoms stop when the motion stops. But for the unlucky ones, the symptoms may sometimes linger for days afterward.

## 🍴 What to Eat

While you're feeling sick, try drinking a carbonated beverage such as ginger ale to help settle your stomach, says Christine Gerbstadt, M.D., R.D., a spokesperson for the American Dietetic Association. You might also try munching on fat-free salted crackers.

As a general rule, try to eat lightly when you're traveling. Eating frequently, too, can help you prevent an empty stomach, which can make motion sickness worse.

Drink a lot of water before and during travel. Water will help you stay hydrated, which in turn will help prevent symptoms of motion sickness.

## 🚫 What Not to Eat

Before and during a trip, avoid high-fat and spicy foods, which can aggravate digestive discomfort during motion sickness. It's also best to avoid sugar because it can cause headaches and irritability. In addition, steer clear of alcohol, which can be dehydrating.

## 💊 Supplements for Motion Sickness

If your motion sickness is severe and you're not able to eat, make sure to take a high-quality multivitamin to get all your essential nutrients. Other supplements that might help relieve motion sickness include the following:

### GINGER

Although studies on the effects of ginger for motion sickness are not conclusive, ginger has been used for centuries in Chinese medicine.

### PEPPERMINT

Another possible treatment is peppermint. Drinking it in a tea or sucking on a peppermint lozenge can sometime relieve the nausea associated with motion sickness.

## 📋 Stay-Healthy Strategies

- **DON'T READ IN THE CAR.** Looking down at a book will tell your eyes you're not moving, even though your inner ears can sense the motion.

- **AVOID LOOKING OUT THE SIDE WINDOWS** of a moving vehicle. It is less disturbing to the inner ear sensors to look out the front window.

- **AVOID CIGARETTE SMOKE.** The fumes from cigarettes can aggravate motion sickness.

- **BREATHE DEEPLY,** but try not to hyperventilate or breathe too quickly, which can worsen motion sickness. Deep breathing will relieve stress and can help calm the symptoms of motion sickness. Make sure to open a window, too, if you can.

- **STEER CLEAR OF STRONG ODORS** before and after travel. Noxious smells may cause or worsen nausea while you're motion sick.

- **GET OUTSIDE.** Stop the car and go for a short walk if you can, or at least open the window. On a boat, go to the upper deck and take in the fresh air.

---

## The Best Seat

No one wants to abandon traveling just because of motion sickness. According to the Mayo Clinic, there are ways you can ease your travels by choosing the right seat or cabin. Here's what they suggest:

- If you're traveling by ship, ask for a cabin in the forward or middle parts of the ship or on the upper deck.

- If you're traveling by plane, ask for a seat over the front edge of a wing. Aim the air vent toward your face.

- If you're traveling by train, take a forward-facing seat near the front and next to a window.

- If you're going by car, ask to drive or sit in the front passenger's seat.

# MULTIPLE SCLEROSIS

MUSCLE WEAKNESS. VISION PROBLEMS. Lack of coordination. For approximately 400,000 people in the United States, these symptoms add up to multiple sclerosis (MS), a potentially devastating neurological condition that affects the central nervous system.

MS is believed to be an autoimmune condition, a disease in which the immune system mistakenly attacks normal healthy tissue. With MS, the immune system attacks myelin, the fatty substance that insulates nerve fibers, making it difficult for nerves to transmit impulses. Damage to the myelin distorts these nerve impulses going to and from the brain, causing miscommunication. These distortions, in turn, produce the symptoms of MS, which include numbness, poor coordination, and tremors. Over time, the damage causes the tissue to harden and scar.

No one knows exactly what causes MS. The condition usually emerges between 20 and 50 years of age. The severity of MS varies widely, and the disease is highly unpredictable, fluctuating between active phases and remissions in which there are no symptoms.

Determining whether you have MS isn't always easy. Many symptoms mimic those of other neurological problems, and it may take several doctor visits to pinpoint whether or not you actually have MS. The condition is also difficult to diagnose because the symptoms vary so much, even within each patient. Diagnosis usually involves the use of magnetic resonance imaging (MRI) to look for multiple patches of scar tissue in several areas of the central nervous system.

Although there is no cure for MS, there are medications that can slow the progression of the disease. Patients may also take steroids to shorten attacks or medications to relieve their symptoms.

The key to living with MS is good management of the symptoms, which may involve physical therapy, exercise, and adequate rest. An important component of managing MS is a healthy diet.

## What It Looks Like

People with MS often notice that their vision is distorted. Some people may lose their vision completely, see double, or become incapable of distinguishing colors. Sometimes there is eye pain involved as well.

MS may also cause difficulties with walking and feeling tactile sensations. People with MS may become uncoordinated and fatigued, and lose bladder and/or bowel control. Many people suffer from tremors, poor balance, and muscle tightness. Some become paralyzed.

In some people, MS results in cognitive problems and emotional difficulties. The condition can cause forgetfulness, difficulty concentrating, mood swings, depression, and irritability.

---

**TIP**

*Give tai chi a try. This ancient Chinese exercise can help promote relaxation, improve balance, and reduce fatigue. It can also lower stress.*

---

## ¶¶¶ What to Eat

Focus on eating a nutrient-rich diet that reduces inflammation, says Andrew Larson, M.D., co-author of *The Gold Coast Cure*. That means eating whole, unprocessed foods that are rich in micronutrients and fiber, namely a lot of fresh fruits, vegetables, and whole grains.

Micronutrients are the antioxidants and phytonutrients that occur naturally in plant foods. Fiber is the undigestible carbohydrate that helps stabilize blood sugar levels, improve digestion, and prevent constipation. Adequate fiber is important for preventing bowel incontinence.

Make sure to also eat foods rich in omega-3 fatty acids, the healthy fat found mostly in cold-water fish such as salmon, trout, and tuna as well as walnuts, flaxseed, and flax oil. Omega-3s can help reduce inflammation, which is a root cause of MS. You can also get omega-3s from enriched eggs.

If you're suffering from fatigue and weight loss as the result of having MS, make sure you're getting enough calories. That doesn't mean going overboard with high-fat, high-calorie foods. Rather, it means eating smaller meals more frequently or noshing on healthy higher-calorie snacks such as fruit, a hard-boiled egg, whole-grain crackers, peanut butter, and low-fat yogurt.

Drink plenty of water too. Resist the urge to restrict fluid intake if you're experiencing loss of bladder control. Inadequate fluids can cause other problems such as difficulties swallowing, dry mouth, loss of appetite, and constipation, which will only aggravate your MS.

Finally, eat foods rich in calcium. Muscle weakness, balance problems, and fatigue can lead to inactivity that will weaken bones. To keep them strong, make sure to eat foods high in calcium, such as low-fat dairy products, broccoli, spinach, tofu, salmon with edible bones, and foods fortified with calcium.

## ⊘ What Not to Eat

Avoid saturated fat, which occurs primarily in animal products such as red meat, dairy products, and butter. Eliminate red meat entirely if possible. If you do eat it, do so in moderation. Cut out all processed foods that contain saturated fat, such as packaged cookies, cakes, and desserts, and omit all dairy products that contain more than 1 percent fat.

You should also cut out foods that contain trans fats. These fats are produced in the hydrogenation of oil and are found in many packaged foods as well as margarine, shortening, and snack foods. An ingredient list that includes partially hydrogenated oil is usually the tip-off that the food contains trans fats.

In addition, restrict your intake of refined flour and sugars, found in pasta, crackers, pizza dough, muffins, bagels, and many other bread-type foods. These foods typically lack in fiber and other nutrients. You also need to avoid foods that contain refined sugars such as high fructose corn syrup, corn syrup, glucose, and sucrose.

Be choosy about the types of vegetable oil you cook with. Certain vegetable oils, including soybean, corn, and safflower, are high in omega-6 fatty acids, which in large quantities can promote inflammation. A better alternative is extra virgin olive oil. Finally, don't drink too much caffeine, which acts as a diuretic. And drink alcohol in moderation—maybe one glass of wine once or twice a week. Alcohol is a depressant and can worsen problems with coordination and aggravate bladder problems.

## ⚇ Supplements for MS

Start with a quality multivitamin, which will help ensure you get all your daily nutrients. But there may be other supplements that can help too. Always talk to your doctor first before taking supplements. Among those to consider are the following:

### CALCIUM AND MAGNESIUM

The lack of exercise sometimes associated with MS can make bones weak. Studies have shown that people with MS have lower bone density. Taking calcium can help strengthen bones. Magnesium will aid with absorption of calcium and help with muscle coordination.

### VITAMIN D

This fat-soluble vitamin helps ensure absorption of calcium. Studies suggest that people with adequate vitamin D intake may be at lower risk for MS.

### ANTIOXIDANTS

Certain antioxidant vitamins and minerals may be able to shield the body from excessive free-radical damage, which may be involved in the destruction of myelin seen in MS. Selenium, vitamin C, and vitamin E all have powerful antioxidant effects. But remember, more is not necessarily better. Be especially careful with vitamin E, which has a blood-thinning effect.

### GAMMA LINOLENIC ACID (GLA)

GLA is a type of omega-6 fat that can help promote anti-inflammatory hormones. It is found in borage oil, evening primrose oil, hemp oil, and black currant oil.

### FISH OIL

Fish oil supplements contain healthy omega-3s—the same kind found in fatty cold-water fish—that can reduce inflammation.

# 🗒 Stay-Healthy Strategies

- **GET EDUCATED.** Arm yourself with knowledge about MS, which is a complex illness. The National MS Society Web site at www.nationalmssociety.org is a good starting place.

- **FIND A GOOD NEUROLOGIST.** Choose a doctor you like who communicates clearly, listens to your concerns, and stays abreast of research in MS. A good doctor will also help you get diagnosed early so that you can begin treatment.

- **MAKE AN EFFORT TO EXERCISE.** Physical activity may be difficult at times, but keep in mind that regular exercise can improve appetite, sleep, and mood. A study in *Neurology* found that people with MS who did yoga every week or who exercised on a stationary bicycle had less fatigue than those who did not do anything active.

- **LEARN TO CONTROL STRESS.** Having MS can be extremely stressful. Developing strategies to manage stress is essential to living with the disease and may even help lessen the symptoms.

## If It Sounds Too Good to Be True…

People with chronic, debilitating illnesses such as multiple sclerosis (MS) are prime targets for unscrupulous snake-oil peddlers. The pain and suffering associated with the disease make you vulnerable to sales pitches that promise to cure you of MS. But the truth is, MS cannot be cured, only controlled. Always do your research before attempting a new treatment. Ask your physician about anything that intrigues you. And be wary of anything that sounds too good to be true. Chances are, it probably is.

# OSTEOPOROSIS

YOU LIKE TO THINK YOU'RE THE PILLAR of good health. You eat lots of fruits and veggies, exercise regularly, and get plenty of sleep. But you may be overlooking your bone health. Over a lifetime, that puts you at risk for osteoporosis, a silent condition with potentially deadly consequences.

Osteoporosis is low bone density, a condition that afflicts about ten million people in the United States, eight million of them women. Each year, approximately 1.5 million American adults suffer an osteoporosis-related fracture. Another thirty-four million people are believed to have low bone mass, or osteopenia, which puts them at risk for osteoporosis.

It's natural for bones to weaken with age. Bones are in the constant process of building up and breaking down. The prime years for building bone occur in adolescence. But eventually, the breakdown outweighs the buildup, especially after menopause, when women lose the protective effects of estrogen. In the five to seven years after menopause, women may lose as much as 20 percent of their bone mass.

Several factors raise your risk for osteoporosis. Some women are cursed with bad genes. A family history of the disease means you're more likely to develop osteoporosis.

Other women never even attain peak bone mass—which occurs around age 30—because they don't get enough calcium or weight-bearing exercise in their youth. If you never reach peak bone mass—the point at which your bones are at their densest—you will begin the weakening process from a lower point, which puts you at risk for osteoporosis.

Many other factors put you at risk for osteoporosis too. Being thin or small-boned and Asian or Caucasian means you're more likely to get the bone-thinning disease. You're also at greater risk if you've had anorexia nervosa, taken medications such as steroids, or experienced a deficiency of estrogen due to an early hysterectomy.

Lifestyle factors play a role as well. Smoking cigarettes, drinking excessive amounts of alcohol, and not getting enough weight-bearing exercise puts you at risk for osteoporosis. But one of the biggest problems is not getting enough calcium and vitamin D in your diet. That's why nutrition plays a major role in the prevention of osteoporosis.

## 🔍 What It Looks Like

People with osteoporosis often look healthy, though it may cause some women to shrink in height or to develop a curvature in the upper spine known as dowager's hump. The disease process happens gradually, and it often isn't until a woman suffers a fracture that she realizes she has osteoporosis. The only way to know for sure whether you have osteoporosis is to have a bone density test.

A bone mineral density test should be given to women based on their risk profile, says the National Osteoporosis Foundation (NOF). The NOF recommends testing all women age 65 and older, as well as younger postmenopausal women with one or more risk factors (besides being white, postmenopausal, and female). Postmenopausal women who have had fractures should also be tested.

## 🍴 What to Eat

Calcium is an essential mineral found in your bones that also helps muscles contract, blood clot, and your heart beat. If you don't get enough calcium from the foods you eat, your body will take calcium from your bones, which will cause them to weaken. That's why adequate calcium intake is so critical, says Lynn Sutton, R.D., C.D.E., a registered dietitian in Albany, New York.

Good sources of calcium include low-fat milk, yogurt, and cheese. An eight-ounce glass of skim milk, for instance, provides 298 mg, while an eight-ounce serving of yogurt delivers 415 mg. An ounce of Swiss cheese provides 219 mg. You can also find calcium in fortified orange juice; canned fish with edible bones; dark green vegetables such as broccoli, kale, and collards; and tofu.

Most women, however, do not get enough calcium, says Charles Hammond, M.D., professor of obstetrics and gynecology at Duke University in Durham, North Carolina. In fact, he says, the average American diet contains only about 500 to 750 mg of calcium, well below the amounts recommended for adults. In reality, women over age 65 should get 1,500 mg a day. If you already have osteoporosis, or if you're postmenopausal and not taking hormone therapy, you should also aim for 1,500 mg. Women between the ages of 25 and 50 should get 1,000 mg a day.

It's also critical to eat foods that contain vitamin D. Getting all the calcium you need won't help if you're not ingesting enough vitamin D, which is needed to help the body absorb calcium. Good dietary sources of vitamin D include fortified milk and cereals, eggs, cheese, salmon, and sardines. Your skin also manufactures vitamin D when it's exposed to sunlight. Spending 15 minutes a day in the sun two or three times a week will satisfy your daily vitamin D needs. But older adults are less able to make vitamin D this way and will surely need supplements to ensure adequate intake.

## 🚫 What Not to Eat

Certain foods may inhibit the absorption of calcium or promote the elimination of it in the urine, both of which will weaken the bones. Too much caffeine from coffee, tea, or soda, for instance, may act as a diuretic and cause you to lose calcium. The same is true of salty foods such as snacks, canned soups, and fast foods, which contain a lot of sodium.

In addition, you should limit your alcohol intake, because consuming more than 7 ounces of alcohol a week reduces bone density and raises your risk for falls and hip fractures. And although fiber is essential for the prevention of many other medical problems, too much of it can inhibit calcium absorption. So continue to eat fiber, but eat it in moderation.

Other substances that decrease absorption include saturated fats, tannins, phytates, and oxalates. Saturated fats are found in animal products such as red meat, whole dairy foods, and butter. Tannins occur in tea and certain grains. Phytates are a compound found in whole grains, bran, and soy that can bind calcium and limit absorption. Oxalates are calcium-binding acids that occur in spinach, rhubarb, beets, and chocolate. Many of these foods contain healthy nutrients, so don't give them up entirely. If you do enjoy them, make sure to take a calcium supplement to compensate for deficits.

You should also steer clear of soda. For starters, soda tends to displace more nutritious drinks such as calcium-rich milk. Soda also contains phosphorous, a mineral that in the right amount is important to bone health, but which in excess will inhibit calcium absorption and promote bone loss.

# ⚙ Supplements for Osteoporosis

Start with a quality multivitamin that will supply the basic nutrients you need for good health. Because you probably won't satisfy your calcium and vitamin D requirements just through food, you'll likely need supplements to help. Here are the main supplements to consider:

## CALCIUM CARBONATE

This type provides the largest percent of elemental calcium and is best taken at meals when the stomach produces more acid. This form is not recommended for people who take medications known as proton pump inhibitors (such as Nexium, Prilosec, or Prevacid), which reduce stomach acids. You should also not take this form of calcium if you are elderly, because aging often reduces your production of stomach acids. Examples of calcium carbonate include Viactiv, Caltrate, Os-Cal, and the antacid Tums.

> **TIP**
>
> *Take your supplements at different times of the day. Your body absorbs only about 500 mg at a time. Take them with meals and snacks that have the least amount of calcium.*

## CALCIUM CITRATE

For people who take drugs that inhibit stomach acids, calcium citrate is a better option. These can be taken at any time. An example of calcium citrate is Citracal.

## VITAMIN D

When choosing a calcium supplement, take one that contains vitamin D to ensure absorption.

## Stay-Healthy Strategies

- **DO THE RIGHT EXERCISES.** Swimming is a great workout, but it does little to strengthen bone. Look for weight-bearing activities that force you to exert your bones against gravity. For bone health, do weight-bearing activities such as walking, jogging, dancing, and strength training. Aim for a 20- to 30-minute weight-bearing workout three to five times a week.

- **QUIT SMOKING.** Cigarette smoking weakens bones, so do what you can to stop.

- **STAY SAFE.** Keep throw rugs off floors and maintain well-lit walkways. A safe environment will prevent falls that can lead to bone fractures.

- **DO IT ALL.** Eating enough calcium isn't enough to prevent osteoporosis. Make sure to include all these strategies for healthy bones.

## Do You Need Medication?

Modern medicine has provided drugs that can actually strengthen bones and slow their loss. Most of these drugs fall under two broad categories. Selective estrogen receptor modulators such as raloxifene (Evista) work by strengthening bone tissue. Bisphosphonates such as alendronate (Fosamax) and risedronate (Actonel), which now comes in a version with calcium, work by slowing bone loss.

Women at high risk for fracture may be prescribed teriparatide (Forteo), a synthetic version of parathyroid hormone, which stimulates bone formation. Always discuss medications and their possible side effects with your doctor before taking them.

# PARKINSON'S DISEASE

MOST OF US TAKE FOR GRANTED our ability to move about, walk, sit, and perform our daily tasks. But each time your body engages in motion, the brain is gathering information and preparing you for the activity. A central area of the brain called the striatum works with other parts of the brain, called the substantia nigra, to send out commands that keep you balanced and coordinated. All this communication occurs without any conscious thought.

Parkinson's disease is a chronic and progressive neurological illness that disrupts this process. It occurs when the nerve cells in the substantia nigra die or become impaired. The destruction and death of these cells depletes the brain of a neurotransmitter called dopamine. Dopamine is a messenger chemical that allows messages to pass from nerve endings down the spinal cord to your muscles, allowing them to move in a smooth, coordinated fashion. Without enough dopamine, your body experiences tremors, clumsiness, difficulty with fine movements, stiffness, and struggles with balance. By the time symptoms emerge, about 80 percent of nerve cells in the substantia nigra have been damaged.

According to the National Parkinson Foundation (NPF), there are 1.5 million people with Parkinson's in the United States, and each year 60,000 new cases are diagnosed. The cause of Parkinson's is unknown; some genes have been identified, and environmental factors are also thought to play a role. The condition is more common in the elderly and affects men and women in almost equal numbers. Most people develop Parkinson's after the age of 65, but in about 15 percent of sufferers, diagnosis occurs before the age of 50.

There is no X-ray or blood test that can confirm you have Parkinson's. Rather, a physician makes a diagnosis after taking a careful history and performing a neurological examination. In some cases, tests and scans may be ordered to rule out other medical conditions.

At this point, there is no cure for Parkinson's disease. Instead, the goal of treatment is to lessen the symptoms and to maintain and improve the patient's quality of life. Treatment for Parkinson's involves medications that replace or mimic dopamine in order to reduce the tremors, stiffness, and slowness. Some people with severe symptoms may be candidates for surgery.

## What It Looks Like

People who have Parkinson's disease have a resting tremor; their movements are frequently slow, stiff, and clumsy. Later in the illness, they may have trouble with balance. In addition to these common symptoms, people with Parkinson's may have a masked facial expression, their speech may be soft and muffled, and their handwriting small and cramped. They may shuffle when they walk. They may have sore, cramped muscles and experience pain and fatigue. About 50 percent of people with Parkinson's may suffer from depression at some point in their illness.

Many people with Parkinson's suffer from constipation. The disease causes the intestines to move more slowly than normal, and many people have difficulties getting enough exercise or drinking enough fluids. Drugs to treat Parkinson's can also cause constipation. In hot weather, constipation may even lead to dehydration.

The type of constipation may vary. The most common type of constipation is difficulty expelling the stool because it is hard, dry, and painful to pass. The longer the stool remains in the gut, the more the water in the stool is reabsorbed into the tissues and the dryer it gets.

Some people may have normal stools but be unable to expel them. This difficulty may be due to a lack of coordination of the sphincter muscles in your rectum. You may also have this problem if you aren't taking enough medication or if the drug is wearing off. To address this problem, try soaking a washcloth in hot water, wringing it out, and applying it to the rectal area. You may also try gently massaging the rectal area with a finger or using glycerin suppositories.

Do not hesitate to call your physician if your constipation is prolonged, as it can lead to serious problems that need urgent medical attention. In Parkinson's, the bowel can twist and cause an obstruction, which, if not treated, can be fatal.

## 🍴 What to Eat

Good nutrition is critical at all stages of Parkinson's disease, but there is no special diet for Parkinson's, according to Susan Calne, C.M., R.N., the NPF outreach coordinator at the Pacific Parkinson's Research Centre in Vancouver, Canada. People with Parkinson's should strive to eat a well-balanced diet that includes a variety of foods from each food group, namely fruits and vegetables, meat and meat alternatives, dairy products, and breads and cereals. But if you have nutrition questions or develop a change in your weight, difficulty chewing or swallowing, or constipation, a consultation with a registered dietitian may be helpful.

For every Parkinson's patient, it's important to get enough calories and protein to prevent weight loss and to maintain muscle strength. Weight loss is common in people with Parkinson's, especially as the disease progresses.

As already noted, one of the most important aspects of diet in regard to Parkinson's is preventing constipation. Constipation is a common problem at all stages of Parkinson's disease, and you need to take early steps to avoid it. A bowel management program should begin from the moment you are diagnosed. (For one program, see the sidebar on page 251 about the Pacific Parkinson's Research Centre bowel management program.)

People with Parkinson's also need to take enough calcium in order to maintain bone density and strength. The deterioration in coordination and muscle strength puts you at greater risk for falls that may lead to fractures, especially if bones are weak. In older people, hip fractures may be fatal. Foods rich in calcium include low-fat milk, yogurt, and cheese, as well as broccoli, kale, spinach, and fortified orange juice. To ensure proper absorption of calcium, it's also essential to get enough vitamin D, which is available in fortified foods such as milk and supplements and is also manufactured in the skin when it's exposed to sunlight.

Make sure to drink plenty of fluids, too, especially if you become dizzy upon standing (orthostatic hypotension) and/or suffer from constipation. It's critical to stay well hydrated in warmer temperatures. In addition to beverages, patients can stay hydrated with smoothies, sorbets, and fruit, which may be easier to swallow. People who feel dizzy when they get out of bed may want to drink a clear liquid, tea, or coffee before rising. Eating more salt can also help orthostatic hypotension. People with Parkinson's

## The Protein Matter

In the early 1980s, some people believed that restricting protein was beneficial for people with Parkinson's disease, especially those who were taking levodopa (Sinemet), the most common medication for Parkinson's. Too much protein interfered with the absorption of levodopa, which often resulted in severe and unpredictable fluctuations in a patient's mobility. Low-protein diets were believed to counter this side effect by improving medication absorption and enhancing the patient's mobility.

Although limiting protein did seem to help a small number of patients who were taking immediate-release levodopa, the diet was generally considered unhealthy in the long-term. After all, people with Parkinson's were at risk for malnutrition. Inadequate amounts of protein also

reduced muscle mass and put patients at greater risk for osteoporosis.

Since then, the low-protein diet has become less popular among health care professionals treating Parkinson's. For one, the debut of controlled-release versions of levodopa has made the medication better tolerated. And experts have also learned that rather than restrict protein, patients may still be able to enjoy it by limiting the amounts they eat in a single sitting or redistributing it throughout the day.

Still, if you insist on trying a low-protein diet, do so under the careful supervision of a registered dietitian and your neurologist. Results should be notable within a week or two. If you do not notice any benefits in that time, discontinue the diet.

and low blood pressure should not be on salt-restricted diets unless they have another medical condition that requires it.

Some people with Parkinson's may have trouble swallowing, a condition known as dysphagia. It might help to eat foods that are hotter or cooler than body temperature, which can trigger muscles in the mouth to chew and swallow. Soft, minced, or pureed foods may also make swallowing easier. For some people who have trouble swallowing thin liquids, viscous fluids and carbonated drinks may be better choices. Drinking ice-cold carbonated drinks with meals or sour foods may help enhance swallowing as well.

The way you eat is also important. Those who are struggling with excessive weight loss may want to try eating smaller, more frequent meals and snacks throughout the day. Some people may benefit from having their meals pre-cut for them, while others may fare better if they eat their meals separately from others, without the worry of keeping others waiting. And because people with trouble swallowing are at greater risk for choking, they should always eat in an upright position and in the presence of a caregiver who knows the Heimlich maneuver.

## What Not to Eat

If you have troubles swallowing, avoid eating foods that are crumbly, sticky, hard, or difficult to chew.

Although people with Parkinson's are more likely to experience weight loss rather than weight gain, those who are overweight should avoid stringent diets. Not eating enough calories can lower energy levels. If weight loss is necessary—as it is in the case of excess weight interfering with mobility—try switching to more nutritious foods and eating healthy portions.

## Supplements for Parkinson's

Taking a high-quality multivitamin will help ensure that you get all the essential nutrients you need. To protect your bones, your doctor may also recommend taking a calcium and vitamin D supplement. But beyond that, supplements are generally not recommended for people with Parkinson's, largely because there are no known benefits.

# A Bowel Management Program

Many patients with Parkinson's suffer from constipation. Here is the Pacific Parkinson's Research Centre bowel management program. Start by doing the suggestions in level 1 and progress to the next level if your symptoms do not improve.

## Level 1

Modify your diet by increasing fiber with whole grains (e.g., rice, oats, and barley) and both soft cooked and raw fruits and vegetables. Try the fruit lax recipe below. Drink six to eight 8-oz. glasses of water or juice daily. Remember that fruits and vegetables contain large amounts of water. Use dried fruit as a sweet snack but pay extra attention to dental hygiene if you start to eat a lot.

Avoid introducing too much bran or bulking agents into your diet too quickly. These products can cause painful cramps, gas, and bloating. If you do want to use some bran, introduce it slowly, one tablespoon at a time, on top of fruit lax or cereal or in baked goods. If you experience gas, consider taking an over-the-counter anti-gas product, available from your pharmacy. Hot peppermint water, made with peppermint oil, can also help, and a hot water bottle or heating pad on the stomach can be comforting.

Consider stool softeners. These remedies coat the stool and make it easier to pass. There are several brands on the market. If you are constipated, use one regularly. You should also take stool softeners if you take medications that contain codeine, such as Tylenol #3.

### Fruit Lax Recipe

Mix up one pound of mixed, dried fruits (your choice; they do not have to be prunes). Put the fruit in a bowl and cover it with cranberry juice and leave to soak overnight. You can also soak the fruit in senna tea, which is available from health food stores and some pharmacies.

Process the mixture in a food processor or blender, but leave it chunky. Some people prefer to cook this recipe and add some molasses. Put it in a plastic tub with a lid and keep in the fridge. Have at least half a cup for breakfast each day.

## Level 2

If you're still constipated after following the recommendations in Level 1 for two days, try adding one tablespoon of psyllium (Metamucil) to juice two to three times a day. Taking psyllium three times a day with plenty of liquid is preferable to taking it all in one dose. You must also be able to maintain an adequate fluid intake (six to eight glasses of water a day) and exercise regularly if you want the bran or bulking agents to work well for you. You should avoid bran (including bran muffins), Metamucil, Prodiem, and other bulking agents if you have difficulty swallowing and/or experience choking episodes.

If the advice in Levels 1 and 2 relieves your constipation, you should continue with the recommendations indefinitely. Levels 3 through 5 are not intended for continuous use.

## Level 3

If you are still constipated after two days, add the following:

- Sennosides, 12–24 mg at bedtime OR
- Bisacodyl, 10 mg at bedtime OR
- Cascara, 5 ml (1 tsp) OR
- Two Senokot tablets

## Level 4

If you remain constipated after one to two days, add the following:

- Lactulose, 15 ml twice daily OR
- Glycerin suppositories (to use one, lubricate the tip with KY jelly and gently insert it while sitting on the toilet)

## Level 5

If constipation persists after one or two days, add a Fleet enema. If this fails, you should contact your physician.

# 🗒 Stay-Healthy Strategies

- **TAKE YOUR MEDICATIONS WITH FOOD.** Taking your drugs on an empty stomach may increase your risk for side effects such as nausea and dizziness.

- **GATHER INFORMATION.** Learn as much as you can about Parkinson's disease and how to live with it. One good source is the NPF, which offers several free brochures on its Web site (www.parkinson.org) on topics ranging from exercise to daily living and mental health.

- **FIND A PHYSICIAN YOU LIKE AND TRUST.** Look for doctors who specialize in Parkinson's and who stay abreast of the latest information. Keep in mind, too, that treating Parkinson's often requires a team approach from several health care professionals. So consider enlisting other health care experts for your medical team, such as a nurse, physical or occupational therapist, registered dietitian, speech language pathologist, and social worker who fully understand Parkinson's.

- **SEEK ADVICE ABOUT THE BEST EXERCISE AND PHYSICAL ACTIVITY** that is most appropriate for your level of disability. Although difficult, movement can still be beneficial.

# PNEUMONIA

PNEUMONIA REFERS TO ANY INFECTION of the lungs that typically occurs when your defenses are down. The infection may come from any of several pathogens, including bacteria, viruses, fungi, and parasites. Most cases are caused by viruses, and often develop after you've had an upper respiratory infection such as a cold.

Together with the flu, pneumonia ranks as the seventh-leading cause of death in the United States. In 2003, for example, about 63,000 people died as a result of pneumonia. Pneumonia is also a common cause of hospitalization, especially among the elderly.

Some people are at greater risk for pneumonia. High-risk groups include the elderly, the very young, and those with underlying health problems such as sickle cell anemia, diabetes, and chronic obstructive pulmonary disease.

Pneumonia itself isn't contagious, but the germs that lead to upper respiratory illnesses are. Preventing these other, less serious upper respiratory illnesses can help prevent pneumonia from developing.

Treatment for pneumonia is usually fluids and rest, but it may also involve antibiotics if bacteria are the cause. With treatment, most cases of bacterial pneumonia are cured within a week or two. Viral pneumonia tends to last longer, while walking pneumonia, caused by mycoplasma (a specific type of microorganism responsible for about 20 percent of all cases of pneumonia), may take as long as six weeks to go away.

## What It Looks Like

The signs and symptoms of pneumonia vary widely depending on the age of the patient and that person's health status. Common symptoms include the following:

- Fever
- Chills
- Cough
- Rapid breathing
- Breathing with grunting or wheezing sounds
- Labored breathing that causes the rib cage to sink inward
- Vomiting
- Chest pain
- Abdominal pain
- Decreased activity

- Loss of appetite
- Bluish or gray color of the lips and fingernails, if extreme

When pneumonia is caused by bacteria, the illness usually comes on quickly with a sudden high fever and unusually rapid breathing. When viruses are the cause, symptoms tend to appear more gradually and are often less severe. Pneumonias caused by mycoplasma often lead to sore throat and headache.

## ▯▯▯ What to Eat

It's important to sustain a healthy weight if you develop pneumonia, says Susan Krantz, M.A., R.D., assistant director of clinical nutrition services for Shore Memorial Hospital in Somers Point, New Jersey. To maintain your strength and body weight, you want to make sure you get plenty of protein. Good sources of protein include lean meats such as chicken, turkey, and fish; low-fat dairy products such as skim milk and yogurt; and legumes, beans, and nuts.

Make sure to get plenty of vitamin A into your diet. Vitamin A is found in brightly colored fruits and vegetables such as carrots, cantaloupes, spinach, sweet potatoes, mangoes, and apricots, as well as fortified milk and cheese.

In addition, eat foods that contain vitamins C and E, which can boost immunity. Good sources of vitamin C include citrus fruits, green and red peppers, strawberries, blueberries, broccoli, kiwi, and spinach. Vitamin E is found in vegetable oils and nuts, especially almonds and hazelnuts. It is also found in wheat germ, seeds, and dark leafy greens.

Make sure to also eat foods that contain zinc, copper, and selenium, minerals that are recommended for strengthening immunity. Zinc is found in lean ground beef, wheat germ, cashews, pecans, and sunflower seeds. Selenium is most abundant in Brazil nuts, cashews, seafood, garlic, brown rice, chicken, and eggs. Copper is found in many types of nuts and seeds as well as seafood, lentils, and mushrooms.

Try eating cold-water fish such as tuna, salmon, mackerel, and herring. These fish contain omega-3 fatty acids that help to combat inflammation, which occurs when the lungs are infected.

Finally, load up on water. Liquids prevent dehydration and will keep the mucus in your lungs loose.

## ⊘ What Not to Eat

Minimize your intake of dehydrating beverages, such as alcohol and caffeinated drinks, including coffee and tea. For some people, too much caffeine can also make it hard to get rest, which is essential for recovery.

## ⁙ Supplements for Pneumonia

Take a high-quality multivitamin that ensures you get all the essential nutrients. Look for those that say "100 percent daily value" on the label.

Some people with pneumonia may not eat enough to get all the nutrients they need from food and may need additional vitamin and/or mineral supplements. But keep in mind that some vitamins and minerals are toxic in large amounts, so always talk to your doctor first before taking supplements.

### VITAMIN A

Vitamin A is an antioxidant that helps combat disease-causing free radicals and boosts immunity. It also helps maintain the integrity of the lining of the lungs.

### VITAMIN C AND E

These vitamins are both antioxidants, which can help prevent infection and free-radical damage.

### ZINC

Zinc is a disease-fighting mineral that may help lower the incidence of pneumonia.

## Stay-Healthy Strategies

- **GET YOUR REST.** Even if you aren't sleeping, resist the urge to do too much when you have pneumonia. It's okay to spend your days resting on the couch.

- **ALWAYS TAKE ALL YOUR MEDICATIONS.** Stopping an antibiotic too soon can cause the infection to return and may make you vulnerable to bacteria that are resistant to some antibiotic medications.

- **SEE YOUR DOCTOR.** Get a prompt and proper diagnosis if you suspect you have pneumonia, and then make sure to keep all your follow-up appointments to monitor your progress.

- **GET VACCINATED.** The pneumococcal vaccine guards against twenty-three types of pneumococcal bacteria and is effective in 80 percent of healthy adults, according to the American Lung Association. A flu vaccine can also help prevent pneumonia by protecting you against the flu, often a precursor to pneumonia.

## Considerations for the Elderly

Older people need to be extra careful if they develop pneumonia. According to the American Academy of Family Physicians, here are some red flags that may signal you need nutritional or lifestyle interventions from a health professional:

- You have an illness or condition that has changed the kind or amount of food you eat.

- You eat fewer than two meals a day.

- You have a poor appetite.

- You eat few fruits, vegetables, or milk products.

- You drink three or more servings of beer, liquor, or wine almost every day.

- You have lost or gained ten pounds in the past six months.

- You're not always able to shop for, cook for, or feed yourself.

- You need assistance with self-care.

# POLYCYSTIC OVARIAN SYNDROME

FOR MANY WOMEN, IRREGULAR PERIODS are nothing new. But for some women, these problems trace their cause to a condition called polycystic ovarian syndrome (PCOS), a common hormonal problem that occurs in women during their reproductive years. PCOS can cause facial hair growth, high levels of insulin in the blood, and infertility. Women with PCOS may be prone to weight gain and hot flashes. PCOS affects 6 to 10 percent of all women of childbearing age.

To understand PCOS, it's helpful to understand something about the ovaries. The ovaries are two small organs located on either side of a woman's uterus. Each ovary has numerous follicles, tiny sacs called cysts, that are filled with liquid that hold eggs. Each month, in healthy women, about 20 eggs start to mature. Usually one becomes dominant, matures, and is released so it can be fertilized, a process known as ovulation. The process triggers the release of progesterone, a hormone involved in menstruation and pregnancy. If the egg is fertilized, then pregnancy results. If it doesn't, menstruation occurs.

In women with PCOS, the ovary doesn't make all the hormones it needs for any of the eggs to become mature. Instead, these eggs become tiny cysts and may form a "string of pearls" on the outside of the ovary. (These cysts are not the same as ovarian cysts, which grow inside the ovary and disrupt ovary function.) Oddly enough, some women with PCOS may not even have these cysts.

What all PCOS sufferers do have in common is that menstruation is irregular or absent. Without the release of the egg, ovulation does not occur and the hormone progesterone is not made. Without progesterone, a woman may have no menstrual cycle or an irregular one. To make matters worse, the cysts produce male hormones known as androgens, which further inhibit ovulation.

No one knows what causes PCOS. Some experts suspect there is a genetic link, because women with PCOS often have a sister or mother with the condition. It's also hard to separate cause from effect. For instance, PCOS appears to be more likely to occur in women who are overweight. But being overweight may actually be a symptom of the condition.

In any case, women with PCOS are at risk for other major health problems such as insulin resistance, diabetes, and heart disease. That's why it's important to get treatment for PCOS, though it cannot be cured. A vital part of any treatment plan is a healthy eating strategy and weight control.

# 🔍 What it Looks Like

Women with PCOS have infrequent menstrual periods, no periods, or irregular bleeding. They may have trouble getting pregnant and suffer from excess hair on their face, chest, stomach, or back. They may also have weight gain, diabetes, high cholesterol, and high blood pressure. Other symptoms include the following:

- Acne, oily skin, or dandruff
- Pelvic pain
- Male-pattern baldness or thinning of the hair
- Dark patches on the skin or skin tags, tiny flaps of skin in the armpits or neck area
- Sleep problems, including sleep apnea, in which you stop breathing for extended pauses during sleep
- Fatigue
- Depression and mood swings

# 🍴 What to Eat

A healthy diet is critical for women who have PCOS and need to maintain or lose weight, says Lynn Sutton, R.D., C.D.E., a registered dietitian in Albany, New York, who specializes in treating people with insulin resistance and diabetes. Women with PCOS should eat a high-fiber diet that includes a variety of fresh fruits and veggies as well as whole-grain foods such as brown rice, oatmeal, and wheat bread. Most experts recommend getting 20 to 35 grams of fiber a day, but women with PCOS should aim for 35 grams a day.

Fiber cannot be digested, but it is a wondrous food in the human diet, especially for PCOS sufferers and people with insulin resistance or diabetes. Soluble fiber, the kind that dissolves in water, is critical because it holds water, which helps slow down digestion and, in turn, slows the release of glucose into the bloodstream. This helps keep blood sugar levels more stable. It also helps lower LDL cholesterol, triglycerides, and high blood pressure, while raising levels of HDL cholesterol. Good sources of soluble fiber include oats, kidney beans, peas, flaxseed, apples, oranges, and carrots.

Insoluble fiber is beneficial because it helps prevent constipation by moving waste more quickly through the colon. Good sources of insoluble fiber include whole-wheat foods, cauliflower, beans, spinach, peas, and apples. As you can see, some foods supply both. Both types of fiber can help minimize weight gain by making you feel full.

Other good sources of fiber include whole grains such as brown rice, whole-wheat bread, and quinoa as well as legumes such as chickpeas, kidney beans, pinto beans, and black beans. When choosing whole-wheat breads, look for those that contain at least two grams of fiber in each serving.

For protein, choose lean meats and fish that are grilled, baked, or broiled. Fish contain omega-3 fatty acids, a healthy type of polyunsaturated fat that can help lower cholesterol, triglycerides, and blood pressure. You can also get omega-3s in flaxseed and walnuts.

Other good sources of protein include seeds, legumes, and soy foods, which contain beneficial plant sterols and stanols. Soy foods come in many forms including tempeh, tofu, edamame, soy milk, and soy burgers.

Try to get your fats from healthy sources, which are foods that contain monounsaturated and polyunsaturated fats. These types of fat can help lower cholesterol. Good sources of monounsaturated fats include olive oil, canola oil, walnuts, avocado, and peanuts. Polyunsaturated fats can be found in safflower, sesame, corn, and sunflower seed oils as well as nuts and seeds.

It's also important to eat a well-balanced mix of all the macronutrients at each meal. Eating complex carbs with lean proteins and healthy fats will help slow digestion, slow the rise of blood glucose, and help you feel full longer.

Pay special attention to portion sizes and calories too. Because losing weight is important when you have PCOS, you should always try to avoid overeating.

## What Not to Eat

For women with PCOS, it's important to reduce fat intake and lower calories in an effort to lose weight, especially if you carry your weight around your waist. To do that, avoid foods high in saturated fats, which occur in animal products such as red meat, whole dairy products, and butter. You should also steer clear of foods with trans-fatty acids, which are often found in packaged foods such as candy bars, cookies, muffins, and crackers. These foods often contain partially hydrogenated oils.

Try to cut out fried foods, too, such as french fries, doughnuts, and fried chicken, which are high in saturated fat and calories. In addition, restrict or eliminate refined foods, which are typically high in sugar. Too much sugar can elevate insulin levels and cause an increase in cho-

lesterol, triglycerides, and blood pressure. That means avoiding white bread, rolls, muffins, and bagels as well as candy bars, desserts, and sugary beverages such as soda.

And if you have high blood pressure as well, avoid high-sodium foods such as potato chips, processed meats, and canned soups. Too much salt has been proven to worsen blood pressure.

## Supplements for PCOS

A quality multivitamin will supply the basic nutrients you need for good health. But you might also consider taking the following:

### NIACIN

Niacin is a B vitamin that occurs in wheat and rice bran and Brewer's yeast. It is also found in whole grains, legumes, fish, and peanuts. As a supplement, niacin may help lower total cholesterol and LDL while increasing HDL.

### GARLIC

This pungent spice may help lower cholesterol and triglycerides. If you want to try garlic supplements, make sure to choose one that has allicin, the most bioavailable form of garlic.

### CHROMIUM

Chromium is a trace mineral that enhances the function of insulin and the metabolism of food.

### PSYLLIUM

Psyllium is a seed husk and soluble fiber that can ensure bowel regularity and lower cholesterol. Talk to your doctor first before taking psyllium, especially if you have food allergies, because some people react to psyllium.

### COENZYME Q10

Your body naturally produces CoQ10, a substance involved in energy production. As a supplement, it may help lower blood pressure, blood glucose, and body weight.

## 📋 Stay-Healthy Strategies

- **RULE OUT OTHER CONDITIONS.** PCOS does tend to mimic other conditions, such as hypothyroidism. Make sure you get properly diagnosed.

- **EXERCISE REGULARLY.** Physical activity will not only promote weight loss but will also improve insulin sensitivity.

- **TREAT YOURSELF KINDLY.** Women with PCOS may become depressed while trying to diagnose and manage their symptoms. Incorporate into your routine rewards that lift your mood.

- **GET SMART.** PCOS is a complex condition with many facts. Learn as much as you can, and you'll feel more empowered.

## Tips from the Biggest Losers

What works best for people who lose forty pounds or more and keep it off? According to Lynn Sutton, R.D., C.D.E., a registered dietitian in Albany, New York, here are some of the most successful weight-loss strategies from the members of the National Weight Control Registry:

- Make sure the timing of your diet—when you decide to start dieting—and the diet you choose are ones that suit you, not someone else.

- Keep fat intake low and protein and carbs moderate.

- Weigh yourself weekly to track success or to detect an increase before it gets out of hand.

- Keep a food log. Writing it down makes you accountable.

- Get aerobic. Walking, biking, running, bowling, and swimming were among the favorite exercises.

- Exercise at least 30 minutes three times a week for maintenance and daily for weight loss.

# PREGNANCY

BEING PREGNANT CERTAINLY ISN'T A DISEASE, but it is a distinct state of health that for most women means a change in their dietary needs. Entire books have been dedicated to the topic, as the mother's nutritional status in pregnancy can play a big role in the health of her baby.

Among the most important needs for pregnant women is folic acid, a B vitamin that can help prevent neural tube defects in the unborn baby. Folic acid can be found in foods, but getting enough often requires taking a prenatal vitamin, which should begin several months before a woman actually becomes pregnant.

Pregnancy begins at conception, when an egg released from the ovary is fertilized by sperm and implanted in the lining of the uterus. Most pregnancies last forty weeks from the time of a woman's last menstrual period (thirty-eight weeks after conception).

During that time, the mother's body goes through major hormonal shifts that prepare her to carry and sustain the baby. Different women are affected differently by these hormonal changes. Some women glide through with relative ease, while others suffer a host of bothersome symptoms including severe mood swings.

For women who have been hoping to get pregnant, discovering that they have conceived can a time of great joy. But pregnancy can also be a time of tremendous discomfort.

## 🔎 What It Looks Like

Most women suspect they're pregnant when they miss a menstrual period. Women who have irregular periods may have a harder time pinpointing their pregnancy. Home pregnancy tests, often followed by a visit to the obstetrician-gynecologist, can usually confirm whether conception actually occurred.

Initially, a woman may not show any outward signs of being pregnant. But internally she may feel distinct changes almost immediately. She may feel more tired than usual. Her breasts may feel more tender and sensitive. The areolas, which are rings around the nipples, may darken and enlarge. She may also start to notice some pangs of nausea, increased urination, and a fullness in her abdomen. Some women become sensitive to smells and tastes of certain foods. Others may have strange cravings, even for foods they normally abhor.

As the months go on, the symptoms may fluctuate. After an initial phase of extreme fatigue, some women start to feel very energetic in their second trimester. The nausea often lifts by then and, thankfully, doesn't return. You will also start to feel bumps and kicks from your baby.

By the third trimester, most women are feeling tired again as the weight of the baby grows. Eventually, the cervix starts to dilate in preparation for delivery.

## 🍴 What to Eat

The basis of a healthy pregnancy is a well-balanced diet that includes an extra 300 calories a day to support the growing fetus, says Mary Jane Minkin, M.D., a clinical professor of obstetrics and gynecology at Yale University School of Medicine and the author of *A Woman's Guide to Sexual Health*. That means eating a diet rich in whole foods such as fruits and vegetables, whole grains, lean proteins, and low-fat dairy foods.

It's important to make sure you get enough folic acid, either in your diet or in a supplement. Inadequate folic acid has been linked to a higher risk for spina bifida, a neural tube defect in which the spine fails to close completely. Folic acid is a B vitamin found in fortified breakfast cereals, breads, and pastas, as well as spinach, navy beans, and wheat germ. Even women who are hoping to conceive should make sure they're getting enough folic acid.

Getting enough calcium is also critical during this time. Women should get 1,000 to 1,200 mg of calcium a day from low-fat dairy foods such as yogurt, milk, and cheese. You can also get calcium from broccoli, dark leafy greens like kale, canned fish with bones, calcium-fortified orange juice, and tofu processed with calcium.

In addition, you need to eat foods rich in iron and zinc, two other major minerals that you'll need more of in pregnancy. Iron will help sustain the increase in blood volume that occurs in pregnancy and is found in legumes, eggs, and lean meats. Eating foods rich in vitamin C such as citrus foods, broccoli, tomatoes, and strawberries will help enhance absorption of iron. Zinc, which is vital to your baby's growth and brain development, is found in whole grains, meat, seafood, and chicken.

Many of these foods are also rich in protein, which Minkin touts as vital to a healthy pregnancy. Good sources include chicken, turkey, beans, tofu, and fish. Protein supplies you with the extra energy you need but is less likely to cause any excess weight gain to stick around after delivery.

## 🚫 What Not to Eat

Limit your intake of caffeine to two cups of coffee or tea a day. Too much caffeine may raise your risk for miscarriages and can rob you of the sleep you need during this time. In addition, you should limit your intake of alcohol to an occasional glass of wine. Most doctors recommend that you give up all alcohol during pregnancy.

Be wary of eating too much food. Ideally, women should gain twenty-five to thirty-five pounds during pregnancy with a single fetus. For some women, the weight gained during pregnancy becomes difficult to shed and can set the stage for ongoing weight problems later in life. So do your best to gain a healthy amount. The key, Minkin says, is to gain the weight by eating the right foods. Weight gained by eating unhealthy foods such as cookies, cakes, and snack foods is more likely to stay with you than pounds accumulated from eating extra healthy foods. And remember, pregnancy is not a time for dieting or for cutting out certain nutrients such as fat, which are vital to your developing baby. Just do your best to eat well.

## ♘ Supplements for Pregnancy

Take a high-quality multivitamin that contains folic acid and calcium to ensure you get the essential nutrients you need. Many doctors will prescribe specially formulated prenatal vitamins just for women attempting to get pregnant or for those who already are. Take your vitamin faithfully by devising strategies to help you remember it every day. And do not take any other supplements without discussing them with your doctor first. Chances are, you won't need to take anything else.

## ☐ Stay-Healthy Strategies

- **EXERCISE REGULARLY.** Getting physical activity every day will help relieve the discomforts of pregnancy, limit your weight gain, and help keep your fetus healthy. Ideally, you should start before you get pregnant.

- **GET ENOUGH SLEEP.** Pregnancy is not the time to fight the body's natural urge for rest. So make time for extra sleep if needed.

- **LIMIT STRESS.** Staying relaxed will help ease any discomforts you have. So do what you can to minimize stress.

- **KEEP IT GOING.** If you've picked up some healthy habits during pregnancy, keep them up afterward, especially if you choose to nurse. Breastfeeding moms, for instance, will continue to need about 500 extra calories each day.

# Heartburn and Hemorrhoids

Two of the most unpleasant side effects of pregnancy are heartburn and hemorrhoids. Relaxed muscles in the digestive tract are the result of an increase in progesterone. Heartburn occurs when stomach acids rise up into the esophagus, causing a burning sensation in your throat. Hemorrhoids are swollen blood vessels around the anus that often accompany constipation, and make it difficult and painful to have a bowel movement.

Certain eating strategies can help alleviate these problems. According to the American Dietetic Association, you can try these tips for heartburn:

- Eat small meals throughout the day instead of large ones
- Walk after you eat
- Eliminate caffeinated and carbonated drinks
- Eat slowly in a relaxed setting
- Elevate your head when sleeping
- Wear loose-fitting clothes

For hemorrhoids, you can try to do the following:

- Drink lots of fluids
- Load up on fiber
- Exercise every day
- Eat dried plums, prune juice, and figs, which are natural laxatives

# PREMENSTRUAL SYNDROME

ALMOST EVERY WOMAN HAS EXPERIENCED premenstrual syndrome, or PMS, at one time or another. Your symptoms might be abdominal cramps or a blue mood. Or maybe you feel swollen and bloated. Many women may be irritable and just not quite themselves. Others may have trouble sleeping.

PMS occurs in the week or two before you get your period, which is known as the luteal phase of the menstrual cycle. The luteal phase lasts about 14 days, starting with ovulation and ending the day before your period. With the onset of menstruation, PMS symptoms usually disappear.

According to the American College of Obstetricians and Gynecologists, premenstrual emotional and physical changes occur in as many as 85 percent of all women during their child-bearing years. Approximately 20 to 40 percent of these women say these days are difficult, and 5 to 10 percent say they interfere with work, lifestyle, or relationships. Most women, however, do not seek treatment for PMS.

No one knows exactly what causes PMS, or why some women are more prone to it than others. It's believed that some women are more sensitive to the hormonal upheaval that occurs during the menstrual cycle. Any woman or girl who has started menstruating may develop PMS.

## 🔎 What It Looks Like

PMS generally includes both physical and emotional symptoms. A formal diagnosis of PMS is usually based on your symptoms, when they occur, and how much they affect your life. Symptoms include the following:

- Mood changes that may include depression, irritability, anxiety, lethargy, and low libido
- Loss of concentration and difficulties remembering
- Breast swelling and tenderness
- Fatigue and trouble sleeping
- Upset stomach, bloating, constipation, or diarrhea
- Headache, migraine
- Changes in appetite or food cravings

- Tension, irritability, mood swings, or crying spells
- Weight gain
- Swelling

Not every woman has every symptom, and symptoms may vary from month to month even for the individual woman. For most women, the key is recognizing that you do suffer from PMS and to develop effective strategies for coping with your symptoms.

## What to Eat

Start with a healthy, well-balanced diet that includes plenty of fruits and vegetables and whole grains, says Mary Jane Minkin, M.D., co-author of *A Woman's Guide to Menopause and Perimenopause* and clinical professor of obstetrics and gynecology at Yale University School of Medicine. These types of foods will help stabilize blood sugar levels and provide plenty of fiber, which may help even out hormone levels.

For protein, eat lean meats such as chicken, fish, and pork. These foods contain vitamin B6, which may help tame the symptoms of PMS. Protein will also promote satiety and may help you better resist cravings.

Try eating foods made of soy as well. Soy products, which include tofu, tempeh, and edamame, contain substances called isoflavones, plant estrogens that act as natural estrogens. A small study in the *British Journal of Nutrition* found that women who ate soy were able to reduce breast tenderness, headaches, cramps, and swelling more than those who took a placebo.

In addition, make sure to get plenty of foods rich in calcium and vitamin D, which may

relieve the symptoms of PMS. Good choices include low-fat yogurt, skim or 1 percent milk, and low-fat cheese. These foods also ensure good bone health.

## What Not to Eat

It isn't easy to resist a craving, but try to limit your intake of foods that are too salty or sweet. High-salt foods will worsen your bloating, which may cause uncomfortable breast tenderness. Foods high in sugar may exaggerate mood swings that result in peaks and dips in energy. Both foods may cause unwanted weight gain.

You should also try to limit or eliminate caffeine, which will only worsen anxiety, tension, or irritability. Avoid drinking alcohol, too, which can also worsen your mood, especially if you're feeling depressed.

## Supplements for PMS

Take a high-quality multivitamin to ensure you're getting all the nutrients you need. Some supplements have been found to help relieve premenstrual symptoms. Supplements you might want to discuss with your doctor include the following:

### VITAMIN B6
Pyridoxine helps the body convert an amino acid called tryptophan into serotonin, the feel-good neurotransmitter. It has long been considered helpful for women with PMS. But keep the dose low (50 to 100 mg, Minkin says), since too much can cause nerve damage.

## VITAMIN E

Although it's not confirmed, some studies have suggested that small doses of vitamin E may help relieve symptoms of PMS.

## MAGNESIUM

Magnesium is a major mineral that helps relax cells in nerves and muscles. One study found that magnesium given over two menstrual cycles helped relieve symptoms of fluid retention such as breast tenderness, weight gain, and bloating in the second month, but not the first.

## EVENING PRIMROSE OIL

The oil of this small yellow wildflower has been used to help treat symptoms of PMS, especially breast tenderness.

## 📋 Stay-Healthy Strategies

- **TRY TO GET ENOUGH SLEEP.** When you're well rested, you're better able to withstand the hormonal fluctuations of your cycle.

- **GET SOME AEROBIC EXERCISE.** Rigorous activity stimulates the production of feel-good endorphins in the brain.

- **TAKE CONTROL OF STRESS.** Make time to meditate, pray, or practice relaxation exercises, which will help buffer you against the mood swings of PMS.

- **IF YOU THINK YOU HAVE PMS,** keep track of your symptoms for several cycles. Having a record will help you pinpoint when the symptoms are most bothersome. It is also helpful to have if you decide to seek medical help.

## PMS Q&A

**Q.** What is premenstrual dysphoric disorder (PMDD)?

**A.** PMDD is a severe, disabling form of PMS. Women with PMDD experience depression, anxiety, tension, insomnia, and persistent anger or irritability. The symptoms are frequently severe enough to result in problems with relationships and carrying out normal activities. Women with PMDD also suffer from physical symptoms such as headache, joint and muscle pain, lack of energy, bloating, and breast tenderness.

According to the American Psychiatric Association, a woman may be diagnosed with PMDD if she's suffered these symptoms for most of her menstrual periods over the past year. She must have at least five of the eleven typical symptoms and at least one of the following symptoms:

- Feeling sad, hopeless, or self-deprecating

- Feeling tense, anxious, or "on edge"

- Marked changeability of mood interspersed with frequent tearfulness

- Persistent irritability, anger, and increased interpersonal conflicts. The symptoms must occur during the week before her period and interfere with daily functioning or social activities.

Treatment for PMDD typically involves the use of antidepressants called selective serotonin reuptake inhibitors (SSRIs), such as sertraline (Zoloft) and fluoxetine (Sarafem).

# PROSTATE ENLARGEMENT

TUCKED BELOW A MAN'S BLADDER is the prostate gland, a reproductive gland that produces fluid for sperm. The prostate is wrapped around the urethra, the canal through which urines passes. In healthy men, the prostate is about the size of a walnut, and urinating is an easy task. But with age, the prostate can become larger, making urination more challenging.

An enlarged prostate is medically known as benign prostatic hyperplasia. The enlargement disrupts the flow of urine, which is how most men first notice that anything is wrong.

The condition becomes increasingly common with age. About half of all men in their 60s suffer from prostate enlargement. By the time men are in their 70s and 80s, the condition affects as many as 90 percent of all men.

The exact cause of prostate enlargement is uncertain, and it's unclear why some men are more affected than others. The only well-defined risk is aging. Some experts believe that prostate enlargement occurs when the amount of active testosterone declines, so that proportionally, there is more estrogen circulating. The excess estrogen stimulates substances in the prostate that promote cell growth.

Others believe that aging causes an increase in the production of a substance called dihydrotestosterone (DHT), which is involved in prostate cell growth.

## What It Looks Like

The degree of prostate enlargement varies from man to man. Some men won't experience any problems at all. But other men may notice changes in the way they urinate. The urine flow may be weak, and it may feel as if you can't completely empty your bladder. Some men may have trouble starting urination, while others may experience frequent stops and starts while urinating.

Prostate enlargement can also increase your need to urinate, and you may have more frequent trips to the bathroom in the middle of the night. Some men notice greater urgency when they feel the need to go. In some cases, prostate enlargement may cause blood in the urine or recurrent urinary tract infections.

Treatment for prostate enlargement depends on the severity of your symptoms and whether they interfere with proper emptying of the bladder. Most men take medications for prostate enlargement, but there are also other therapies and surgeries that can help reduce the size of the prostate.

## ᵉᵉⁱ What to Eat

Eat foods high in zinc, an antioxidant mineral that is essential to good prostate health. One of the best sources is pumpkin seeds. Zinc is also found in meats, seafood, whole grains, wheat germ, sunflower seeds, eggs, and milk.

Another good food to eat is lycopene-rich tomatoes, even in tomato sauce. Lycopene is a phytochemical that's been found to decrease the incidence of cancer cells in the prostate. Lycopene may also inhibit the growth of normal prostate cells, thereby preventing enlargement.

## What Not to Eat

Avoid soy products such as tofu, tempeh, and miso, which contain plant estrogens that could stimulate prostate growth. In addition, avoid alcohol and caffeine, diuretics that can cause excessive urination.

## Supplements for Prostate Enlargement

Take a high-quality multivitamin to ensure overall health. Other supplements to consider taking include the following:

### SAW PALMETTO

This herbal remedy taken from the American dwarf palm tree is well known for its beneficial effects on prostate enlargement. But be patient: Saw palmetto takes about six weeks to work.

### AFRICAN PYGEUM

This herbal remedy comes from an evergreen tree grown in South Africa. It's been used for centuries in Europe as a treatment for prostate enlargement and may relieve the urinary difficulties associated with the condition.

### ZINC

This major mineral enhances a man's overall prostate health and may help relieve some of the enlargement.

### NATURAL TESTOSTERONE

Ask your physician about taking natural testosterone to help boost the ratio of testosterone to estrogen. You'll need to get this at a holistic pharmacy.

# 📋 Stay-Healthy Strategies

- **GET CHECKED OUT.** Do not try to diagnose your prostate problems without seeing a doctor for an exam and diagnosis.

- **EXERCISE REGULARLY.** Physical activity can help lessen the symptoms of prostate enlargement.

- **DON'T HOLD IT.** Urinate whenever you feel the urge.

- **WATCH YOUR FLUID INTAKE.** Don't drink too much at once and avoid drinking too many fluids in the two hours before bedtime.

## What's the PSA Test?

By a certain age, most men become familiar with the PSA test, which tests for a protein called prostate-specific antigen. The protein is produced by cells in the prostate gland and acts as a marker for prostate cancer.

In healthy men, the PSA levels in the blood are low. But with age, PSA levels may rise. Sometimes the higher PSA levels are an indication of prostate cancer, but not always. Other times, they're an indication of benign prostate conditions such as prostatitis, an inflammation of the prostate. In any case, a high PSA level usually alerts the doctor that more testing may be needed, especially if a digital rectal exam detects abnormalities on the prostate.

Normal PSA levels are considered to be between 0–4.0 ng per milliliter, but there is no absolute value that applies to all men. Rather, your risk for prostate cancer goes up as the values go up. Your PSA levels are also influenced by other factors such as infection, medications, and age. Only a biopsy of the prostate can confirm whether you have cancer. Consult your doctor to decide when and whether to get a PSA test.

# PSORIASIS

FOR SOME PEOPLE, PSORIASIS MAY SEEM like just a cosmetic problem, a disease that creates lesions on the skin. But in reality, psoriasis is a serious health condition that can have a significant impact on a patient's quality of life.

Psoriasis causes patches of skin to become inflamed. These patches are called lesions, and they vary widely in terms of severity. Some people are afflicted by just a few, while others may have them on large areas of skin. Fortunately, most cases of psoriasis tend to be mild. But about 25 percent of sufferers have moderate to severe forms of the disease.

Psoriasis affects more than 4.5 million people in the United States. The condition typically begins between the ages of 15 and 35 and occurs equally in both men and women. Though the sight of the psoriatic lesions may make some people uncomfortable, the disease is neither contagious nor a sign of infection.

The cause of psoriasis is a mystery, but experts believe there is a genetic component involved. A child whose parent has psoriasis has a 10 percent chance of getting the disease too, says the National Psoriasis Foundation. If both parents have it, the risk goes up to 50 percent.

Experts are also fairly certain that the immune system is involved in psoriasis. For reasons that are unclear, the immune system somehow triggers the excessive growth of skin cells. Normal skin cells mature and fall off the body surface in 28 to 30 days. Psoriatic skin cells, on the other hand, take just three to four days to mature and rise to the surface. And instead of falling off the surface, the cells gather and form the lesions characteristic of psoriasis.

Psoriasis alternates between flare-ups and remission, periods when the disease is inactive. The disease may be triggered by stress, injury to the skin, sunburn, scratches, certain infections, and medications such as antimalarial drugs, lithium, and certain beta-blockers. Other triggers may include weather, diet, and allergies. But what triggers the condition in one person may have no effect in another person.

Treatment for psoriasis often involves a combination of topical ointments or medications. Finding the right medications often takes time, and every patient needs to experiment to find the best combination.

# What It Looks Like

Psoriasis is most likely to appear on the scalp, knees, elbows, and lower back, but it can develop anywhere, including the palms of the hands, the fingernails, the face, and even the genitals. The lesions are often symmetrical, meaning if a lesion appears on the right side, it will appear in roughly the same place on the left side.

There are actually five distinct forms of psoriasis. Plaque psoriasis, the kind that produces scaly lesions, is the most common and accounts for about 80 percent of all cases. Sufferers usually experience raised, red lesions that are covered with silvery-white scales. It may start with red bumps and become itchy or burn. The skin also becomes dry and painful. Other forms are as follows:

- Guttate, which is characterized by small dot-like lesions

- Pustular, which causes weeping lesions and intense scaling

- Inverse, which produces inflammation

- Erythrodermic, which creates intense shedding and redness of the skin

There are no special blood tests or diagnostic exams for diagnosing psoriasis, only the careful examination of a physician. If the condition is severe, it can lead to infection, poor circulation, and dehydration.

## Psoriatic Arthritis

Some people with psoriasis will develop psoriatic arthritis, a specific type of arthritis that occurs in about 23 percent of psoriasis patients, according to the National Psoriasis Foundation. Psoriatic arthritis resembles rheumatoid arthritis but is generally milder.

People with psoriatic arthritis have stiff joints and inflammation in the tissue around the joints. Psoriatic arthritis can affect the fingers and toes and may involve the neck, lower back, knees, and ankles. In severe cases, psoriatic arthritis can be disabling and cause irreversible damage to joints.

## ¶¶ What to Eat

Focus on eating foods that diminish inflammation, says Amy Neuzil, N.D., a naturopathic physician in Austin, Texas. One of the best choices is fatty fish such as mackerel, salmon, herring, and sardines, which contain omega-3 fatty acids. A study found that people with psoriasis who ate fatty fish for six weeks experienced an 11 to 15 percent reduction in their symptoms. Certain spices and seasonings also have an anti-inflammatory effect. These foods include garlic, ginger, and turmeric.

Make sure to also eat plenty of fruits, vegetables, and whole grains too. In general, these foods are rich in antioxidants, which can lower systemic inflammation. In particular, focus on those with deep hues, such as dark leafy greens, blueberries, and beets.

Fruits and vegetables have another benefit—they're rich in fiber, which helps the body process toxins and reduce inflammation. Studies have suggested that a vegan or vegetarian diet may be better for people with psoriasis. In particular, vegans—who eat no animal products at all in their diet—tend to have a lower incidence of psoriasis.

Whatever you eat, try to maintain a healthy weight. People who are overweight generally have worse symptoms of psoriasis. If you're overweight at the time of diagnosis, look for ways to lose weight.

## 🚫 What Not to Eat

Avoid foods made with white sugar, which can trigger inflammation in the body. Other inflammatory foods include refined flour, red meat, alcohol, and foods that are made with hydrogenated oils, artificial sweeteners, and artificial colors. These substances promote inflammation, which is the root cause of psoriasis.

Some people with psoriasis may suffer from food allergies. The best way to find out whether you're affected by a particular food is to do an elimination diet. Eliminate a food for about two weeks, then reintroduce it into your diet and see if you experience a reaction.

Also, drink alcohol in moderation. Alcohol, especially in excess, can trigger psoriasis and worsen your symptoms.

## 💊 Supplements for Psoriasis

Consider taking a high-quality multivitamin for overall health, then check with your doctor before starting any supplement. When considering supplements, do not take any vitamin C beyond what's in the multivitamin, Neuzil says. Vitamin C stimulates a substance in the body called cyclic GMP, which is involved in skin turnover and is already high in people who have psoriasis. Some supplements to consider include the following:

### FISH OIL

Taking fish oil can help reduce inflammation. But if you're on a blood thinner such as warfarin (Coumadin) or aspirin, be sure to talk to your doctor first, because too much fish oil can cause bleeding.

### FLAXSEED OIL

Flaxseed oil is an anti-inflammatory agent just like fish oil. But some people cannot convert it into the active substance needed to reduce inflammation, so fish oil is generally preferred.

### PROTEOLYTIC ENZYME

A proteolytic enzyme–enzymes that gobble up proteins–taken on an empty stomach will enter the bloodstream and digest any inflammatory particles.

### CHROMIUM

Chromium can help relieve your symptoms and tame any sugar cravings.

### SELENIUM

The excessive turnover of skin in psoriasis can make some sufferers deficient in this essential mineral.

### ZINC

Zinc is another mineral that can help tame inflammation while boosting the immune system.

## Stay-Healthy Strategies

- **REDUCE STRESS.** Too much stress can trigger a flare-up or worsen itching. Learn a relaxation technique and practice ways to change your thinking in order to reduce stress.

- **CONTROL THE ITCH.** Constant scratching can worsen your condition and make your skin bleed. To minimize itching, keep your skin moist by applying moisturizers as soon as you step out of the bath. You can also try applying a cold compress or soaking in an oatmeal bath.

- **LEARN YOUR TRIGGERS.** Whether it's cold winter weather or stress on the job, find out what sets off your symptoms. Then develop strategies to eliminate them.

- **COPE WITH DIFFICULT EMOTIONS.** Visible lesions can cause anxiety, low self-esteem, and depression. If your psoriasis is making it hard for you to cope, consider talking to a mental health professional.

# RAYNAUD'S PHENOMENON

IT'S NORMAL FOR BLOOD VESSELS TO CONSTRICT when they're exposed to cold temperatures; that's the body's natural way of preserving heat by preventing heat loss to the extremities. But in people who have Raynaud's phenomenon, the blood vessels undergo vasospasms that severely reduce circulation to the extremities. This reduction in blood flow causes fingers—and sometimes toes and the tip of the nose—to turn white, blue, and purple, before turning red during recovery.

Raynaud's phenomenon comes in two forms. For some people, it is a primary disorder with no underlying disease and symptoms that are generally mild. The primary form usually begins before the age of 30. Others have the secondary form of the disease, which is the result of another illness such as scleroderma or rheumatoid arthritis. The secondary form is typically more severe and tends to occur after age 30.

Raynaud's can affect almost anyone but is generally more common among women. The condition is triggered by cold temperatures but also by stress, abrupt changes in temperature, and cigarette smoking. In some people, even a stroll through the freezer section of a supermarket can trigger an attack.

There is no cure for Raynaud's, though some people can get relief with the use of medications that improve blood flow. The best way to cope with the condition is to prevent attacks by dressing warmly, using gloves and hand warmers, and reducing stress. If you do experience Raynaud's, try to warm up the affected body parts quickly. Persistent, severe Raynaud's can cause a reduction in blood flow severe enough to injure or kill the involved tissues.

## ⑪ What to Eat

Besides eating a well-balanced diet to ensure healthy immune function and blood vessels, make sure to eat foods that contain omega-3 and omega-6 fatty acids, healthy fats that can reduce inflammation and improve blood flow, says Jacob Teitelbaum, M.D., author of *Pain Free 1-2-3*. Good sources include cold-water fish such as tuna, salmon, herring, and mackerel.

It's also important to get enough magnesium. Magnesium plays several roles in the body. It signals muscles and blood vessels to relax and contract and helps maintain nerve and muscle cells. Foods that contain magnesium include legumes, spinach, pecans, peanut butter, and whole grains.

# What Not to Eat

Avoid eating too much refined sugar—the kind found in sodas, desserts, and fruit juices—which can worsen inflammation.

Limit your intake of caffeine, which is found in coffee, tea, and sodas. Caffeine increases vasoconstriction. You should also avoid alcoholic beverages. Alcohol may make you feel warm initially, but after a brief spell of blood vessel dilation, you'll experience a drop in overall body temperature that can lead to vasoconstriction.

# Supplements for Raynaud's

Take a high-quality multivitamin to ensure you get your essential nutrients. Other supplements you might want to consider include the following:

## MAGNESIUM

Taking magnesium as a supplement can help relax the spastic blood vessels that cause pain and numbness in the extremeties.

## FISH OIL AND FLAXSEED OIL

Both these oils can help thin the blood and improve blood flow, mainly in people with the primary form of disease. But again, avoid these products if you're already taking an anticoagulant.

# Stay-Healthy Strategies

- **STAY WARM.** Do whatever you can to prevent an attack of Raynaud's, even if it means wearing gloves in warm weather or using oven mitts to retrieve items in the freezer.

- **MANAGE STRESS.** Stress is a trigger for Raynaud's, so do what you can to minimize stressful events in your life. Consider taking up a relaxation exercise such as meditation, prayer, or tai chi.

- **EXERCISE REGULARLY.** Physical activity, especially the aerobic kind, can help improve overall blood flow in the body. Exercise is especially beneficial for people suffering from primary Raynaud's.

- **GET CHECKED.** Raynaud's can be a sign of another more serious disorder such as scleroderma. So talk to your doctor if you are suffering from Raynaud's. You may need to undergo blood tests to determine whether you have another disease that warrants treatment.

# The Art of Staying Warm

It isn't always easy to keep Raynaud's at bay. In some sufferers, the condition can strike even in the summer. But there are steps you can take to minimize your attack and to stay warm.

Start by keeping extra clothing in your car. An extra jacket or sweatshirt can help you trap body heat when temperatures drop or you enter an air-conditioned restaurant. You should also keep a pair of spare gloves in your purse, car, or desk. Although you may be uncomfortable wearing gloves at your office or in the supermarket in the summer, they are one of your best weapons against chilly temperatures.

Consider purchasing chemical warmers that you can clutch in your hand when you feel cold. These hand warmers are often used by outdoor enthusiasts who engage in winter sports.

Wear a hat. A hat is one of the best ways to preserve body heat. And make sure to dress in layers. Many companies now make undergarments that you can easily wear under sweaters.

Other ways to warm up include drinking a hot beverage, washing your hands under warm water (with rubber gloves if it's hot water), and circling your arms backward as if preparing to throw an underhand pitch.

# RHEUMATOID ARTHRITIS

EVERY DAY, TWO MILLION PEOPLE in the United States awaken to the pain of rheumatoid arthritis (RA), an autoimmune disease that causes inflammation in the lining of the joints. The affected joints are typically warm, swollen, and painful, and often experience a decrease in the range of motion.

RA belongs to a family of rheumatic disorders that also includes lupus, scleroderma, and fibromyalgia. These conditions afflict the body's connective tissues. At the same time, RA is an arthritic condition, which means it causes the joints to become inflamed. As an autoimmune condition, RA is characterized by a malfunction of the immune system in which antibodies attack otherwise healthy tissue, in this case the lining of the joints.

Most RA sufferers are women. Many are first diagnosed between the ages of 30 and 55, though the incidence tends to increase with age. The disease occurs in all races and ethnic groups and can begin in childhood and young adulthood. The prevalence is slightly higher among Pima and Chippewa Indians and slightly lower among African-Americans living in rural settings.

## What It Looks Like

The signs and symptoms of RA can vary significantly from one patient to the next. RA can cause mild to severe pain in and around the joints. It can also cause a reduction in your range of motion. Some people who have RA are plagued by persistent fatigue or a low-grade fever. As a result, sufferers may experience depression brought on by the frustrations of having RA.

RA tends to involve specific joints, including the metacarpophalangeal joints, which are the first row of knuckles down from the wrist, and the proximal interphalangeal joints, which are the second row. In addition, it tends to afflict the first row of joints on the toes down from the ankle, called the metatarsophalangeal joints.

Most people with RA will notice morning stiffness or stiffness after prolonged periods of inactivity. About a third will develop rheumatoid nodules, bumps below the skin that may be as small as a grain or as big as a golf ball.

RA is most likely caused by a combination of genetics and environment. There appears to be a genetic predisposition toward developing RA in people who have a gene called the human leukocyte antigen complex, which is involved in immune function. But experts believe that RA may also be triggered by environmental factors, including infection, hormones, cigarette smoking, stress, and occupational hazards, such as asbestos, asphalt, and vibration.

# 🍴 What to Eat

According to Harry Fischer, M.D., co-author of *What to Do When the Doctor Says It's Rheumatoid Arthritis*, one of the best things you can do for RA is to maintain a healthy weight. Excess weight imposes a greater burden on your joints and can worsen your pain. So a well-balanced diet filled with plenty of nutrient-rich foods is critical.

Among the best foods you can eat is fish that contain omega-3 fatty acids that can reduce the pain and swelling in RA. Studies of two specific acids—eicosapentaenoic acid (EPA) and docosahexaenoic acid (DHA)—have been shown to reduce the number of swollen joints and morning stiffness. Good options include salmon, sardines, mackerel, herring, anchovies, and lake trout.

Fresh fruits and vegetables are also important. These foods contain antioxidants—vitamins A, C, and E—that are believed to shield the body from free-oxygen radicals that cause disease. Some experts believe that the joint damage in RA is caused by excessive amounts of free radicals in the joints. Beta carotene, which forms vitamin A, and vitamin C are found in fruits and vegetables. Vitamin E is found in grains, vegetable oils, and nuts.

In addition, you need adequate calcium, a mineral found in dairy products, fortified foods, and leafy greens, that helps counter the breakdown of bone. Many people who have had RA for a long time take corticosteroid medications such as prednisone, which raises the risk of osteoporosis. People with RA are also at greater risk because the pain can prevent them from getting enough

exercise. In addition, your risk goes up if you're female, have a slim build, and have a family history of osteoporosis.

It's also important to get enough phosphorous in your diet if you have RA. Like calcium, phosphorous helps strengthen bone. Phosphorous can be found in virtually all foods but is most prevalent in protein-rich foods such as milk, meat, poultry, fish, eggs, legumes, and nuts.

To ensure that calcium and phosphorous are properly absorbed, eat foods that contain vitamin D. Vitamin D is found in fortified milk and also made in the skin when it is exposed to sunlight. Preliminary research suggests that vitamin D may have a protective role in RA. It may also help relieve joint and muscle pain in people who are vitamin D–deficient.

In addition, people who have RA tend to have lower levels of vitamin B6, or pyridoxine, a B vitamin found in whole-grain cereals, fish, bananas, and peanut butter. One study found that as levels of vitamin B6 decreased, the activity, severity, and pain of RA increased.

Without enough vitamin B6, your body has a hard time breaking down an amino acid called homocysteine, which has been associated with heart disease and stroke. Experts believe the inflammation in RA causes a reduction in vitamin B6, which is why it's essential to get enough in your diet.

Finally, people with RA who take methotrexate need to make sure they get enough folic acid. Folic acid works with vitamin B12 to produce hemoglobin in red blood cells, and in pregnant women it can help lower the risk for neural tube defects in the developing fetus. In addition, folic acid lowers levels of homocysteine, an amino acid that has been associated with heart disease. Folic acid, also called folate or folacin, is found in leafy greens, legumes, fortified cereals, and enriched grain products such as macaroni, bread, cornmeal, rice, and flour. People who take methotrexate to treat RA may be at risk for deficiency of folic acid and require supplementation.

## What Not to Eat

It would be simple if there were certain foods that triggered RA, however, there is no scientific evidence to prove that specific foods can worsen your symptoms. But even without proof, many people believe that certain foods and food additives worsen their pain. Foods that potentially aggravate RA pain include tomatoes, corn, pork, oranges, milk, and any foods that contain gluten.

If you think a certain food is aggravating your RA symptoms, you may consider trying an elimination diet. Removing a food from your diet, then gradually introducing it back in small quantities and watching for symptoms may help you identify a food culprit. Before attempting an elimination diet, talk to your doctor or a registered dietitian. Eliminating a food that supplies important nutrients—the calcium and vitamin D in milk, for instance—means that you'll need supplements or another food to replace the missing nutrients.

In general, you should also avoid foods that promote weight gain. Foods that are rich in saturated fat, such as red meat, butter, and whole dairy products, and those high in trans-fatty acids, such as processed foods, should also be restricted. In addition, you should be careful about drinking alcohol, which is not only high in calories and void of nutrients, but can also cause dangerous

### Can Glucosamine and Chondroitin Sulfate Help RA?

For years, people who have osteoarthritis have reaped the benefits of these two supplements, which can help alleviate the pain and stiffness caused by wear and tear on the cartilage. But glucosamine and chondroitin sulfate generally don't help people with RA, whose pain and stiffness is brought on by inflammation.

interactions with certain RA medications.

## Supplements for RA

Taking a quality multivitamin can ensure you get the essential nutrients you need. But there are also some other supplements that may have some benefit in taming the inflammation of RA:

### FISH OIL

Studies have found that fish oil may alleviate the pain and swelling of RA, especially in mild cases. But fish oil supplements do not help relieve RA pain any better than nonsteroidal anti-inflammatory drugs (NSAIDs) do, and they do not slow the progression of disease.

If you do decide to take fish oil supplements, consult your doctor first. Fish oil can cause the blood to become thinner, and combining it with NSAIDs, aspirin, or blood-thinning medications such as warfarin (Coumadin) or heparin may cause excessive bleeding. In addition, some fish oils may be high in fat-soluble vitamins (A, D, E and K), which can cause toxic effects in the body if allowed to build up.

## GAMMA LINOLENIC ACID (GLA)

GLA is an omega-6 fatty acid that may also have anti-inflammatory effects. It is found in supplements such as evening primrose oil, black currant oil, and borage oil. Like fish oil, it also has a blood thinning effect. You should talk to your doctor before taking supplements with GLA.

## SELENIUM

Selenium is a trace mineral found in soil that acts as an antioxidant. People who have RA generally have lower levels of selenium in their blood. Preliminary studies suggest that selenium may help relieve symptoms by controlling free-radical damage. Selenium is found in an array of foods including Brazil nuts, seafood, rice, and beef.

## FOLIC ACID

People who are taking methotrexate should consult their doctor about the need for supplementation with folic acid. Even low doses of methotrexate can deplete folate stores and cause side effects that resemble folate deficiency.

## HERBAL REMEDIES

According to the Arthritis Foundation, there are other anti-inflammatory supplements that might reduce the pain and swelling of RA:

- **BOSWELLIA** is an herb used in the traditional Ayurvedic medicine of India. When combined with turmeric and zinc or ginger and ashwagandha, it may relieve inflammation.

- **BROMELAIN** is an enzyme in pineapple juice that breaks down protein and relieve pain and inflammation.

- **GRAPESEED** comes from the seeds of grapes from a woody vine native to Asia minor. Preliminary evidence shows it may strengthen connective tissue.

- **GREEN TEA** comes from the leaves of the tea plant in southeast Asia. The tea contains polyphenols, which are antioxidants that combat inflammation.

- **THUNDER GOD VINE** comes from the leaf and root of a vine-like plant in Asia. Studies have shown it may suppress the immune system and relieve the pain and inflammation of RA.

## Stay-Healthy Strategies

- **SEEK TREATMENT FOR RA.** This condition is best treated aggressively with a combination of disease-modifying antirheumatic drugs such as methotrexate or biologic response modifiers such as etanercept (Enbrel).

- **TRY TO EXERCISE IF POSSIBLE.** Not moving can aggravate your pain, weaken muscles, and cause increasing stiffness in your joints. It can also worsen depression.

- **GET YOUR SLEEP.** Good sleep combats fatigue, helps you cope with pain, and boosts your energy. Not enough sleep can cause depression.

- **LEARN TO DO THINGS IN NEW WAYS.** On the job and at home, learn to adjust the objects you use and the way you move so that you lessen pain and reduce strain on your joints.

# ROSACEA

OUR FACES REDDEN FOR MYRIAD REASONS: a hot day, too much sun, an embarrassing moment. But for some people, reddening of the facial skin is a medical problem known as rosacea.

Rosacea is a common inflammatory skin disease that occurs in approximately fourteen million adults. The condition is especially common in people with fair complexions and seems to be more prevalent in people with a tendency to blush. But unlike blushing, rosacea causes the skin to redden for extended periods of time, often an hour or more. Eventually, people with rosacea may have permanently red skin. In some people it may cause sensitivity and inflammation of the eyes. Rosacea may also affect the nose, causing the nose to become large and bulbous, a condition known as rhinophyma. The late comedian W.C. Fields became famous for his bulbous nose, which was actually a case of rhinophyma.

Most people develop rosacea after age 30. As the condition progresses, the redness worsens, often causing pimples, bumps, and visible blood vessels to appear on the face. Rosacea seems to be more common in women, but it is more severe when it occurs in men.

The symptoms of rosacea are triggered by different factors in different people. Some people react to spicy foods, others to extreme temperatures. Still others experience rosacea when they're under stress. Some people report a worsening of symptoms during strenuous exercise, menopause, and drinking alcohol. The symptoms typically alternate between periods of remission and flare-up.

People who have rosacea may be vulnerable to depression and anxiety over the changes in their appearance. They may develop low self-esteem and suffer the consequences in their professional and personal lives.

Unfortunately, there is no cure for rosacea, only treatment and control of the symptoms. Rosacea sufferers need to be treated by dermatologists, who may prescribe a topical antibiotic. More severe cases may require treatment with an oral antibiotic. In extreme cases, surgery may be required to reduce the size of a bulbous nose.

Regardless of the severity, rosacea benefits from a healthy lifestyle, which includes a good diet.

## 🔍 What It Looks Like

At its earliest stages, people with rosacea will notice a tendency to blush or flush, though it often comes and goes. The redness typically appears on the chin, forehead, cheeks, and nose. After a while, the redness may persist and resemble a sunburn that refuses to go away. Over time, as the condition progresses, small red bumps or pustules that resemble acne may develop, but they won't be accompanied by blackheads. The facial skin may burn, sting, or itch. Many people also develop tiny but visible blood vessels on the face. And in some people, the skin may become dry and rough and develop raised red patches called plaques.

In some cases the eyes become involved, causing what is called ocular rosacea. The eyes may feel irritated and appear watery or red. In addition, the eyelids may become red and swollen, and sufferers may become prone to styes, infections in the glands of the eyelid. If the eye involvement is severe and untreated, it may result in corneal damage and vision loss.

## 🍴 What to Eat

Load up on fresh fruits and vegetables, which will help on several fronts, says Christine Gerbstadt, M.D., R.D., a spokesperson for the American Dietetic Association. Fruits and veggies are rich in fiber, which can help reduce transit time, the amount of time between the ingestion of food and its elimination. Insoluble fibers, commonly known as roughage, don't dissolve in water, but instead soak it up, which adds bulk and softness to stool and helps move waste through the colon.

Good sources of insoluble fiber include whole-wheat foods; wheat, oat, and corn bran; veggies such as cauliflower and green beans; flaxseeds; and the skins of fruits and root vegetables. To make a high-fiber diet more tolerable, drink a lot of fluids (preferably water), which will help reduce transit time.

Another good food to eat is cold-water fish, which contain omega-3 fatty acids that can help tame inflammation. Good choices include salmon, tuna, and trout. You can also get omega-3s from flaxseed oil.

And because treatment for rosacea often involves antibiotics, make sure to eat unsweetened yogurt that contains *acidophilus* cultures. These probiotics will help restore the healthy bacteria destroyed by antibiotics.

## 🚫 What Not to Eat

Avoid any foods or beverages that can cause the skin to redden. That means eliminating spicy foods, alcoholic beverages, and hot foods and drinks, such as soups, coffee, and tea. Spices that trigger rosacea symptoms include chili powder, white and black pepper, and cayenne.

Consider cutting back or eliminating caffeine. Caffeine is a stimulant that can make some people anxious, which can trigger rosacea.

Some people experience a flare-up of symptoms from eating specific foods. A survey by the National Rosacea Society found that some people are bothered by chocolate, tomatoes, yogurt, cheese, meats prepared in marinade, and citrus fruits. The best way to figure out your triggers is to keep a diary that notes what you ate and any subsequent symptoms. Check out the National Rosacea Society Web site at www.rosacea.org/patients/materials/checklist.html for a patient diary checklist that you can download.

## 💊 Supplements for Rosacea

Taking a quality multivitamin can provide you with the essential nutrients you need. You might also consider taking the following:

### HYDROCHLORIC ACID

Some experts believe that people with rosacea are deficient in hydrochloric acid, an acid in the stomach that aids digestion. The amount of acid often lessens with age. Always consult a physician before taking hydrochloric acid supplements, because taking too much can damage the stomach lining.

### VITAMIN C

An extra dose of this antioxidant vitamin can help enhance immunity.

### PROBIOTICS

*Lactobacillus acidophilus* is a healthy bacteria that can help improve skin health and restore the bacteria killed off by treatments with antibiotics.

## 📋 Stay-Healthy Strategies

- **EXERCISE IN MODERATION.** High-intensity workouts can provoke reddening in people with rosacea. You might also consider breaking up your exercise into shorter intervals.

- **CLEANSE YOUR FACE GENTLY WITH NONABRASIVE CLEANSERS AND LUKEWARM WATER.** Avoid any skin products that aggravate your condition, including those that are scented.

- **BEWARE OF THE BLUES.** Having rosacea can be emotionally upsetting. If you suspect you have depression, seek professional help.

- **WATCH THE WEATHER.** Wear sunscreen whenever you're outdoors and avoid extreme temperatures, which can aggravate rosacea.

### Medical Conditions Can Trigger Rosacea

Whether it's a cold or the hot flashes of menopause, certain medical conditions are known to set off a flare-up of rosacea. In women, menopause may be the first time that rosacea emerges. Rosacea has also been linked to high blood pressure. But if your symptoms are accompanied by itching, troubles breathing, or diarrhea, call your doctor.

# SCLERODERMA

IN A SOCIETY THAT PUTS A PREMIUM on clear complexions and smooth, unwrinkled skin, any illness that attacks the skin can be devastating—physically and psychologically. For some people, the skin may actually harden and become painful in a condition known as scleroderma.

Scleroderma, also called systemic sclerosis, is a complex illness that comes in several forms, each with differing levels of severity. It is an autoimmune disease, meaning that there is a malfunction of the immune system in which healthy tissue comes under attack. It is a disease of the body's connective tissue, namely the skin, tendons, and bones. At the same time, scleroderma is a rheumatic condition characterized by inflammation and/or pain in the muscles, joints, or fibrous tissues.

The term *scleroderma* is a Greek term, literally meaning "hard skin." In its localized form, hard tight skin is often the extent of the disease. But in its systemic form, the problems are more complex and may involve vital organs such as the lungs, kidneys, and heart. Each of these two broad categories has three different types, with varying degrees of severity and types of skin or organ involvement. Careful diagnosis by a skilled rheumatologist is often necessary to determine the extent of each case.

The basic problem in scleroderma is the overproduction of collagen, the primary protein in the body's connective tissue. In the skin, it is responsible for both strength and elasticity. Without it, skin wrinkles.

Experts believe that scleroderma occurs when the immune system stimulates cells called fibroblasts to produce too much collagen. The buildup of collagen creates thickened connective tissue around skin cells and internal organs. In milder forms of the disease, the buildup is confined to the skin and blood vessels. In systemic forms, it can interfere with the normal functioning of the skin, blood vessels, joints, and internal organs.

Every patient has her own symptoms, with varying degrees of severity. Some cases are mild, while others may be life-threatening. The severity of disease depends on the organs that are involved and the extent of that involvement, as well as the accuracy and speed of diagnosis and effectiveness of treatment.

According to the Scleroderma Foundation, scleroderma affects approximately 300,000 people in the United States. Nearly a third of them have the systemic form, with the rest having the localized form. The disease is much more common in women than in men, but it can be found in almost every age group. Most people are first diagnosed between the ages of 25 and 55.

No one knows exactly what causes scleroderma. Although the condition is not directly inherited, experts believe there may be a genetic predisposition in some families that have other autoimmune diseases such as lupus and celiac disease. But the disease is not contagious, and it remains rare for two close family members to have the disease.

## What It Looks Like

Some people with scleroderma have hardening of the skin. Others develop calcinosis, calcium deposits on the fingers, behind the forearms, and on the buttocks that sometimes become painful. Many people have Raynaud's phenomenon, a condition in which the blood vessels in the hands—and often the toes or tips of the nose or ears—constrict abnormally in reaction to cold or extreme temperatures, stress, or certain activities. As a result, the fingers and toes may react with extreme sensitivity to the cold, sometimes even when temperatures are normal or warm.

Some people may notice they have difficulties swallowing, which indicates the disease has affected the esophagus. Swallowing problems may first be noticed as heartburn.

Other people may have painful joints. More severe cases of the disease may involve other organs including the lungs, heart, and kidneys, which is why regular examinations are important. Like other autoimmune diseases, the symptoms may alternate between flare-ups and remission.

## What to Eat

If you can, try to eat a diet rich in antioxidants, which will keep your immune system strong. Fruits, vegetables, and whole grains are all good sources of these nutrients, as well as fiber, which will keep constipation at bay. If you can't tolerate raw fruits and veggies, consider cooking them first.

Make sure you eat enough calcium, especially if you're taking steroids as part of your treatment, says Lise Gloede, R.D., C.D.E., a nutrition consultant in Arlington, Virginia. Calcium will keep bones strong and help stave off osteoporosis. Good sources of calcium include low-fat milk, yogurt, cheese, and dark leafy greens. Make sure to also get enough vitamin D, which is essential for the absorption of calcium. Vitamin D occurs in fortified foods such as milk and soy milk.

It's also important to drink a lot of water, especially with meals. Water will help foods to go down and also help to prevent constipation. In people whose esophageal function is affected by scleroderma, water is essential to help move the food downward.

The way you eat is just as important, if not more so, than the types of food you eat. If you're experiencing problems with motility of food—it's moving slowly down the throat and into the stomach—try eating softer foods such as apple-sauce and mashed potatoes. You can also purée foods such as chicken and dip drier foods, such as bread, into milk. Get into the habit of sitting down for your meals and always eat slowly. Make sure to chew your food well.

Try eating four to six smaller meals instead of two or three large ones. Large meals are more likely to stay in the stomach longer and are more likely to irritate your symptoms of reflux.

## What Not to Eat

Limit your intake of alcohol, caffeine, chocolate, and carbonated beverages, which can stimulate the production of stomach acid. You should also steer clear of highly acidic foods such as citrus fruits, tomatoes and tomato sauces, and onions. All these foods can stimulate stomach acids that can reflux into the esophagus.

Avoid eating too close to bedtime, because that will prevent you from taking advantage of gravity to encourage food to move downward.

## Supplements for Scleroderma

Take a high-quality multivitamin that supplies 100 percent of most vital nutrients. Beyond that, most people with scleroderma should avoid taking supplements because they may interact with other medications.

## Stay-Healthy Strategies

- **CONSULT A REGISTERED DIETITIAN** for an individualized nutrition plan tailored to your specific needs, symptoms, and medications. Check out the American Dietetic Association's Web site at www.eatright.org for registered dietitians in your area.

- **STAY AS ACTIVE AS POSSIBLE.** Exercise can help you maintain your physical functioning and preserve your independence. If necessary, talk to a physical therapist about specific exercises for you.

- **MANAGE STRESS.** Too much stress can trigger a flare-up, and in people with Raynaud's it can cause the blood vessels in the fingers to constrict. So find a relaxation exercise you enjoy and develop ways to cope with your daily stressors.

- **FIND A PHYSICIAN YOU TRUST.** Having scleroderma often means frequent doctor visits. Work with a doctor who can orchestrate all the screenings you need and who is well-versed in scleroderma.

## Get Educated

Getting a diagnosis for scleroderma can be tricky. It often takes years before you even go to the doctor with your symptoms, assuming that a little heartburn is normal or that many people have Raynaud's. Both these assumptions have some truth to them, but if symptoms persist, you should discuss them with your doctor.

Once you go to your doctor, there are often several blood tests and X-rays involved. If it turns out you do have scleroderma, the information can be overwhelming and confusing.

The best thing to do is to learn as much as you can about the disease. You'll learn, for instance, that sometimes the skin will thin out on its own and that many cases of limited scleroderma do not progress beyond where you're at now. You'll also better understand why you need so many screenings. But get your information from reputable sources such as www.scleroderma.org, the Web site of the Scleroderma Foundation.

# SEASONAL AFFECTIVE DISORDER

SOME PEOPLE WELCOME THE COOLER MONTHS of winter as a time for skiing, cozy indoor gatherings, and the chance to escape the heat. But for some people, the cooler spells also bring a depressive condition known as seasonal affective disorder.

Seasonal affective disorder—often called SAD—is just as the name implies: a type of depression that coincides with the seasons. Most SAD sufferers have what is called winter depression, which usually begins in late fall or early winter and goes away by summer. Less commonly, some people have summer depression, which begins in the late spring or early summer, then disappears by winter. Experts believe that SAD is related to changes in the amount of daylight during different times of the year.

According to the American Academy of Family Physicians, winter SAD affects as many as half a million people in the United States. Another 10 to 20 percent of Americans may experience mild SAD. Like depression, the condition is more common in women than in men. SAD is also uncommon in people under age 20. The risk for SAD goes down with age and is more common in northern climates.

People with SAD may undergo treatment with light therapy, which involves spending daily time in front of a specially devised light box. But some people may benefit from therapy or the use of antidepressants.

## What It Looks Like

Not everyone with SAD has the same symptoms. Those who have winter depression may notice a change in appetite that includes cravings for sweet and starchy foods. They may also gain weight and notice a decline in energy levels. Some people suffer fatigue and have a tendency to sleep too much. They may have trouble concentrating and feel overly irritable, sensitive, and isolated. People who have summer depression may experience poor appetite, weight loss, and insomnia.

All SAD sufferers may experience the classic signs of depression, such as feelings of guilt and hopelessness, a loss of interest or pleasure in activities you used to enjoy, and physical problems such as headaches. SAD tends to recur year after year, often at about the same time of year.

## 🍴 What to Eat

Like depression sufferers, people with SAD tend to crave carbohydrates, which trigger the release of the feel-good neurotransmitter serotonin, says Lisa Dorfman, M.S., R.D., a licensed psychotherapist and spokesperson for the American Dietetic Association. But it's important to choose your carbs carefully and to make sure to eat a lot of complex carbohydrates such as fruits, vegetables, and enriched whole-grain foods. These foods contain B vitamins, magnesium, zinc, and other antioxidants, as well as fiber, and will help you feel full longer than simple carbs such as bagels and pasta.

Balance out your carbs with some protein, which will help prevent lethargy. For instance, spread some peanut butter on a slice of toast, or add grilled chicken to your whole-wheat pasta. The combination will help you feel fuller and prevent the highs and lows that come with eating carbs alone.

People with SAD also need to get enough folate, a B vitamin that may be deficient in people with depression. Good sources include spinach, lentils, and peas. In addition, they should eat foods rich in tryptophan, an essential amino acid that aids in the production of serotonin, a feel-good neurotransmitter that is involved in regulating mood. Good sources of tryptophan include poultry, bananas, dairy products, and peas.

Make sure to eat cold-water fish such as salmon, tuna, and mackerel, which are rich in omega-3 fatty acids. These healthy fats are important for proper brain function. Some studies have found that these healthy fats may help relieve depression.

## 🚫 What Not to Eat

Limit foods high in saturated fats such as red meat, cheese, butter, and rich desserts. Although depression can cause cravings for these foods, they ultimately make your body sluggish and fatigued. The same is true for all kinds of sugar, even the natural variety. Sugary foods deliver a quick jolt of energy, but then cause a crash that depletes energy and leads to fatigue, which can worsen your symptoms.

Some individuals should also avoid aspartame, the artificial sweetener commonly known as Equal or NutraSweet. Studies have found that aspartame may affect the proper function of serotonin. If you develop a headache, fatigue, lethargy, or anxiety after consuming aspartame, discontinue its use.

Finally, avoid drinking alcohol and caffeine. Alcohol is a depressant that causes dehydration, which can lead to fatigue. Caffeine is a stimulant, and, in excess, it can cause anxiety, irritability, and exhaustion.

## Supplements for SAD

Start by taking a quality multivitamin, which will ensure you're getting the essential nutrients you need. Before taking any supplement talk to your doctor. Some remedies may interact with antidepressant medications. Possible supplements include the following:

### SAM-E

SAM-e, or adenosylmethionine, is a natural substance that may relieve depression and fatigue. It helps produce and regulate hormones that affect mood. But any benefit requires very high doses, and it can be quite expensive.

### ST. JOHN'S WORT

Although highly regarded in Europe as a treatment for depression, experts in the United States say it is effective only for mild depression. And be careful: St. John's wort should never be taken with other antidepressants, and it may interact with other medications.

### 5-HTP

5-HTP is a form of tryptophan that can help boost levels of serotonin. Taking it at bedtime may help promote sleep, and higher doses may relieve depression. But it should never be taken if you're on antidepressants.

### B COMPLEX VITAMIN

The B vitamins are involved in the healthy metabolism of neurotransmitters. Some of these vitamins may be deficient in people with depression.

### FISH OIL

Fish oil supplements contain omega-3 fatty acids, which may help with proper brain function. But check with a doctor if you're on a blood-thinning medication such as warfarin (Coumadin).

## Stay-Healthy Strategies

- **CONSULT WITH A REGISTERED DIETITIAN** about your food habits and eating behaviors. A nutrition expert can evaluate your diet, identify excesses and deficiencies, and spot food interactions that may be playing a role in your depression.

- **HEAD OUTDOORS.** Being in natural daylight can sometimes help relieve the depression. So try taking a walk even on crisp, wintry days.

- **EXERCISE REGULARLY.** Physical activity is a natural mood booster, so try to do something active every day.

- **LET IN SOME DAYLIGHT.** Rearrange your rooms and offices, if possible, so that you spend more time near windows and get more sunlight.

# Surviving the Holiday Blues

For some people, the holiday season is a joyous time, filled with family gatherings, social events, and acts of charity. But the high expectations of the season create a difficult time for other people who may suffer from a condition experts call the holiday blues.

Although the holiday blues may be worsened by winter weather, they're more often caused by the stress and high expectations that come with the holidays. The weeks leading up to the actual holidays are often filled with obligations and demands that some people may find taxing and draining. Some people may become depressed by all the activity and react with symptoms of stress such as headaches, overeating, and troubles sleeping. Those who don't have close family ties may sink into a real depression, fueled by loneliness.

Here are some strategies from the National Mental Health Association to help you navigate this difficult time of year:

- Keep expectations realistic. Avoid setting out with lofty goals, only to find yourself overwhelmed. Learn to pace yourself.

- Get organized. Plan your purchases in advance and make lists. Prioritize the important activities. Be realistic about what you can and cannot do.

- Shift your focus from the day to the season. The season of giving is just that, so try spreading out activities over a period of weeks to decrease your stress and boost your enjoyment.

- Keep in mind that the holidays do not mean that feelings of sadness or loneliness will just go away. Learn to accept these sentiments, even if you don't express them.

- Live in the moment. Don't dwell on how your holiday used to be. Accept that life brings changes. You might also try looking toward the future.

- Perform acts of charity. Volunteering some time to help others can often improve a blue mood.

- Enjoy activities that are free, such as driving around to look at holiday decorations, going window shopping without buying, or making a snowperson with children.

- Avoid excessive drinking, which will only increase your feelings of depression.

- Celebrate the holidays in a new way this year. Create a new tradition or ritual that you truly enjoy.

- Spend time with supportive and caring people. Reach out and make new friends or contact someone you have not heard from for awhile.

- Make time for yourself. Taking time out to recharge your batteries—however you choose to do it—can help you enjoy the season a little more, especially if you let others share in the responsibilities.

# SHINGLES

MOST ADULTS CAN STILL RECALL the itchy aggravation of chicken pox. Today, the incidence of chicken pox has been significantly reduced with the varicella vaccine, an inoculation that shields you from chicken pox. But in older adults, the virus can sometimes be reactivated and emerge as a disease called shingles.

Shingles is characterized by an outbreak of rash or blisters on the skin. It is caused by the varicella-zoster virus, the same virus that causes chicken pox and is a member of the herpes virus family. Experts believe the virus lies dormant in your body after your initial bout of chicken pox, which means anyone who has had chicken pox is at risk for shingles.

Over the course of an 85-year lifetime, one in seven people will experience shingles. Those who are more likely to experience a recurrence include those with compromised immune systems, such as people who take steroids and those who are undergoing chemotherapy. People who have undergone organ transplants are also at greater risk because they must take drugs to suppress their immune systems. In addition, people with HIV infection are more susceptible. Some experts believe high levels of stress can raise your risk too.

Experts believe that during the original battle with the varicella-zoster virus, some particles leave the skin blisters and move into the nervous system. When the varicella-zoster virus is reactivated by stress, infection, or illness, the virus moves back down the long nerve fibers to the skin, resulting in the blisters that we describe as shingles.

The severity and duration of an attack is influenced by age: The older you are, the more severe the attack. But the severity of shingles can be reduced by immediate treatment with antiviral drugs, such as acyclovir, valcyclovir, or famcyclovir. Antiviral drugs may also help prevent the painful after-effects of shingles, called postherpetic neuralgia. This condition can cause severe pain that can linger for as little as a month or as long as several years.

One way to prevent shingles is by getting a shingles vaccine called Zostavax. The vaccine was just approved by the U.S. Food and Drug Administration in 2006 for people age 60 and older who have had chickenpox. Researchers found that the vaccine reduced the expected number of cases of shingles by half and dramatically reduced the severity and complications in people who still got the disease. Keep in mind that the shingles vaccine is a preventive therapy. It will not work as a treatment for those who already have shingles or postherpetic neuralgia.

## 🔍 What It Looks Like

Shingles typically starts with burning or tingling pain in or under the skin. Sometimes it may start with numbness. Some people may also develop fever, chills, headache, or upset stomach.

After a few days, a rash resembling that of chicken pox will emerge on the skin. These are typically small, fluid-filled blisters that appear on the now-reddened skin. The blisters are typically accompanied by severe pain that is often intense and unrelenting. The rash is most likely to appear on the back, trunk, chest, head, face, neck, and lower part of the spine.

For most people, the lesions eventually heal and leave no scars. The pain subsides within three to five weeks. However, shingles is a serious health threat that can lead to postherpetic neuralgia, an extremely painful condition that can trigger depression. The same people who are at greater risk for shingles are also at greater risk for postherpetic neuralgia.

For some people, shingles can occur more than once. If it does, it typically strikes at a different location. Those who have recurrent shingles may be infected with a related herpes simplex virus, not the varicella-zoster virus.

## 🍴 What to Eat

Boost your immunity by eating a lot of fresh, unprocessed foods such as fruits, vegetables, and whole-grain foods, says Amy Neuzil, N.D., a naturopathic physician in Austin, Texas.

Eat foods rich in B vitamins, which are essential for healthy nerves. B vitamins thiamin and vitamin B12 are especially beneficial to include in your diet. Good sources of thiamin include lean pork, whole-grain bread, legumes, nuts, and seeds. Vitamin B12 is found in animal products such as seafood, meat, poultry, eggs, and milk.

Make sure to eat foods that contain magnesium too. Magnesium is a major mineral that promotes healthy nerves. Good sources of magnesium include spinach, peanut butter, legumes, nuts, whole grains, and lima beans.

It's also important to eat foods that are rich in L-lysine, an amino acid that may block the activity of the herpes virus. L-lysine occurs in beans, fish, red meat, and dairy products.

### Is Shingles Contagious?

Yes and no. An adult cannot catch shingles from someone else who has it. You also can't get shingles just by being near someone who has chicken pox. But the shingles rash can cause chicken pox in someone who has never had chicken pox before.

## ⊘ What Not to Eat

Steer clear of foods that promote inflammation, such as saturated fats and refined carbohydrates. Saturated fats are found in red meat, butter, and whole dairy products. Refined carbohydrates include most packaged goods and white breads.

You should also stay away from foods that contain an amino acid called arginine, which helps promote the replication of the virus. These foods include peanuts, almonds, raisins, nuts, and seeds, as well as anything with chocolate.

Avoid drinking too much caffeine or alcohol, which, in excess, can weaken immunity.

## ⚬ Supplements for Shingles

Take a high-quality multivitamin to ensure overall health and well-being. You might also consider taking the following:

### L-LYSINE
L-lysine has long been regarded as a treatment for any type of a herpes infection. It works by inhibiting replication of the herpes virus and is best taken on an empty stomach.

### AVENA SATIVA
*Avena sativa* is oat straw, which is available as an herbal remedy. It may help reduce inflammation associated with shingles.

### LICORICE
Licorice contains anti-inflammatory and antiviral substances that can relieve the pain and inflammation of shingles.

### COLOSTRUM
Colostrum is the nutrient-rich liquid that mammals produce before lactation. Bovine colostrum may help bolster immunity.

### REISHI MUSHROOMS
Reishi mushrooms are believed to strengthen the immune system. If you choose to eat them as a food, make sure to wash them thoroughly.

### CAPSICUM ANNUUM
This is a topical cream made from cayenne pepper. As a cream, it can reduce the pain and viral activity associated with shingles.

## 📋 Stay-Healthy Strategies

- **GET TREATED EARLY.** Early diagnosis and prompt treatment with antiviral medications can lower your risk for postherpetic neuralgia. If you notice any symptoms, contact your doctor immediately.

- **MAKE SURE TO SLEEP.** A good night's sleep will strengthen your immune system and make you better able to tolerate the pain while you heal.

- **CONSIDER ACUPUNCTURE.** This ancient Chinese medicine may help relieve the pain associated with shingles.

- **RELIEVE YOUR STRESS.** It isn't easy living with chronic pain, but stress can make it worse. Develop strategies to reduce your stress, such as meditation, deep breathing, or progressive muscle relaxation exercises.

# SJOGREN'S SYNDROME

FOR SOME PEOPLE, DRY EYES AND A DRY MOUTH are the result of a dry, windy day; not enough liquids; or perhaps rigorous exercise. But others may have these problems every day, especially if they're suffering an autoimmune condition known as Sjogren's syndrome. The disease, which is pronounced SHOW-grinz, is named for the Swedish doctor who first described the condition in 1933.

In Sjogren's syndrome, white blood cells attack the moisture-producing glands of the eyes and mouth, causing excessive dryness. About half the time, Sjogren's occurs alone in what is known as primary Sjogren's. The rest of the cases are secondary Sjogren's because they occur simultaneously with another connective tissue disease such as lupus, rheumatoid arthritis, scleroderma, or polymyositis.

Sjogren's is one of the most prevalent autoimmune disorders in the United States and affects as many as four million people. Ninety percent of all patients are women, with an average age of onset in the late 40s. But the disease does occur in men and can begin at other ages.

Treatment often involves close attention to the eyes and mouth with help from over-the-counter remedies that can promote moisture. Artificial tears, for instance, can help keep eyes lubricated, while mouth gels can moisten the mouth. But in some cases, you may need prescription medications.

## What It Looks Like

Dry eyes and mouth are the most obvious symptoms of Sjogren's, but you may also experience swelling, trouble swallowing and chewing, a dry cough, and cavities. Some people develop oral yeast infections, also known as thrush. Others may have a dry nose and throat. The condition can also cause severe fatigue and pain, depending on the organs that are affected.

Although the symptoms are most noticeable in the eyes and mouth, Sjogren's also affects the rest of the body. The kidneys, gastrointestinal tract, blood vessels, and other vital organs can all become dry, causing fatigue and, in some cases, pain.

No two patients ever have the same constellation of symptoms, as Sjogren's affects every person differently.

## ⍾⍾ What to Eat

Eat a healthy, well-balanced diet to ensure proper immune function, says Jacob Teitelbaum, M.D., author of *Pain Free 1-2-3*. It's also important to eat foods that contain omega-3 fatty acids, the healthy fats that can reduce inflammation, which is involved in the autoimmune response. Foods that contain these fats include cold-water fish such as tuna, salmon, herring, and mackerel. These foods help not just the inflammation, but they can also relieve dry eyes and mouth.

Make sure to also get enough magnesium, a major mineral. Magnesium is an antispasmodic that can help relax muscles and maintain nerve and muscle cells. Foods rich in magnesium include legumes, spinach, pecans, peanut butter, and whole grains.

---

### TIP

*If you have Sjogren's syndrome and plan to become pregnant, tell your doctor first. A certain antibody in your blood may put your unborn baby at risk for heart problems. You'll need to discuss this with your doctor.*

---

## ⊘ What Not to Eat

Don't eat refined sugar, which is found in sodas, desserts, and fruit juices. Refined sugar can worsen inflammation.

Limit your intake of caffeine and alcohol, which can cause dehydration that only causes more dryness in your eyes and mouth. Caffeine is found in coffee, tea, and sodas.

## ⚇ Supplements for Sjogren's

Take a high-quality multivitamin to ensure you get your essential nutrients. Other supplements you might want to consider include the following:

### FISH OIL AND FLAXSEED OIL

Both these oils can help reduce inflammation. But you should avoid these products if you're already taking an anticoagulant such as warfarin (Coumadin), which could cause excessive bleeding.

### MAGNESIUM

Taking magnesium as a supplement can help relax the muscles that are affected by Sjogren's.

## ⍰ Stay-Healthy Strategies

- **USE A HUMIDIFIER.** Humidifiers can keep the environment more comfortable, especially in the winter when the heat is on.

- **SIP WATER REGULARLY** for dry mouth.

- **VISIT YOUR DENTIST REGULARLY.** People with Sjogren's are more vulnerable to cavities.

- **EXERCISE REGULARLY** to relieve the fatigue caused by Sjogren's.

# STRESS

STRESS MAY NOT BE CONSIDERED A DISEASE, but it is certainly an affliction for many people these days. Long commutes to hectic jobs. Family obligations. A jam-packed calendar. By the end of the day, you may not be sick, but you certainly feel the stress in your tense shoulders, aching head, and extreme fatigue.

In reality, stress is a normal response to an event that poses a threat to our well-being and safety, a fight-or-flight reaction that helped our ancestors dodge saber-toothed tigers. The stress reaction braces us to tackle these situations and enhances the odds of our survival.

These days, stress is less likely to come from a giant tiger and more apt to be the result of long hours on the job, relationship difficulties, or the ongoing juggling act that seems so common in modern families. Some events, such as a painful divorce, the death of a loved one, or moving to a new city are naturally stressful. But even happy events can cause stress and anxiety—think of wedding planning or giving birth. You can also get stressed out from excessive worrying.

Not everyone feels the same amount of stress. Some people are just naturally easygoing and better able to shrug off life's most difficult moments or challenges. Others are easily stressed—even a long line at the bank can set off the stress response.

For some people, stress can become chronic and a serious health problem. Some experts believe stress plays a big role in heart disease, cancer, and diabetes. Living with chronic stress keeps stress hormones elevated, which means your body is in a perpetual state of fight-or-flight, even when there is nothing to run from and your body isn't moving. But your body doesn't know that and remains in a constant state of stress.

## 🔎 What It Looks Like

Stress has many effects on the body. According to Kathleen Hall, a stress expert, the founder of the Stress Institute, and the author of *A Life in Balance*, stress can cause blood vessels to narrow, increase your risk for stroke, and lower your immune defenses. Stress also impairs short-term memory, causes fatigue, and increases blood pressure and respiration.

Other signs and symptoms of stress include the following:

- Difficulty sleeping
- Changes in appetite

- Panic attacks
- Muscle tenseness and soreness
- Frequent headaches
- Gastrointestinal problems
- Prolonged feelings of sadness or worthlessness

You may notice that you have cravings for fats and carbohydrates that can deliver quick energy. Eating too much of these foods, however, will encourage your body to stockpile the fat in your belly, where you have a ready supply of energy in the event of a real emergency. The problem occurs when the fat isn't burned up, which is what happens when the stress comes from sources that don't require energy, such as our fretful minds.

## ¶¶¶ What to Eat

A healthy, well-balanced diet is the best pre-scription for times when you're seriously stressed, Hall says. Among the best foods are those that contain vitamin C, which some stud-ies have found help to decrease the physical effects of stress, such as reducing blood pressure and lowering the production of cortisol. Good sources of vitamin C include blueberries, straw-berries, broccoli, and tomatoes. These foods con-tain antioxidants that can help combat disease.

When you do have a carb craving, reach for whole grains, which will keep you full longer. Make sure to also eat foods high in B vitamins, especially B6, such as turkey, tuna, sunflower seeds, and bananas. B6 is involved in the produc-tion of serotonin, the feel-good hormone, and helps produce a calming effect.

Be sure to also drink a lot of water, which is naturally cooling and relaxing. Water will help flush out any toxins that may be taxing your body.

The way you eat matters too. When you're overly busy, you may be tempted to skip meals. Don't. Instead, make sure to schedule regular meals and to eat a normal amount at each sitting. Plan exactly what you're going to eat and where you'll eat it. Planning prevents last-minute runs to fast food restaurants where you're less likely to eat well. Having a regular schedule of meals will also help you feel in greater control. In addition, it's a good idea to tote around some healthy snacks to keep you fortified and to prevent mindless nibbling.

---

### TIP

*Don't let stress make you fat. Many people are vulnerable to overeating when they're feeling stressed out. Learn to take control of stress so you don't overindulge and make the wrong food choices.*

---

## What Not to Eat

You might be craving them, but it's best to steer clear of foods high in sugar, such as chocolate, which will ultimately increase your stress. The initial jolt of energy is always followed by a crash that depletes energy and causes fatigue.

You should also avoid caffeine and alcohol, which may worsen your stress. Too much caffeine can heighten anxiety and insomnia and also cause dehydration, which will tire you out even more. Alcohol is a depressant that, in excess, can keep you from getting the sleep you need. It is also a diuretic that can cause dehydration.

## Supplements for Stress

To make sure you're getting all the nutrients you need, take a multivitamin. You might also consider taking the following:

### VITAMIN C

Studies have shown that high doses of vitamin C can help keep you healthy during times of stress.

### B COMPLEX VITAMIN

A formulation that includes all the essential B vitamins can help produce a calming effect.

### MAGNESIUM

Magnesium is a major mineral that can promote relaxation in the muscles and help tame the effects of stress.

### CALCIUM

Calcium is a major mineral that has a calming effect on the nervous system.

## Stay-Healthy Strategies

- **GET REGULAR EXERCISE.** Physical activity is the ultimate stress buster because it releases feel-good endorphins. Even a short 10-minute stroll can help.

- **ALTER YOUR THINKING.** It isn't easy, but a lot of stress comes from how we view our circumstances. Some people may see a job loss as an opportunity. Others may view it as a major catastrophe.

- **FACE UP TO FEARS.** Conquering situations that make you nervous can help eliminate stress. So if public speaking gives you the jitters, try joining a club that forces you to do it more regularly.

- **BOOK RELAXATION INTO YOUR DAY.** Whether it's a yoga class or meditating at home, make time to rest and relax. Take a nightly bath, spend time socializing, or pursue hobbies that you really enjoy.

- **DITCH PERFECTION.** Trying to do it all or striving for perfection will set you up for stress. So learn to let go, say no, and focus on what's most important to you.

- **LEARN TO SAY NO.** Women, in particular, have a hard time saying no when someone asks them to bake brownies, take on an extra assignment, or look after someone. Practice ways in which to assert yourself in difficult situations and learn to pick and choose your activities wisely.

# The Body Under Stress

Imagine walking alone through a park late at night. Suddenly, you hear footsteps behind you. Your pace quickens and your heart begins to race. Your senses go into high alert.

These responses are the result of chemical changes inside your brain where the hypothalamus releases corticotropin-releasing hormone (CRH). It is your physical reaction to a potential threat. CRH, in turn, triggers the release of norepinephrine, epinephrine, and cortisol, three hormones that work together to help prepare the body to fight or flee.

With help from these hormones, you become stronger, more agile, and ready to react. You may also become more focused. Internally, your body is mobilizing reserves of fat and carbohydrates for immediate energy, so if the mysterious person grabs for your purse, you're ready to fight or chase him.

Now assume the person walking behind you passes by, and you realize he's simply running to catch a bus. The threat disappears. Your heart rates slows, and you feel calmer. Inside your body, while the other hormones have stopped exerting their effects, cortisol remains, acting on the brain to halt the production of CRH to stop stress response.

In these situations, cortisol is a good thing, a vital hormone that prepares you to cope with a threat. When the stressful event vanishes, cortisol also helps bring a halt to the body's stress response.

# STROKE

EXPERTS CALL IT A BRAIN ATTACK—a medical condition much like a heart attack except that it occurs in the brain and blocks blood flow to this most vital organ. Every 45 seconds in this country, someone has a stroke. Every year, there are about 700,000 strokes, killing nearly 157,000 people. It is the nation's third-leading cause of death behind cancer and heart disease. Strokes are particularly common among African-Americans, who are almost twice as likely to experience a brain attack than Caucasians. They are also more common in men, the elderly, and people with a family history of stroke. Unfortunately, recurrence is common: Approximately 25 percent of people who have a stroke will have another one within five years.

In reality, there are three types of stroke. Most people who have a stroke suffer an ischemic stroke. An ischemic stroke is the result of atherosclerosis, in which a clogged artery obstructs blood flow to the brain. In some cases, the blockage occurs in the blood vessel that leads to the brain, which is called cerebral thrombosis.

In others, a clot forms elsewhere—usually in the heart and the large arteries of the upper chest and neck—and then breaks off and travels to the blood vessels of the brain, a situation known as cerebral embolism. Eventually, the traveling clot gets lodged in a vessel too narrow to pass through. An embolism can also be the result of atrial fibrillation, an irregular heartbeat that can lead to the development of a clot near the heart.

Some people may experience a hemorrhagic stroke, which is a less common form. A hemorrhagic stroke is the result of a weakened blood vessel that ruptures and bleeds. The rupture is usually the result of abnormally formed blood vessels or the ballooning of a weakened part of a blood vessel.

Transient ischemic attacks (TIAs) are a third type of stroke. These relatively minor strokes occur for short periods of time and then go away on their own. TIAs are generally a warning sign that you are at risk for a major stroke.

For the people who survive, a stroke can create a host of physical problems. Many survivors suffer from a lack of coordination, balance, and flexibility, and experience severe pain. If the brain's language processing centers are affected, a survivor may have difficulties with speaking, writing, and reading. Swallowing may be impaired. Memory may be faulty, and problem-solving skills may be diminished. Some survivors may have personality changes. Others experience depression and apathy.

Many of the same medical conditions that raise your risk for heart disease also put you at risk for stroke. These include high blood pressure, high cholesterol, inactivity, a poor diet, and cigarette smoking. Being overweight also elevates your risk, as does drinking alcohol and using illicit drugs. Having another condition that affects the arteries makes a stroke more likely as well.

While you certainly can't change your gender or ethnic makeup, or turn back time, you can take steps to lower your risk for stroke by adopting healthy lifestyle practices. An essential part of that is a well-balanced diet that promotes a healthy weight.

## 🔍 What It Looks Like

Identifying a stroke is essential. A stroke is a medical emergency, and getting treatment quickly is important to your survival. According to the American Stroke Association, the following are the warning signs:

- Sudden numbness or weakness of the face, arm, or leg, especially on one side of the body

- Sudden confusion, trouble speaking or understanding

- Sudden trouble seeing in one or both eyes

- Sudden trouble with walking, dizziness, loss of balance, or coordination

- Sudden, severe headache with no known cause

Anyone who has these symptoms should call 911 immediately. Prompt treatment can make an enormous difference in whether you survive and how well you fare after a stroke.

### Why the Rush?

If you think you're having a stroke, getting to a hospital quickly is imperative. Once there, you'll most likely be given a clot-busting drug that can dissolve the clot. But in order for the drug to be most effective, it needs to be administered as soon as possible.

## 🍴 What to Eat

People at risk for stroke—or who want to prevent another one—should focus on eating a diet that lowers risk factors, says Marie Savard, M.D., author of *The Body Shape Solution for Weight Loss and Wellness*. The diet should be geared toward reducing high cholesterol and high blood pressure and getting blood glucose under control if you have diabetes. A critical component of the eating plan should be losing weight and reducing waist size.

To meet these goals, make sure to eat fish rich in omega-3 fatty acids, which may lower your risk for stroke. Good choices include salmon, tuna, and mackerel. Omega-3s are also found in walnuts, flaxseed, and fortified foods including peanut butter and breakfast cereal.

Incorporate a colorful array of fruits and vegetables so your body gets a lot of phytonutrients and antioxidant vitamins. Fruits and veggies provide fiber as well. Soluble fiber, the kind that dissolves in water, will help slow down digestion and keep blood sugar in check. It also helps reduce LDL cholesterol (the bad kind), triglycerides, and high blood pressure, while raising levels of HDL cholesterol (the good kind). Soluble fiber is found in oats, kidney beans, peas, flaxseed, apples, oranges, and carrots.

But don't leave out insoluble fiber, which can help prevent constipation. Both types of fiber also help minimize weight gain by making you feel full. Insoluble fiber is found in whole-wheat foods, cauliflower, beans, spinach, peas, and apples. As you see, some foods supply both. Other good sources of fiber include whole grains such as brown rice, bulgur wheat, and quinoa.

For protein (as well as fiber), eat legumes such as chickpeas, kidney beans, pinto beans, and black beans. Other good sources of protein include chicken, fish, and soy products. Soybean foods come in many forms including tempeh, tofu, edamame, soy milk, and soy burgers.

Aim to eat primarily monounsaturated fats, which are healthier and less damaging to the arteries than saturated fats. Good sources of monounsaturated fats include avocados, almonds, nuts, pecans, and olive or canola oil.

## What Not to Eat

High blood pressure is a major risk for stroke, so avoid foods high in sodium, such as canned soups, packaged meals, and processed meats such as hot dogs, pastrami, and bologna. Be careful in restaurants—especially fast-food eateries—which tend to load up their food with salt.

Avoid foods high in saturated fats, which occur primarily in animal products such as red meat, dairy products, and butter. All fats contain a lot of calories, so learn to substitute whole dairy and butter with skim versions and consider using margarine spreads made of plant stanols in place of butter. Also try to restrict or limit fried foods, which are typically cooked in high-fat, high-calorie oils.

You should also steer clear of foods that contain trans-fatty acids, which are often found in packaged foods such as candy bars, cookies, muffins, and crackers—the kinds commonly found in vending machines. Beware of any food that contains partially hydrogenated oils, which form trans-fatty acids.

In addition, try to restrict or eliminate foods high in sugar, which can raise insulin levels and cause an increase in cholesterol, triglycerides, and blood pressure.

## Supplements for Stroke

Consider taking a quality multivitamin, which provides the basic nutrients you need, especially on days when you don't eat as well. You might also consider taking the following:

### FISH OIL

Studies show that omega-3 fatty acids offer protection against any form of cardiovascular disease, including stroke. If you're on blood-thinning medication, talk to your doctor first, because fish oil may increase your risk for bleeding.

## CERTAIN B VITAMINS

Taking folic acid and vitamins B6 and B12 may help reduce homocysteine levels, a substance that has been implicated in the development of cardiovascular disease.

## MAGNESIUM

Magnesium is an essential mineral that may help lower blood pressure, relax blood vessels, and promote healthy contractions of the heart.

## PSYLLIUM

Psyllium is a seed husk and a soluble fiber that can help regulate bowels and lower cholesterol. Talk to your doctor before taking psyllium, especially if you have food allergies, because some people react to psyllium.

## ASPIRIN

Research has shown that one baby aspirin a day can prevent heart attack in men and stroke in women. Talk to your doctor before starting on aspirin, which can cause a number of side effects including stomach irritation and bleeding.

## Stay-Healthy Strategies

- **WATCH YOUR WEIGHT.** Make an effort to lose weight and to maintain a healthy weight. Learn to control portions, read food labels, and make healthy food choices.

- **KNOW YOUR BLOOD PRESSURE.** High blood pressure raises your odds of having a stroke, so try to keep yours low with regular exercise and a healthy diet.

- **STOP SMOKING.** Women who smoke and use oral contraceptives are at a higher risk for stroke.

- **EXERCISE EVERY DAY.** Try to make sure you do some form of physical activity, be it walking, yardwork, or bicycling. The key is to be active whenever you can.

### For Women Only

According to the National Stroke Association, women sometimes experience stroke symptoms that men won't. These include the following:

- Sudden face and limb pain
- Sudden hiccups
- Sudden nausea
- Sudden general weakness
- Sudden chest pain
- Sudden shortness of breath
- Sudden palpitations

# TEMPOROMANDIBULAR JOINT

MOST PEOPLE DON'T GIVE A THOUGHT to their temporomandibular joint. But every time you talk, chew, yawn, or laugh, you're exercising this important joint, which connects the upper jaw to the lower jaw. In some people, the temporomandibular joint may become stiff, tender, or painful. These symptoms add up to a condition known as temporomandibular joint disorder, or TMJ.

TMJ typically occurs when you grind and clench your teeth at night, a condition called bruxism. The grinding and clenching is believed to be the result of unrelieved daytime stress. But other factors can also cause TMJ, including arthritis, too much gum chewing, and misalignment of the teeth.

According to the TMJ Association, TMJ affects more than ten million people in the United States, most of them women in their childbearing years. Research suggests that hormones may be one reason why women are more vulnerable.

Treatment for TMJ may involve several strategies, depending on the severity of your condition. But most times, you can get relief on your own without major medical intervention. Massaging the joint can help relieve the tension for some people, while others may do better with the application of heat or cold. Still others may need anti-inflammatory medications to relieve the pain. You may also need to break certain habits that are causing the pain, such as clenching your teeth. Severe cases of TMJ, however, may require surgery.

## What It Looks Like

TMJ can produce any of several symptoms in varying degrees of severity. The symptoms of TMJ may come and go, depending on factors such as your stress levels and even the weather.

A majority of patients with TMJ will experience headaches and dizziness. Many of them also have facial pain, which is often worsened by opening and closing the jaw. Others notice ear pain without any signs of infection. The ear pain may be accompanied by a feeling of fullness in the ears. People with TMJ may also notice ringing in their ears, a condition known as tinnitus.

In some people, TMJ causes sounds in the jaw area. You may notice grinding, crunching, or popping sounds, a condition known medically as crepitus.

## What to Eat

People who have TMJ should eat softer foods that don't strain the jaw muscles and bones, says Christine Gerbstadt, M.D., R.D., a spokesperson for the American Dietetic Association. Try to eat foods that are soft, even puréed, if your condition is severe. Good choices include soups, stews, oatmeal, steamed vegetables, and fruit smoothies.

To help inhibit inflammation, consider eating foods rich in omega-3 fatty acids. These healthy fats are found in cold-water fish such as tuna, salmon, herring, and mackerel, as well as nuts and flaxseed.

It's also important to watch the way you eat. Cut your foods into smaller pieces. Avoid taking large bites that force excessive chewing. These habits can all place a strain on the temporomandibular joint.

## What Not to Eat

Avoid foods that are hard to chew, which will only aggravate your TMJ pain. Foods such as crunchy cereals, well-done meats, and chewy bagels can overwork the jaw muscle and cause tension and pain in the jaw. If you chew gum, you may have to stop.

Limit your intake of foods that aggravate inflammation, such as those high in saturated fat. These foods include red meat, whole dairy products, and rich desserts, as well as refined carbs such as muffins, crackers, and cookies.

## Supplements for TMJ

Take a high-quality multivitamin to get all the essential nutrients you need. You might also consider taking the following:

### MAGNESIUM
This major mineral relaxes the muscles and may help alleviate some of the tension in the jaw.

### CALCIUM
Calcium has a similar relaxant effect and also helps keep bones, including those in the jaw, strong.

### B COMPLEX VITAMIN
The B vitamins play a role in maintaining healthy nerves and alleviating stress that can cause the grinding that leads to TMJ.

## Stay-Healthy Strategies

- **GET FITTED FOR A MOUTH GUARD.** Wearing the guard to bed every night can help protect against the clenching and grinding that results in TMJ.

- **DEVELOP STRESS-REDUCTION STRATEGIES.** Stress can be a major factor behind TMJ. So find ways to cope with stressful situations and make time to relax.

- **CONSIDER BIOFEEDBACK.** Biofeedback is an alternative treatment for stress that involves training the mind to control physiological functions. It may help TMJ sufferers learn to relax their jaw muscles.

- **GIVE YOGA A TRY.** Yoga is an exercise that involves proper breathing, movements, and a series of postures called asanas. Regular practice helps train you to become more sensitive to sensations in your body.

# ULCERATIVE COLITIS

ULCERATIVE COLITIS (UC) is a type of inflammatory bowel disease (IBD) in which the colon becomes inflamed. Unlike the other type of IBD, Crohn's disease, which can affect any part of the gastrointestinal tract, UC involves only the colon. But the symptoms of the two conditions are similar, and diagnosis to determine which one you have can sometimes be a challenge.

With UC, the colon mucosa, or inner lining of the colon, becomes inflamed and develops small open sores, or ulcers, that bleed and produce pus and mucus. The inflammation typically occurs in the rectum and involves parts of or the entire colon. The inflammation causes the colon to empty frequently and leads to diarrhea, abdominal pain, and blood in the stools.

No one knows for sure what causes UC, but experts believe the immune system is involved, just as it is in Crohn's disease. An abnormal response by the immune system to substances in the intestines triggers a defensive effort by the body's white blood cells. This inappropriate response creates inflammation that becomes chronic when the immune system doesn't shut down.

UC affects about 500,000 people in the United States, and the incidence is equally split between males and females. Most people are diagnosed in their mid-30s, though the condition can develop at any age. The disease definitely has a genetic link; it is more common in people of Jewish descent and less so among African-Americans.

Although the condition can be treated with medications, some people eventually need surgery to remove the colon.

## What It Looks Like

UC begins with increasingly loose stools that eventually become diarrhea. The diarrhea may occur suddenly or develop gradually. Often, the diarrhea is bloody and accompanied by severe abdominal pain and cramping. Sufferers often feel an urgent need to have a bowel movement.

Some people also experience significant loss of appetite and weight loss. If the bleeding is severe, the person may develop anemia. Children with severe cases may experience delayed development and stunted growth. In more serious cases, there may be skin problems, eye inflammation, joint pain, and liver problems.

Not everyone will suffer serious symptoms— approximately half of all patients have mild cases. Symptoms also tend to come and go, alternating between periods of activity and remission.

It's easy to confuse UC with infections that cause diarrhea. Stool samples may be needed to detect infectious causes of diarrhea. In addition, your doctor may do a sigmoidoscopy—a diagnostic exam that involves inserting a long thin tube into the anus—to view the lower end of the colon and the rectum—or a colonoscopy to view the entire colon. During the procedure, the doctor will look for ulcers, inflammation, and bleeding.

## IBD Is Not IBS

It's easy to confuse inflammatory bowel disease (IBD) with irritable bowel syndrome (IBS). The acronyms are similar, and the symptoms are even a lot alike.

But in reality, these are two distinct disorders. IBS is a disorder that has no inflammation but rather involves excessive muscle contractions in the colon. It is sometimes called spastic colon or nervous colitis.

IBD actually includes two conditions: ulcerative colitis or Crohn's disease. Both are chronic diseases that involve inflammation in the intestines.

## ¶¶¶ What to Eat

There's no single diet that benefits everyone with UC, but a healthy, well-balanced diet is helpful for staying well, says Jeannie Moloo, R.D., a nutritionist in Sacramento, California, and the co-author of *The No-Salt, Lowest Sodium* cookbook series. Try to eat fresh, unprocessed foods such as fruits, vegetables, and lean proteins, including chicken and fish. Cold-water fish may be especially beneficial because they contain omega-3 fatty acids that help reduce inflammation.

People with UC need to drink plenty of fluids too. Any disease that causes diarrhea puts you at greater risk for dehydration. Practice sipping rather than gulping, which can introduce air into your system and create discomfort.

During a remission, eat as many fruits, veggies, and lean proteins as you possibly can. Maximizing your calorie and protein intake during a remission will ensure you maintain your weight and help you replenish your nutrient stores. Make sure to also eat fermented foods such as sauerkraut, miso, and kimchi, which can help boost healthy microorganisms in the digestive tract and restore it to good health. Choose fermented foods that have not been heated, so that the healthy microorganisms are still thriving.

# What Not to Eat

Steer clear of foods high in saturated fat, such as red meat, butter, and pork, which can worsen inflammation. For the same reason, you should also avoid fried and greasy foods as well as foods high in sugar.

Some experts may recommend doing an elimination diet to figure out which foods aggravate any symptoms. An elimination diet involves cutting out allergenic foods such as wheat and dairy, then gradually reintroducing them and noting any symptoms. But keep in mind that what may appear to trigger UC one time may not have anything to do with the underlying disease. "A patient may wind up restricting his diet unnecessarily, especially when he is already limited in nutrient intake from flare-ups," Moloo says.

During a flare-up, avoid any foods that aggravate your digestive tract. That means steering clear of bulky grains, alcohol, spicy foods, and milk, which can increase diarrhea and cramps. During a flare-up, or if you have strictures–tight bands that constrict the anal opening–you should also eliminate high-fiber foods, such as raw fruits and vegetables, beans, seeds, and nuts, which can create gas and aggravate your symptoms.

## Supplements for UC

Having UC puts you at risk for malnutrition, so take a quality multivitamin to get the essential nutrients. Nutrients that may become deficient include vitamin B12, folate, vitamin D, selenium, magnesium, calcium, potassium, zinc, and iron. Deficiencies will depend in part on the severity and location of the inflammation. You should talk to your doctor about your particular case.

But some supplements may help minimize flare-ups and improve your condition. These include the following:

### VITAMIN C

This antioxidant vitamin may help lower the incidence of flare-ups.

### FISH OR FLAXSEED OIL

These oils are rich in omega-3 fatty acids, which might help reduce the inflammation and aid in healing the irritated membrane.

### PREBIOTICS AND PROBIOTICS

These supplements work together to promote the growth of healthy bacteria. Prebiotics are sugars that stimulate the growth and activity of good bacteria in the colon called *Bifidobacteria*. Probiotics are healthy bacteria such as *Lactobacillus acidophilus* that help balance intestinal microflora and may help relieve the symptoms of UC.

### PSYLLIUM

Psyllium is a seed husk and a soluble fiber that may help prevent flare-ups of UC. One study compared it to mesalamine, a drug for IBD, and found psyllium was just as effective.

### BROMELAIN

Bromelain is a naturally occurring substance in pineapple that can help reduce inflammation.

## Stay-Healthy Strategies

- **PRACTICE RELAXATION.** Doing yoga, qi gong, or meditation can help relieve stress, which worsens UC.

- **GET REGULAR EXERCISE.** Physical activity can lessen your symptoms and reduce your stress levels.

- **GET A COLONOSCOPY.** People with UC are at greater risk for colon cancer, so get regular colonoscopies.

- **LEARN ABOUT YOUR CONDITION.** Read up on UC. Knowing as much as you can will help you better cope with this disease.

### Consider the Specific Carbohydrate Diet

People who suffer from ulcerative colitis may benefit from the Specific Carbohydrate (SC) Diet, which was popularized in the book *Breaking the Vicious Cycle* by Elaine Gottschall. The SC Diet involves eating few or no carbohydrates and instead focuses on eating foods that contain monosaccharides, carbohydrates that are rapidly absorbed.

The SC Diet is based on the premise that sicknesses such as UC, Crohn's disease, and candidiasis are caused by an imbalance of intestinal flora. The diet allows you to eat most fresh, raw, or frozen vegetables; legumes; unprocessed meats; natural cheeses low in lactose; homemade yogurt; most fruits; and select oils including olive, coconut, soybean, and corn.

But it prohibits many other foods, including all sugars except honey; all starchy foods such as bread, potatoes, yams and pasta; all milk products except homemade yogurt; all grains; and canned vegetables. It also bans canola oil, mayonnaise, ice cream, candy, chocolate, and products that contain baking powder.

The diet is intended to restore balance to your digestive tract and tame the bacterial overgrowth that is making you sick. Over time, the diet is believed to heal the gut, which will in turn relieve your symptoms. For more information, see page 75 or check out www.scdiet.org and www.breakingtheviciouscycle.org.

# ULCERS

FOR YEARS, ULCERS WERE THOUGHT to be the result of excessive worry and stress. But it turns out that these sores, which occur on the lining of your digestive tract, are actually the result of a bacteria called *Helicobacter pylori*, or *H. pylori*.

Ulcers can occur anywhere in your digestive tract, which consists of the esophagus, stomach, duodenum (the first part of the intestines), and intestines. Most ulcers develop in the duodenum and are called duodenal ulcers. Those that develop in the stomach are called gastric ulcers. Ulcers located in the esophagus are called esophageal ulcers. You might also hear the term "peptic ulcer," which refers to sores on the lining of the stomach or duodenum.

Peptic ulcers are extremely common. According to the National Institutes of Health, one in ten Americans develops an ulcer at some time in his or her life. Although *H. pylori* is often a cause of peptic ulcers, they can also be caused by long-term use of nonsteroidal anti-inflammatory drugs (NSAIDs) such as ibuprofen and aspirin. In rare cases, cancerous tumors in the stomach or pancreas can cause ulcers. Although stress and spicy foods do not cause ulcers, they can make them worse.

*H. pylori* is a type of bacteria that afflicts about 20 percent of people under age 40 and half of all people over age 60. Most people with *H. pylori* do not develop ulcers, and experts are not sure why some people do while others don't. Experts aren't even sure how *H. pylori* is contracted, but it may be through contaminated food or water. *H. pylori* has also been discovered in saliva, so it's possible that it spreads through kissing or the sharing of utensils and straws.

In people who do develop ulcers, *H. pylori* weakens the surface of the stomach and duodenum, allowing acid to reach the more sensitive lining underneath. The combination of the acid and the bacteria irritate the lining and cause the formation of the ulcer.

## What It Looks Like

Not everyone with ulcers experiences symptoms, and some people may have very mild symptoms. In people with ulcers who do have symptoms, there is often abdominal discomfort that feels like a dull, gnawing ache. The pain may come and go for several days or weeks, and it is common two or three hours after a meal or in the middle of the night, when the stomach is empty. Eating relieves the pain, as do antacid medications. Ulcers may also cause weight loss, bloating, burping, nausea, vomiting, and a weak appetite.

In some cases, ulcers can be quite serious. Some ulcers may cause perforation, in which the ulcer goes through the stomach or duodenal wall. Ulcers can also break a blood vessel and cause bleeding. Sometimes, an ulcer can get in the way of food trying to leave the stomach, causing obstruction. These problems may cause sharp, sudden, and persistent stomach pain; black or bloody stools; or vomit that contains blood or resembles coffee grounds. All these symptoms warrant immediate medical attention.

## ¶¶¶ What to Eat

Eat a diet high in fiber, which can help lessen the risk for ulcers and speed healing if you already have one, says Jacob Teitelbaum, M.D., author of *Pain Free 1-2-3*. A high-fiber diet lowers the acidity of your stomach. Fiber is found in fruits, vegetables, and whole grains. Cruciferous veggies such as broccoli may be especially beneficial because they contain a substance called sulforaphane, a compound that has been found to inhibit *H. pylori*. Another good choice is cranberries, which contain flavonoids that can guard against ulcers.

Add more spices to your diet. Contrary to what you may have heard, some spices may actually help inhibit or destroy *H. pylori*. Garlic, for instance, has been found to have an antibiotic effect on *H. pylori*. Another study found that aqueous extracts of plants for cumin, ginger, chili, borage, black caraway, oregano, and licorice actually killed *H. pylori*, while extracts of turmeric, borage, and parsley were able to prevent the bacteria from adhering to parts of the stomach.

Make sure to also drink plenty of water. Consuming large amounts of water may help relieve the pain.

## 🚫 What Not to Eat

Restrict your intake of foods and seasonings that stimulate the production of stomach acid. You'll know it's happening if you experience heartburn. Foods that simulate stomach acid include milk and dairy products, black pepper, chili powder, cloves, soda, and caffeinated drinks, as well as decaffeinated versions. Do not drink alcohol either, because that can irritate the digestive tract. In addition, avoid coffee—even decaf— because the acids in coffee can be severe irritants.

Check for food allergies, which can aggravate your symptoms. Do an elimination diet that removes suspected foods from your diet and then reintroduce them gradually. If you notice a worsening of symptoms, avoid that food.

## 🌾 Supplements for Ulcers

Take a multivitamin to ensure that you are getting the essential nutrients. You might also consider taking the following:

### CRANBERRY EXTRACT
Cranberry products can help treat *H. pylori* infections that lead to ulcers.

### DGL

A licorice extract called deglycyrrhizinated licorice may reduce the growth of *H. pylori*.

### PROBIOTICS

Healthy bacteria such as *Lactobacillus* can inhibit and even kill *H. pylori*.

### MASTIC GUM

Mastic gum is an herbal remedy used in Mediterranean foods that has been found to kill *H. pylori*.

### CHAMOMILE

Drinking chamomile tea may help promote the healing of ulcers. Chamomile also has a relaxing effect that can help reduce stress.

## Stay-Healthy Strategies

- **QUIT SMOKING.** Cigarettes can prevent proper healing and make you more vulnerable to recurrent infections.

- **SEE YOUR DOCTOR.** Only a doctor can diagnose whether you have ulcers. Your doctor can also prescribe antibiotics that will kill the *H. pylori*.

- **REDUCE STRESS.** Find effective ways to better cope with the stress in your life. Consider doing relaxation exercises such as yoga or meditation to help you relax.

- **STEER CLEAR OF NSAIDS AND ASPIRIN.** Read medication labels carefully and be on the look-out for ibuprofen and aspirin in cough and cold remedies.

---

## *H. Pylori:* A Common Infection

If you've just learned you have an ulcer and that you're infected with *H. pylori*, you're not alone. Approximately half of the world population is infected with *H. pylori*. And in the United States, half of all people older than age 50 have *H. pylori*.

Ulcers are just one problem that this bacteria can cause. According to the Heliobacter Foundation, studies suggest that *H. pylori* is also involved in stomach cancer and may also be responsible for the worsening of rosacea, chronic fatigue syndrome, and chronic halitosis.

# URINARY TRACT INFECTIONS

URINARY TRACT INFECTIONS (UTIs) are a common problem, accounting for more than eight million doctor visits a year. The condition is especially common in women, whose anatomy makes infections more likely. For starters, women have a shorter urethra, the canal through which urine passes, meaning the bacteria doesn't have far to go before causing an infection. To make matters worse, the urethra is located near the rectum, making it easy for bacteria from the feces to infect the urethra.

The urinary system is composed of the kidneys, ureters, bladder, and urethra, which together help remove waste from your body. First the waste is filtered from your blood through the kidneys. The urine is then carried along tubes called ureters and deposited in the bladder, where the urine is stored. When the urine builds up and you feel the urge to urinate, the urine is eliminated through the urethra. Any of these body parts can become infected, but most infections occur in the urethra and the bladder.

The average adult passes about a quart and a half of urine each day. But the amount of urine varies from day to day, depending on what you eat and drink, any medications you take, and your overall health. At night, the amount of urine produced is about half of what is produced during the day.

Infections of the urinary tract are the second most common type of infection in the body, according to the National Institutes of Health. Some people are more prone to UTIs than others. Some women become susceptible during menopause or pregnancy and from having sexual intercourse.

Illness can raise your risk for UTIs too. People who have diabetes are more susceptible to UTIs, as are people who have suppressed immune systems. Elderly people who require catheters or tubes in the urethra or bladder may have more frequent infections as well. Men who have enlarged prostates are more likely to have UTIs. Anyone with an abnormality in the urinary tract is also more vulnerable to UTIs, including infants and children.

Unfortunately, recurrence of UTIs is common. About 20 percent of women who have one UTI will go on to have another, and 30 percent of them will have yet a third or more. Among women who have three UTIs, 80 percent will go on to have more. Usually, the type of bacteria causing each subsequent infection will differ from the previous one. It appears that some women have cells in their urethra that allow bacteria to attach more readily.

## 🔍 What It Looks Like

Not everyone with a UTI has symptoms, but most people will experience at least some symptoms. Women may feel pressure above the pubic bone, while some men may experience a feeling of fullness in the rectum.

Most people with symptoms will notice changes in their urination. Some people may experience a frequent urge to urinate. Others may feel pain or burning near the bladder or urethra, either while you're urinating or even when you're not. Others may try to urinate, only to pass a tiny amount of urine. The urine itself may look milky or cloudy, or even reddish if blood is present.

The symptoms you experience also depend on where the infection is located. For instance, an infection in the bladder or urethra typically doesn't cause a fever. But if you have a fever, the infection may be in the kidneys. A kidney infection may also cause pain in the back or side below the ribs, nausea, or vomiting. Pregnant women are generally more susceptible to kidney infections.

In children, UTIs are more likely to cause a fever, often with no other symptoms. Infants may be extremely irritable and may not eat normally. You may also notice changes in the child's urinary pattern.

## 🍴 What to Eat

The best foods for UTIs are cranberries and cranberry juice, says Marilyn Tanner, R.D., a spokesperson for the American Dietetic Association. Cranberries contain a substance called proanthocyanidins that help reduce the bacteria in your urinary tract.

Drinking cranberry juice may even help prevent infections. However, if you're taking warfarin (Coumadin), check with your doctor before drinking a lot of cranberry juice. Cranberry juice may interact with warfarin and cause excessive bleeding, and your doctor may need to adjust your dosage or schedule more frequent blood tests to monitor it.

It's also important to drink plenty of water to flush out bacteria. Drinking a lot of water will also dilute the concentration of your urine and cause more frequent urination. Urinating more often means the bacteria will spend less time in your urinary tract.

You can also use your diet to help create a more acidic environment in your urinary tract. To do that, try eating yogurt that contains live *acidophilus* cultures. Eating fruits and vegetables rich in vitamin C can also promote more acidity, which will help prevent infections too. Good sources include strawberries, citrus fruits, red bell peppers, kiwi, and broccoli.

## 🚫 What Not to Eat

Avoid foods and beverages that contain caffeine, which can be dehydrating. You should also steer clear of spicy foods, as well as those that are processed or refined. All these types of foods are more likely to aggravate your infection.

Avoid foods and drinks high in sugar, including soda and fruit juices. Sugar encourages the proliferation of bacteria and weakens immunity.

## 💊 Supplements for Urinary Tract Infections

Taking a quality multivitamin can help ensure you get all the necessary nutrients. You might also consider taking the following:

### CRANBERRY EXTRACT

Cranberry prevents bacteria from binding to the lining of the bladder wall, thereby guarding against infection.

### VITAMIN C

This antioxidant can help strengthen your immunity and make your urine more acidic. A more acidic environment prevents the growth of bacteria.

### D-MANNOSE

If you have recurrent bladder infections, the natural sugar D-Mannose can prevent most of them, and it can even eliminate acute infections.

### UVA URSI

This herbal remedy, also known as bearberry, contains a substance called arbutin that may help relieve and prevent infections.

## 📋 Stay-Healthy Strategies

- **DON'T HOLD YOUR URINE.** Urinate whenever you feel the urge.

- **WIPE FROM FRONT TO BACK** after bowel movements.

- **URINATE AFTER HAVING SEX** to remove bacteria.

- **AVOID USING THE DIAPHRAGM** if you're prone to UTIs. Women who use the diaphragm tend to get more infections. Ask your doctor about other birth control choices.

# What's Urinary Incontinence?

Most people have good control over when they urinate—it's often a conscious decision, and you can hold off for a short while if you can't get to a bathroom immediately. But approximately thirteen million people in the United States suffer from a condition called urinary incontinence, in which they lose control over urination. The condition can be embarrassing and distressful, and in extreme cases, can make it difficult for sufferers to leave the house.

Many factors can cause urinary incontinence, and a urinary tract infection is just one of them. Certain medications such as calcium-channel blockers, antidepressants, and antihistamines can lead to urinary incontinence. An enlarged prostate in men can cause it too. Urinary incontinence is also more common in people who are obese, diabetic, and disabled as well as people who smoke.

The good news is that urinary incontinence can be treated with medications, behavioral changes, or various procedures. You do not have to learn to live with it. So talk to your doctor if you suffer from urinary incontinence.

# UTERINE FIBROIDS

HEAVY PERIODS. ABDOMINAL CRAMPS. BACK PAIN. If you're cursed with troublesome fibroids, you may be among the 25 percent of all women who experience these symptoms. In reality, fibroids are extremely common and may affect as many as 70 percent of all women by the age of 40. Not everyone knows they're there.

Uterine fibroids are tumors or growths that occur within the wall of the uterus. These growths are almost always benign, and they can vary significantly in size. Small ones may be as tiny as an apple seed, while large ones can grow to the size of a grapefruit.

No one knows exactly what causes these non-cancerous growths of the uterus. Surges in estrogen, like those during pregnancy, appear to fuel their growth in younger women under the age of 35. Decreases in estrogen, like those during menopause, can cause fibroids to shrink, but this is not always the case. Some women over 35 will experience a growth in their fibroids as their estrogen levels decline.

Fibroids are more common during the child-bearing years and also more likely to occur in African-American, Asian, and Mediterranean women, as well as women who are overweight or who have never given birth. Most women will start experiencing symptoms between the ages of 35 and 50.

Fortunately, women today have several options for treating fibroids. Treatments for fibroids vary depending on the location of the growths and the severity of the symptoms. Some women may opt to do nothing except to have the fibroids monitored by their OB/GYN. Others may take oral contraceptives and progestin-only pills, which shut down your period and suppress excessive bleeding.

If the fibroid is larger, your doctor may prescribe a gonadotropin agonist hormone to shrink the fibroids and lessen the bleeding to prepare for surgery. Long-term use of these drugs, however, can lower bone density and cause menopausal symptoms such as hot flashes and vaginal dryness. But once the drug is discontinued, the fibroids grow back.

In some women, various medical and surgical procedures are necessary to remove the fibroids. A myomectomy will remove the fibroids, while a hysterectomy removes the entire uterus. Women with smaller fibroids may get an endometrial ablation, in which the fibroids are removed by shaving away the endometrial lining using heat, laser technology, electricity, or freezing techniques. A myolysis involves inserting an electrical needle or freezing device into the uterus through a small incision in the abdomen to destroy the blood vessels feeding the fibroids.

Fibroids may also be removed with a nonsurgical procedure called uterine artery embolization, in which small plastic beads are inserted into an artery so that they cut off blood flow to the fibroids and cause them to shrink. Still another technology is the ExAblate 200, which destroys fibroids by using an magnetic resonance imaging (MRI) machine to aim high-intensity ultrasound waves at a woman's fibroids. This technology is still very new and requires more testing before it will be in common use.

## What It Looks Like

Whether they cause symptoms depends on where they're located. Fibroids that grow in the wall of the uterus or on the outside of the uterus may cause no problems at all, even if they're large. You won't know you have them unless they're detected during a pelvic exam or by imaging techniques.

If they're located in the uterine wall and grow into the cavity, they can cause heavy, prolonged menstrual bleeding that can lead to anemia. They can also cause irregular bleeding, pelvic and lower back pain and pressure, difficulties urinating, and an enlarged abdomen. In some women, albeit rarely, fibroids can cause infertility and miscarriage.

## What to Eat

Women with uterine fibroids do better if they eat a diet that boosts their immune system, says Thomas Lyons, M.D., medical director of the Center for Women's Care and Reproductive Surgery in Atlanta and co-author of *What to Do When the Doctor Says It's Endometriosis*. That means eating an abundance of fresh fruits and vegetables, which will enhance immunity with disease-combating antioxidants. These foods are also rich in fiber, which can help prevent and ease gastrointestinal problems that occur with fibroids, such as constipation and hemorrhoids.

Make sure to eat foods rich in B vitamins. The B vitamins help the liver metabolize estrogen. Maintaining a healthy balance of estrogen can help relieve the symptoms of fibroids.

It's also important to maintain a healthy weight if you suffer from fibroids. Fat cells produce estrogen, which will worsen symptoms. Watch your portions and calorie intake.

## What Not to Eat

Steer clear of saturated fats, which are found in red meat, whole dairy products, and butter. These fats contain prostaglandins that can worsen any pain you may be experiencing. Make sure to get your calcium from other sources such as leafy greens, fortified cereals, and supplements.

In addition, stay away from foods rich in sodium. Too much salt will promote premenstrual bloating and could potentially make your fibroid problems worse.

Also avoid alcohol, caffeine, and sugar. These substances promote inflammation and can make your pain worse. Alcohol also stresses the liver and, in excess, can cause nutritional deficiencies that may lower your immunity.

# 💊 Supplements for Fibroids

Take a quality multivitamin to make sure you get all the essential nutrients. Other supplements you might want to consider taking include the following:

### VITAMIN C
This potent antioxidant builds your immune system and may help relieve any cramps and bloating.

### B VITAMIN COMPLEX
The B vitamins help the liver metabolize estrogen. In particular, vitamin B6, or pyridoxine, may help relieve premenstrual syndrome and heavy menstrual bleeding.

### EVENING PRIMROSE OIL
This herbal remedy contains the essential fatty acid gamma linolenic acid (GLA), which helps relieve the symptoms of endometriosis.

# 📋 Stay-Healthy Strategies

- **LEARN ABOUT FIBROIDS AND YOUR TREATMENT OPTIONS.** In some cases, you may simply need to treat the symptoms. In others, you may need to treat the fibroids.

- **REDUCE YOUR STRESS.** Too much stress weakens immunity, which may cause more symptoms of fibroids.

- **TRY OVER-THE-COUNTER ANALGESICS FOR PAIN RELIEF.** If they don't work, talk to your doctor about taking something stronger.

- **ALWAYS TALK TO YOUR OB/GYN** if you notice any abnormalities in your menstrual periods.

## Fibroids Q&A

**Q.** Does uterine embolization destroy my chances of getting pregnant? What about myomectomy?

**A.** Many women who undergo embolization are done with having children, so the answer to this question isn't completely known. But so far, getting pregnant doesn't appear to be a problem. The concerns instead have focused on the safety of pregnancy. In some embolized women who have become pregnant, the baby did not grow properly or the fetus was abnormally positioned. After delivery, embolized women also had a higher incidence of hemorrhage. Some women who undergo embolization also experience ovarian failure, in which the ovaries no longer release eggs or hormones. Ovarian failure also produces symptoms of early menopause such as bone loss, vaginal dryness, and hot flashes.

Unlike a hysterectomy, a myomectomy preserves a woman's ability to get pregnant. But the delivery may require a C-section because the uterine wall is often weakened, and labor may be too rigorous. In some cases, myomectomy can cause scarring, which can lead to infertility.

# VAGINAL YEAST INFECTIONS

SOONER OR LATER, ALMOST EVERY WOMAN suffers from a vaginal yeast infection, an irritating condition caused by a fungus called *Candida albicans*. In healthy women, it's perfectly normal to have yeast inhabiting the vagina in small numbers. The naturally acidic environment of the vagina keeps the numbers of yeast from growing. But if the environment becomes less acidic, the yeast may replicate, eventually causing an infection.

Many factors influence the acidity of your vagina. Your monthly period, pregnancy, antibiotics, birth control pills, steroids, and having diabetes can all cause the vagina to become more acidic. Excess moisture and irritation also stimulate the growth of yeast.

Yeast infections are extremely common. In fact, it's believed that three-quarters of all women will have at least one yeast infection at some time in their lives. Fifty percent of women have more than one infection in their lives.

## What It Looks Like

Women who have had yeast infections in the past are usually familiar with the symptoms right away. Often, the first sign is itchiness and burning in and around the vagina and vulva, the skin around the vagina. Some women may develop a white vaginal discharge that resembles cottage cheese. They may also experience pain during sex or swelling in the vulva.

Because some women can easily recognize the symptoms of a yeast infection, many now can purchase over-the-counter vaginal suppositories without going to see a doctor. But if you are not familiar with the symptoms or have some question as to whether it's truly a yeast infection—they have similar symptoms to some sexually transmitted diseases—it's always best to see your doctor before getting any treatment.

Although vaginal yeast infections are not considered a sexually transmitted disease, you can infect your partner. Men who have sex with women who have a vaginal yeast infection may notice some burning after intercourse or notice a slight rash on the penis.

Women who suffer from recurrent bouts of vaginal yeast infections may want to talk to their doctor about candidiasis, a more systemic version of yeast overgrowth.

## 🍴 What to Eat

According to Michael McNett, M.D., owner and medical director of a multidisciplinary fibromyalgia treatment center in Chicago and co-author of *The Everything Health Guide to Fibromyalgia*, the right diet can diminish your incidence of yeast infections. For starters try to eat unsweetened yogurt every day. Choose yogurts that contain *acidophilus* cultures, the healthy bacteria that can help keep yeast in check.

For overall health, eat a diet rich in fruits and vegetables. To reduce the growth of yeast, focus on low-starch vegetables such as broccoli, cauliflower, celery, cabbage, leafy greens, brussels sprouts, squash, asparagus, radishes, onions, tomatoes, bell peppers, and green beans. Eat carrots, beets, peas, avocado, turnips, parsnips, and eggplant in moderation because they contain more starch.

In addition, eat whole grains, which are low in sugar. Good choices include brown rice, wild rice, millet, oatmeal, oat bran, barley, wheat, rye, and corn.

Virtually all meats are safe, but the best varieties are the lean ones, such as chicken, fish, and turkey. Other healthy foods include legumes such as lentils, beans, and peas, which are rich in fiber and protein.

If you enjoy fruit, limit your intake to just two small servings a day. Eat them at different times of day to minimize the amount of sugar (fructose occurs naturally in fruit) you consume in one sitting.

Finally, consider drinking pau d'arco tea, a type of tea derived from the inner bark of a South American tree. The tea acts as an antifungal and antibacterial remedy and may aid in your recovery.

---

### When It's Not a Yeast Infection

Signs and symptoms of a vaginal yeast infection may actually belong to another culprit. Conditions that mimic yeast infections include bacterial vaginosis, trichomoniasis, and atrophic vaginitis.

Bacterial vaginosis is a common infection that occurs when vaginal bacteria grow out of control. The telltale sign is a foul-smelling discharge.

Trichomoniasis is a sexually transmitted disease caused by a parasite. It is often accompanied by a thick yellow-green or gray-colored discharge.

Atrophic vaginitis occurs after menopause, when a reduction in estrogen levels causes the vaginal tissues to become thinner and drier, which causes pain, itching, and burning.

# What Not to Eat

Cut back your intake of simple carbohydrates such as cookies, cakes, and other products that contain refined sugar, which feed the yeast and encourage their growth.

Steer clear of any food that is highly concentrated with sweeteners, natural or artificial. That means you should avoid anything made with refined sugar, artificial sweeteners (including aspartame), dehydrated cane juice, honey, corn or maple syrup, molasses, and malt.

Reduce your intake of foods that contain yeast, including breads, pastries, pizza crust, beer and wine, and anything that contains vinegar such as ketchup, pickles, and certain salad dressings. In addition, avoid foods that contain mold, such as aged cheese and mushrooms.

To enhance overall health, avoid eating fast foods, junk foods, and soft drinks, which are generally loaded with empty calories—calories with no nutritional value. The goal is to build up your health and immunity.

# Supplements for Vaginal Yeast Infections

Take a daily multivitamin to get the essential nutrients you need for good health. Consider adding a supplement that contains *Lactobacillus acidophilus*, the friendly bacteria (probiotic) that helps inhibit yeast growth and restore balance.

Women who suffer from repeated infections may want to consider a supplement to enhance their yeast-fighting efforts. Recurrent vaginal yeast infections may signal candidiasis (see the Candidiasis chapter on page 72). Women with candidiasis may have weakened immune systems and may have a harder time fighting off other fungal infections, including those in the vagina. Possible supplements include the following:

### CAPRYLIC ACID

Caprylic acid is a fatty acid that has antifungal powers. It may lessen the ability of the yeast to grow and proliferate.

### GARLIC

This aromatic spice helps fight infection and enhances immunity. Look for supplements that contain allicin, the active ingredient.

### UVA URSI

Uva ursi is an herbal remedy better known for combating urinary tract infections. It acts like an astringent and can kill bacteria.

### BERBERINE

Berberine is an herbal treatment for yeast and fungus infections caused by *Candida albicans*.

## BORIC ACID

Suppositories of boric acid may provide relief for women who suffer chronic yeast infections.

## FRUCTOOLIGOSACCHARIDES

Fructooligosaccharides are sugars that feed *acidophilus*, the healthy bacteria, and may help promote their growth without stimulating more yeast.

## 📋 Stay-Healthy Strategies

- **GIVE THE VAGINAL AREA BREATHING ROOM.** Avoid tight-fitting or synthetic-fiber clothes, and always wear cotton underwear. Do not wear pantyhose or leotards every day.

- **DRY THE GENITAL AREA AFTER A BATH OR SHOWER** with a blow dryer set on low or cool.

- **ALWAYS WIPE FROM FRONT TO BACK** after using the toilet. This will help prevent the bacteria that normally live in your rectum from getting into your vagina.

- **CHANGE OUT OF WET SWIMSUITS** or other damp clothes as soon as you can.

- **DO NOT USE DOUCHES, FEMININE HYGIENE SPRAYS, OR DEODORIZED TAMPONS OR SANITARY PADS.**

- **CONSIDER VINEGAR AND WATER DOUCHES** to boost vaginal acidity, which will diminish yeast levels.

# VARICOSE VEINS

EVERY DAY OF YOUR LIFE, your arteries and veins work together to transport blood to and from your heart. Your arteries transport oxygenated (and therefore bright red) blood away from your heart to the rest of your body. The veins bring back unoxygenated blood (which is blue) to your heart and lungs so it can be oxygenated and then recirculated. But when the veins lose their elasticity and can't pump blood back toward the heart, you may develop varicose veins, a common condition that can result in unsightly veins on the legs.

Varicose veins occur primarily in the legs, where the veins face the challenges of gravity. For the veins to work properly, muscle contractions in the lower legs act as tiny pumps. The process is helped along by tiny valves in your veins that open to allow blood to go back toward your heart. Then they shut to prevent the blood from flowing backward.

With age, the veins lose their elasticity and stretch out, causing the valves to lose their ability to close properly. As a result, blood that should head toward your heart may flow backward into your legs. When the blood pools in your veins, the veins become large and twisted.

Some people are genetically predisposed to having varicose veins, but they can also be caused by pregnancy. Pregnancy increases the volume of blood in your body by up to a third, and the weight of the growing uterus can compress the veins that pass through the pelvis, leading to blockage and backup. Many women first notice varicose veins during late pregnancy,

when the weight of the growing fetus puts pressure on the veins in the legs and the extra progesterone relaxes the muscles of the veins.

Varicose veins affect approximately 60 percent of all Americans. The condition is especially common among older women. Approximately all adults over the age of 50 have varicose veins.

Over time, varicose veins can become bigger and more serious. Some people may develop blood clots or sores and ulcers near the area of the varicose vein. Treatment may involve self-help measures or surgical procedures that can close or remove veins.

## What They Look Like

Many women are familiar with the unsightly vision of large, twisted veins in their legs and feet. The veins are often dark purple or blue. Though varicose veins can appear anywhere on your leg, they are most likely to occur in the back of your knees or on the inside of your legs and ankles.

In most cases, varicose veins are simply a cosmetic problem. But in others, they may produce aches and discomfort, or even other medical problems. You may feel a burning, throbbing, itching, or cramping sensation in your lower legs, and you may also notice swelling. Sometimes sitting or standing too long will make them feel worse.

In some cases, varicose veins may lead to more serious problems. If blood in the veins deep in your leg becomes stagnant from pregnancy or prolonged sitting, for instance, you may notice significant swelling. Any sudden swelling, painless or not, requires immediate medical condition, as it could be a sign of a blood clot.

## Spider Veins, Not Varicose

Spider veins resemble spider webs with short, jagged lines and are similar to varicose veins, but much smaller. They're more likely to be closer to the skin's surface and are often red or blue. They occur on the legs, but can also be found on the face. Spider veins vary in size, and most times they do not need treatment.

## ♦♦♦ What to Eat

Load up on fruits, vegetables, and whole grains, says Marie Savard, M.D., author of *The Body Shape Solution for Weight Loss and Wellness*. These foods are naturally rich in fiber, which can help keep constipation at bay. Constipation can strain varicose veins that are already under extra pressure. These foods also contain vital nutrients that can help keep your blood vessels healthy.

## ⊘ What Not to Eat

Avoid foods high in saturated fat and trans-fatty acids, which will cause unwanted weight gain. According to Savard, women with pear-shaped bodies who are overweight are more prone to varicose veins. Too much fat in the hips and thighs will put pressure on the veins in your legs.

Try to stay away from high-sodium foods. Too much salt in the diet will promote water retention and worsen any swelling. Foods that have a lot of sodium include canned foods, processed foods, and deli meats. When buying canned or packaged foods, look for labels that say "no sodium" or "low sodium."

Also, limit your intake of sugar and refined carbohydrates, such as cakes, cookies, bagels, and muffins. These types of food tend to promote weight gain.

Finally, do not drink alcohol or caffeine in excess. Too much of either substance will cause dehydration, which can worsen varicose veins.

## 💊 Supplements for Varicose Veins

Take a quality multivitamin to ensure adequate intake of vital nutrients. You might also consider taking the following:

### BUTCHER'S BROOM

This herbal remedy is known to improve circulation in the legs by strengthening the collagen in your blood vessels. Always talk to a doctor before taking it because it may worsen your high blood pressure.

### BILBERRY

Bilberries grow on low-growing shrubs and are an herbal treatment that may improve circulation by strengthening capillaries.

### HORSE CHESTNUT

Popular in Europe, this herbal remedy may strengthen blood vessels and boost circulation.

### GRAPE SEED EXTRACT

Grape seed extract is derived from grape seeds and contains antioxidants that help promote healthy blood vessels.

## 📋 Stay-Healthy Strategies

- **EXERCISE REGULARLY.** Walking is a great option that improves leg and vein strength.

- **MAINTAIN A HEALTHY WEIGHT.** Too much weight causes pressure on the veins in your legs.

- **CHOOSE SUPPORTIVE CLOTHING.** Wear elastic support hose and avoid anything that is too tight on the waist, groin, or legs.

- **DON'T SIT STILL OR STAND FOR TOO LONG.** Get up and move even when you're traveling. If you have a job that requires standing for long periods of time, try shifting your feet.

### Sclerotherapy

Sclerotherapy is the most common treatment for both spider veins and varicose veins. The procedure involves injecting a solution into the vein that causes the walls of the vein to swell, stick, and become sealed. As a result, the blood flow is cut off and the vein gradually becomes scar tissue. After a while, the vein will fade altogether.

Most patients have significant improvement with sclerotherapy, though the procedure sometimes needs to be repeated. Sclerotherapy does not require anesthesia and can be done in the doctor's office.

# VOMITING

WHETHER A STOMACH BUG, MOTION SICKNESS, or a serious hangover, everyone would agree: Vomiting is an unpleasant experience. Vomiting is a symptom of any of several conditions that range from the relatively minor (a viral infection) to the serious (an intestinal blockage).

In any case, vomiting occurs when the normal digestive processes go in the opposite direction. Rather than pushing food through the stomach into the intestines, the process reverses itself, and the contents of the stomach (and even the intestines) are expelled. At one time or another, almost everyone experiences the ugly and unfortunate results of this reversal of events.

Many disorders and medical conditions can trigger vomiting. Common causes include the following:

- Gastroenteritis, an inflammation of the stomach lining and intestines caused by a viral infection or bacteria

- Inner ear disturbance

- Headaches or migraines

- Medications, especially those for cancer

- Hormones, such as those present during pregnancy

- Toxins in the blood that have been introduced by alcohol, drugs, and even nicotine

- Peptic ulcers—open sores on the lining of the stomach, upper small intestine, or esophagus

that are often brought on by bacteria and cause pain.

## 🔍 What It Looks Like

Many bouts of vomiting are preceded by nausea, an uneasiness in the tummy that makes you feel like you might throw up. Some people may feel weak and turn pale as well. Vomiting itself is the expulsion of your stomach contents.

## 🍴 What to Eat

Chances are, you won't want to eat in the initial hours after vomiting. That's fine. Your system probably welcomes the reprieve. But if the nausea returns, try nibbling on some dry, salted crackers, says Lynn Sutton, R.D., C.D.E., a registered dietitian in Albany, New York.

If you don't vomit again, and as you slowly start to recover, start taking small sips of water or sucking on some ice chips. The fluids will help you stave off dehydration, which is always a risk when vomiting or experiencing diarrhea. If you do not vomit after that, try sipping clear liquids such as water, apple juice, flat ginger ale, weak tea, broth, or jello.

When your appetite returns, go slow. Start with bland foods such as crackers, rice, bananas, applesauce, or toast. Consider adding oatmeal or another hot cereal. Slowly reintroduce others foods, such as cooked vegetables, plain turkey or chicken, and sherbet.

Also eat foods that are lukewarm, not cold or hot. Start with small meals, rather than a single large one. And if your nausea is aggravated by certain odors, try to eat in a room that is aroma-free.

## What Not to Eat

Avoid dairy products, which can unsettle the stomach. The same is true of any food that is fried, greasy, too sugary, or spicy. Also, do not ingest foods or drinks that contain caffeine, because they promote urination and the loss of salt and other electrolytes.

## Vomiting in the Animal Kingdom

Humans are easily nauseated at the sight and smell of another person's vomit. But in the wild, it's not unusual at all for other animals to vomit for survival.

According to Wikipedia, the online encyclopedia, whales vomit every seven to ten days as part of the digestive process and to eliminate nondigestible things they've swallowed. Cats are notorious for vomiting hairballs, and dogs often vomit from eating grass.

Owls vomit as a way to get rid of the bones and fur of their prey that they can't digest. Other birds regurgitate in order to feed their young. Some birds vomit when wounded or threatened.

## ℘ Supplements for Vomiting

Most cases of vomiting do not require supplementation. Rather, treatment of any kind is aimed at the underlying cause. The exception is ginger, a pungent root used for spicing up food. Ginger is often recommended to relieve nausea and vomiting. But you should not use ginger or any other remedy without first consulting a physician, because it may interact with other medications.

## ⎙ Stay-Healthy Strategies

- **GET SOME REST AND RELAXATION.** Trying to be active will worsen nausea.

- **SEE A DOCTOR** if the vomiting persists for more than two days. See a doctor immediately if you see blood in your vomit or if you have severe headache or stiff neck, lethargy, confusion, and rapid breathing or pulse. Vomiting with diarrhea, a fever over 101°F, and confusion also warrants an immediate visit to your physician.

- **CHILDREN SHOULD PROBABLY SEE A DOCTOR SOONER,** depending on their age and the presence of other symptoms. Children younger than six should get to a doctor if the vomiting lasts more than a few hours. Older kids should go if they vomit for more than one day.

- **BEWARE OF DEHYDRATION.** Becoming dehydrated is the biggest problem with vomiting. Look for signs in young children, such as the absence of tears, dark or infrequent urination, dry mouth, irritability, and rapid heartbeat. Adults may have excessive thirst, dry mouth, little or no urination, and severe weakness, dizziness, or lightheadedness.

# WARTS

WITCHES AREN'T THE ONLY ONES TO GET WARTS—in fact, almost everyone has a wart at one time or another. Warts are noncancerous skin growths caused by viruses in the human papillomavirus (HPV) family. They can appear anywhere on your body from the tops of your hands to the insides of your mouth to the rectal area. The location of your wart depends in part on the type of HPV you're infected with.

Some people are naturally more resistant to the HPV viruses and don't seem to get warts as easily as other people. Warts can be contagious if a healthy person touches the wart on the skin of an infected person. You do not get warts from touching a toad. It's also possible to transmit warts by touching objects that an infected person has touched. Warts on the genitals are highly contagious and can be transmitted during oral, vaginal, or anal sex. For more information on genital warts, see the Herpes chapter on page 179.

In some cases, warts will eventually disappear on their own, though it may take months or even years. Others are more stubborn and require medical treatment. But getting rid of the wart is always important. Some warts are cosmetically disturbing and embarrassing. Others may bleed and cause pain. Without treatment, you also risk the wart spreading to other areas of your body or infecting other people.

Treating skin warts may involve applying an over-the-counter salicylic acid or covering the wart with duct tape, as warts deprived of air and sun exposure sometimes die without the need for further treatment. More difficult warts will require a doctor's treatment, which may involve applying cantharidin, a medication, or cryotherapy, the freezing of the wart with liquid nitrogen. In some cases, you may require surgery to have the wart removed by excision.

## What It Looks Like

There are actually several types of skin warts, each with its own distinct appearance and location. Common warts typically develop on the hand, especially around the nail. These warts are gray or flesh colored. They're typically raised from the skin surface and covered with rough, hornlike projections.

Plantar warts occur on the bottom of the foot, which is called the plantar. They usually occur on the heel and the metatarsal heads, just behind the toes. Plantar warts usually grow into the skin, not outward like common warts. Pressure on the foot can eventually lead to a covering over the wart that resembles a callus. Because they do grow into the skin, plantar warts can be more difficult to treat.

Flat warts are usually on the face and the back of the hands, but they can also occur on the arms or legs. They usually appear as small, flat bumps about a quarter-inch in diameter. They may be pink, light brown, or light yellow in color. Flat warts can sometimes spread with shaving. Some flat warts have fingerlike projections.

## ⑪ What to Eat

Warts are sometimes a sign of reduced immunity, so strengthen your defenses by eating a lot of fresh, unprocessed foods such as fruits, vegetables, and whole-grain foods, says Fred Pescatore, M.D., a physician who uses nutrition to treat patients and the author of *The Hamptons Diet Cookbook*.

Eat foods that are rich in L-lysine, an amino acid that may block the activity of HPV. L-lysine occurs in beans, fish, red meat, and dairy products.

## ⊘ What Not to Eat

Avoid foods that contain arginine, an amino acid that may enhance HPV. These foods include peanuts, almonds, raisins, nuts, and seeds, as well as anything with chocolate.

Steer clear of foods and beverages that weaken immunity, such as caffeine, alcohol, and foods rich in sugar.

## ⚬ Supplements for Warts

Take a high-quality multivitamin to ensure overall health and well-being. You might also consider taking the following:

### L-LYSINE

L-lysine has long been regarded as a treatment for herpes infections, which are also caused by HPV. It works by inhibiting replication of the herpes virus.

### ZINC

Taking a supplement of this essential mineral may help speed up the recovery of a wart.

### NATURAL ANTIVIRAL REMEDIES

Certain plants contain substances with antiviral properties. These herbal remedies may help reduce the incidence of genital sores and prevent their recurrence. Among them are the following:

- **GARLIC OIL.** This pungent spice helps eliminate the virus that causes warts.

- **OLIVE LEAF EXTRACT OR OIL.** The oil and extract from the olive tree contains phytochemicals that help fight disease.

- **OREGANO OIL.** This oil, which is derived from oregano, a Mediterranean plant, is a potent germ fighter.

- **LEMON BALM.** This herb contains terpenes and tannins, substances in plants that may have antiviral properties.

- **LAURIC ACID.** This fatty acid that occurs naturally in human milk and coconut milk and is available in a supplement called monolaurin.

- **VITAMIN E OIL.** Vitamin E is a potent antioxidant that, as an oil, may help speed healing of skin warts.

## Stay-Healthy Strategies

- **RESIST THE URGE TO PICK AT WARTS.** Picking can cause the wart to spread elsewhere.

- **WASH HANDS AFTER TREATING A WART.**

- **STAY DRY.** Keeping hands and feet affected by warts dry will help prevent the virus from growing.

- **TREAT WARTS SOONER RATHER THAN LATER.** Prompt treatment is your best defense against recurrent warts and can help prevent their spread.

## Poison Your Warts

One treatment used on warts is cantharidin (Cantharone), a poisonous chemical compound secreted by many species of the blister beetle, and most notably by the Spanish fly. The toxin is secreted by the male blister beetle and transmitted to the female during mating. The substance is then used to cover the eggs as a way to protect them from predators.

Applying diluted cantharidin to a wart is extremely painful and often causes inflammation and blistering. But the substance is extremely potent, even against warts that have not responded to salicylic acid. In some cases, more than one application is required.

# WHAT TO EAT FOR HEALTHY LIVING

KNOWING WHAT TO EAT FOR WHAT AILS YOU can definitely help you feel better when you're sick, even if it doesn't cure you of the disease. But even if you're not sick, healthy eating can be just as important. In fact, it's actually more important because it can prevent you from getting some of these conditions. It can also help you maintain a healthy weight, enjoy higher energy levels, and live an overall higher quality of life.

The truth is, eating well should never be something you start doing when you find out you're sick. Ideally, it should be something you're taught to do during childhood. Once you reach adulthood, it should be an ongoing habit, performed every day, much in the same way you brush your teeth, walk your dog, and pay your bills. But that's an ideal situation.

No doubt, we are fortunate to live in an era of abundance, where food is plentiful and choices abound. The problem lies in the choices that most people make. When given all these options, many people simply make the wrong choices on a regular basis. They choose potato chips instead of an apple. They opt for doughnuts instead of whole-grain cereal. They pick up fast food for dinner instead of making a homemade meal.

The sad result is an epidemic of obesity. In fact, two-thirds of the U.S. population is now overweight or obese. In turn, the growing weight problems are creating a host of other health problems, including diabetes and heart disease.

In reality, a healthy diet isn't all that complicated. It simply means a well-balanced mix of foods that are rich in essential nutrients, eaten in reasonable portions on a regular basis. It even means enjoying dessert on occasion.

In the course of writing this book, it became apparent that certain nutritional mantras are well worth repeating, even when you aren't feeling the aches of arthritis, battling PCOS, or dealing with the weight gain of hypothyroidism. Consider these the dictums of healthy eating.

## Indulge in Fruits and Vegetables

You can never go wrong with a diet rich in fruits and vegetables, and the more colorful the mix, the better. These foods are nature's pharmacy. They are abundant in antioxidant vitamins and minerals and rich in fiber, all of which play essential roles in good health.

But it isn't always easy to load up on fruits and vegetables, especially when it comes to feeding children who frequently prefer less-healthy fare. And sometimes—let's be honest—a juicy hamburger is just much more tantalizing than a spinach salad.

The key, then, is to get these vegetables into your diet whenever possible, even if you need to rely on stealth tactics to appease finicky kids. Top that burger with onions, tomato, and dark leafy greens. Make your own pizza with extra sauce and sprinkle on some broccoli, peppers, or spinach. When making tacos, replace half the ground meat with beans.

If you think fresh veggies are too time-consuming to prepare, try stocking up on frozen ones, says Milton Stokes, R.D., a spokesperson for the American Dietetic Association. Frozen veggies are just as nutritious as fresh ones, and they may be actually more so because they were picked and frozen at peak freshness, he says. Add them to soups, salads, pastas, stews, and sauces. "It's a great way to boost he nutrient profile of something that may not be stellar, such as chicken noodle soup or pizza," Stokes says.

## Choose Your Fats Wisely

For years, fat has been demonized and blamed for its role in making Americans overweight. But in reality, fat is a vital macronutrient, essential for the proper function of the brain and nervous system and for healthy growth. The problem is that many of us eat too much of the wrong type of fat.

One of the worst types of fat is the saturated fats. These are the fats found in red meats, whole dairy foods, and butter, and anything else made with these foods, such as cakes, cookies, and ice cream. Eaten in abundance, they become a serious health hazard that promotes weight gain, inflammation, and disease.

Another unhealthy kind of fat is the transfatty acids. These are the fats produced during the hydrogenation process of oil. Hydrogenating oil gives processed foods a longer shelf life. But inside the body, the trans fats behave much like saturated fats, increasing cholesterol and raising your risk for heart disease.

So rather than satisfy your fat needs with rich desserts or high-fat meats, try eating cold-water fish such as salmon, tuna, mackerel, and herring, which have healthy omega-3 fatty acids. Omega-3 fatty acids have been linked to improvements in eye health, arthritis, and immunity.

## Watch Your Sugar

Sugar has become omnipresent in the American diet. Besides the obvious sources, it's in packaged foods, sauces, salad dressings, yogurt, and breakfast cereals. But most foods high in sugar are full of empty calories—they supply your body with energy but offer no other nutritional benefit.

It's especially important to watch your intake of sugary soft drinks and juices. These are packed with added calories and are often a major culprit in unwanted weight gain. So if possible, opt for calorie-free drinks, such as water and teas sweetened without sugar.

## Limit Caffeine

Many of us can't start the day without our morning java. The jolt of caffeine gives a kick-start to our day. But drinking too much caffeine has many deleterious effects on our health, the worst being its impact on our sleep. Too much caffeine, especially late in the day, makes restorative sleep a challenge for many people.

Without adequate sleep, our health suffers significantly. On a day-to-day basis, we are more irritable, more easily stressed, and less able to concentrate. Over time, our immune systems are weakened. People who are constantly sleep-deprived are also more vulnerable to weight gain, which creates a host of other health problems.

## Three a Day

It's tempting to skip meals, especially if you're trying to lose weight, or if you're in a frantic rush or trying to finish a project. But skipping meals—especially breakfast—is never a good idea. Eating breakfast jumpstarts your metabolism and gives you the energy you need to start your day. And research shows that people who eat breakfast do better at losing weight than people who don't.

Skipping other meals is also a bad idea, no matter how tight a deadline or how busy you are. In fact, most experts recommend eating at least three meals a day, or even four or five small ones. According to Jeannie Moloo, R.D., a nutritionist in Sacramento, California, and the co-author of *The No-Salt, Lowest Sodium* cookbook series, you should eat something every four hours simply to maintain energy. A steady supply of energy will also prevent binges later on because you won't be ravenous with hunger.

## Enjoy Protein

Foods rich in protein should be eaten at every meal, Moloo says. Protein helps you feel full and supplies much-needed vitamins and minerals. It also helps maintain muscle mass. When choosing protein, consider sources other than lean meats, such as legumes, nuts, seeds, and soy foods.

## Eat Fermented Foods

A diet that contains fermented foods can help enhance immunity and bolster digestive health. These foods nourish the body with live bacteria, which supply the digestive tract with numerous beneficial enzymes as well as antibiotic and anticarcinogenic substances. The primary by-product of fermentation is lactic acid, which not only preserves the vegetables and fruits being fermented but encourages the proliferation of healthy flora in the digestive tract. These foods include unpasteurized sauerkraut, miso, yogurt, and quality kefir.

## Alcohol in Moderation

There's nothing wrong with an occasional glass of wine with dinner, a beer with the boys, or an after-dinner cordial. The problem is drinking too much, too often, which can cause all sorts of maladies ranging from malnutrition to breast cancer.

So make sure to drink alcohol in moderation. For women, that means no more than one drink a day, and men, two drinks a day. A drink is 5 ounces of wine, 12 ounces of beer, or 1.5 ounces of 80-proof spirits. "If you do not drink, do not start," advises Christine Gerbstadt, M.D., R.D., a spokesperson for the American Dietetic Association.

## Maximize Variety

Even the healthiest eater can get in a food rut of eating the same foods every day. After all, most of us are creatures of habit. But eating a variety of foods ensures that you get a variety of nutrients.

Try eating chicken for dinner one day, fish the next, and bean chili the next. Apples may be your favorite fruit—and you know that they're good for you—but so are other fruits, such as strawberries, peaches, grapes, and oranges. Learn to cook healthy foods you like in new and different ways. Doing so will encourage you to keep eating these foods and give your taste buds a treat.

## Portions Count

Somewhere along the way, moderation went out of style. In its place came a biggest-bang-for-your-buck mentality that included all-you-can-eat buffets and super-sized meals of fast food. Bigger became better because you were getting more for your money. But these great values came at a price of another kind: your health.

Getting back to eating reasonable portions may be a challenge for people accustomed to heaping mounds of pasta, giant 8-oz. hamburgers, and pizzas smothered in cheese. But eating moderate portions is critical if you want to maintain a healthy weight.

Start by shrinking portions gradually. Order the regular hamburger instead of the larger one. Reduce the amount of cheese you put on your pizza. Serve your pasta on a smaller plate and drink beverages from smaller glasses. Then, pay attention to your internal cues and sensations. Eat slowly, and learn to stop when you feel full. Remind yourself that there's always another occasion to enjoy the food you're eating.

## Live Healthfully

Eating well isn't something that just exists on its own. It's a habit that goes hand-in-hand with a healthy lifestyle, Stokes says. To ensure that you eat well, it's important to also tackle other health challenges in your life. For many people, that means getting a handle on your stress, quitting smoking, sleeping more, and getting more exercise.

Making these changes, however, isn't a quick fix. Change takes time, patience, and serious commitment and effort. The good news is that tackling one unhealthy habit can often set off a ripple effect that will make you healthier in other areas of your life. Once you notice how much better you feel when you exercising more regularly, you'll be less apt to reach for those late-night chips. Once you get a better handle on stress at your job, you won't be as tempted to overeat every night at dinner.

So what are you waiting for? If you're ready to eat a better diet, start today, one small habit at a time. Ditch that afternoon soda. Switch to whole-wheat bread on your sandwiches. Learn to snack on fruit, not cookies. The changes in the way you feel will reinforce your efforts and encourage you to find other ways to improve your diet.

Good luck!

# RESOURCES

## Books

American College of Obstetricians and Gynecologists. *Guidelines for Women's Healthcare.* 2d ed. Washington, D.C.: ACOG, 2002.

American Institute for Cancer Research. *Nutrition after Fifty.* Washington, D.C.: AICR, 2005.

Balch, James F., M.D., and Mark Stengler, N.D. *Prescription for Natural Cures.* Hoboken, NJ: John Wiley and Sons, 2004.

Balch Phyllis A. *Prescription for Nutritional Healing.* 3d ed. New York, NY: Avery, 2000.

Dorfman, Lisa. *The Tropical Diet.* Miami, FL: Food Fitness International, 2004.

Duyff, Roberta Larson. *American Dietetic Association Complete Food and Nutrition Guide.* 2d ed. Hoboken, NJ: John Wiley and Sons, 2002.

Fallon, Sally. *Nourishing Traditions.* Winona Lake, IN: New Trends Publishing, 1999.

Feinberg, Todd, M.D., and Winnie Yu. *What to Do When the Doctor Says It's Early-Stage Alzheimer's.* Gloucester, MA: Fair Winds Press, 2005.

Feingold, Ben M.D. *Why Your Child is Hyperactive.* New York, NY: Random House, 1974.

Fischer, Harry, M.D., and Winnie Yu. *What to Do When the Doctor Says It's Rheumatoid Arthritis.* Gloucester, MA: Fair Winds Press, 2005.

Better Homes and Gardens. *Food for Health and Healing.* Des Moines, IA: Meredith Corporation, 1999.

Friedman, Theodore C., M.D., and Winnie Yu. *The Everything Health Guide to Thyroid Disease.* Avon, MA.: Adams Media, 2007.

Gottschall, Elaine. *Breaking the Vicious Cycle.* Kirkton, ON: Kirkton Press, 1994.

Haas, Elson, M.D., and Daniella Chace. *The New Detox Diet: The Complete Guide for Lifelong Vitality With Recipes, Menus, and Detox Plans.* Berkley, CA: Celestial Arts, 2004.

Hall, Kathleen. *A Life in Balance: Nourishing the Four Roots of True Happiness.* New York, NY: AMACOM, 2006.

Katz, Sandor. *Wild Fermentation: the Flavor, Nutrition, and Craft of Live-Culture Food.* White River Junction, VT: Chelsea Green Publishing Company, 2003.

Larson, Andrew, M.D., and Ivy Larson. *The Gold Coast Cure: The 5-Week Health and Body Makeover, A Lifestyle Plan to Shed Pounds, Gain Health and Reverse 10 Diseases .* Deerfield Beach, FL: Health Communications, Inc., 2005.

Lipski, Elizabeth. *Digestive Wellness.* New York, NY: McGraw Hill, 2005.

LoFrumento, Mary Ann, M.D. *Simply Parenting: Understanding Your Newborn and Infant.* Chatham, NJ: Halo Productions, 2004.

Lyons, Thomas, M.D., and Cheryl Kimball. *What to Do When the Doctor Says It's Endometriosis.* Gloucester, MA: Fair Winds Press, 2003.

Minkin, Mary Jane, M.D. *A Woman's Guide to Menopause and Perimenopause.* New Haven, CT: Yale University Press, 2004.

Minkin, Mary Jane, M.D. *A Woman's Guide to Sexual Health.* New Haven, CT: Yale University Press, 2005.

Moloo, Jeannie. *The No-Salt Lowest Sodium* cookbook series. New York, NY: St. Martin's Press, 2002 and 2003.

Murray, Michael T., Joseph Pizzorno, and Lara Pizzorno. *The Encyclopedia of Healing Foods.* New York, NY: Atria Books, 2005.

Murray, Michael T. *Encyclopedia of Nutritional Supplements.* Rocklin, CA: Prima Publishing, 1996.

Pescatore, Fred M.D. *The Allergy and Asthma Cure.* Hoboken, NJ: John Wiley and Sons, 2003.

Pescatore, Fred M.D. *The Hamptons Diet Cookbook.* Hoboken, NJ: John Wiley and Sons, 2006.

Pescatore, Fred M.D. *Thin for Good: The One Low-Carb Diet that Will Finally Work for You.* Hoboken, NJ: John Wiley and Sons, 2000.

Reader's Digest. *Fight Back with Food.* Pleasantville, NY: Reader's Digest Association, 2002.

Rosenfeld, Isadore, M.D. *Doctor, What Should I Eat?* New York, NY: Random House, 1995.

Savard, Marie, M.D. *The Body Shape Solution for Weight Loss and Wellness.* New York, NY: Atria Books, 2005.

Smolin, Lori A., and Mary B. Grosvenor. *Nutrition: Science and Applications.* Orlando, FL: Saunders College Publishing, 1994.

Stevens, Laura J. *12 Effective Ways to Help Your ADD/ADHD Child.* New York, NY: Penguin Group, 2000.

Teitelbaum, Jacob, M.D. *Pain Free 1-2-3.* New York, NY: McGraw-Hill, 2006.

Waterford, Kathleen. *The Skin Cure Diet: Heal Eczema from the Inside Out.* Lincoln, NE: iUniverse, Inc., 2005.

Yu, Winnie and Michael McNett, M.D. *The Everything Health Guide to Fibromyalgia.* Avon, MA: Adams Media, 2006.

Yu, Winnie, Melvin Stjernholm, M.D., and Alexis Munier. *What to Do When the Doctor Says It's Diabetes.* Gloucester, MA: Fair Winds Press, 2004.

# Articles

Adebamowo, C.A., et al. "High school dietary dairy intake and teenage acne." *Journal of the American Academy of Dermatology* 52, no. 2 (February 2005): 207–14.

Akhondzadeh, S., et al. "Zinc sulfate as an adjunct to methylphenidate for the treatment of attention deficit hyperactivity disorder in children: a double blind and randomized trial." *BMC Psychiatry* 4, no. 9 (April 8, 2004). Available online at www.pubmedcentral.nih.gov.

Al-Gurairi, F.T., et al. "Oral zinc sulphate in the treatment of recalcitrant viral warts: randomized placebo-controlled clinical trial." *British Journal of Dermatology* 146, no. 3 (March 2002): 423–31.

Alm, J.S., et al. "Atopy in children of families with an anthroposophic lifestyle," *The Lancet* 353, no. 9163 (May 1999): 1485–88.

Altura, B.M., et al. "Tension headaches and muscle tension: is there a role for magnesium?" *Medical Hypotheses* 57, no. 6 (December 2001): 705–13.

Arias, Elizabeth. "National Vital Statistics Report." Centers for Disease Control and Prevention 53, no. 6 (November 10, 2004): 1–39.

Arnold, L.E., et al. "Serum zinc correlates with parent- and teacher-rated inattention in children with attention-deficit/hyperactivity disorder." *Journal of Child and Adolescent Psychopharmacology* 15, no. 4 (August 2005): 628–36.

Avisar, R., et al. "Effect of coffee consumption on intraocular pressure." *The Annals of Pharmacotherapy* 36, no. 6 (June 2002): 992–5.

Bailey, E.E., et al. "The use of diet in the treatment of epilepsy." *Epilepsy and Behavior* 6, no. 1 (February 2005): 4–8.

Basson, Marc D. Constipation. http://www.emedicine.com (accessed February 3, 2006).

Bertone-Johnson, E.R., et al. "Calcium and vitamin D intake and risk of incident premenstrual syndrome." *Archives of Internal Medicine* 165, no. 11 (June 2005): 1246–52.

Biederman, M.E., et al. "Case-control study of attention-deficit hyperactivity disorder and maternal smoking, alcohol use, and drug use during pregnancy." *Journal of the American Academy of Child and Adolescent Psychiatry* 41, no. 4 (April 2002): 378–85.

Bodnar, L.M., and Wisner, K.L. "Nutrition and depression: implications for improving mental health among child-bearing-aged women." *Biological Psychiatry* 58, no. 9 (November 1, 2005): 679–85.

Brody, S., et al. "A randomized controlled trial of high dose ascorbic acid for reduction of blood pressure, cortisol, and subjective responses to psychological stress." *Psychopharmacology* 159, no. 3 (January 2002): 319–24.

Bryant, M., et al. "Effect of consumption of soy isoflavones on behavioural, somatic and affective symptoms in women with premenstrual syndrome." *The British Journal of Nutrition* 93, no. 5 (May 2005): 731–9.

Calle, E.E., et al. "Overweight, obesity, and mortality from cancer in a prospectively studied cohort of U.S. adults." *New England Journal of Medicine* 348, no. 17 (April 24, 2003): 1625–38.

Calne, S.M., and Kumar, A. "Nursing care of patients with late-stage Parkinson's disease." *Journal of Neuroscience Nursing* 35, no. 5 (October 2003): 242–51.

Carol, Ruth. "Rosy Cheeks could be rosacea." *Dermatology Insights* 3, no. 1: 23–4.

Cerhan, J.R., et al. "Antioxidant micronutrients and risk of rheumatoid arthritis in a cohort of older women." *American Journal of Epidemiology* 157, no. 4 (February 15, 2003): 345–54.

Chandrasekaran, S., et al. "Effects of caffeine on intraocular pressure: the Blue Mountains Eye Study." *Journal of Glaucoma* 14, no. 6 (December 2005): 504–7.

Collier, P.M., et al. "Effect of regular consumption of oily fish compared with white fish on chronic plaque psoriasis." *European Journal of Clinical Nutrition* 47, no. 4 (April 1993): 251–4.

Coulter, I.D., et al. "Antioxidants vitamin C and vitamin E for the prevention and treatment of cancer." *Journal of General Internal Medicine* 21, no. 7 (July 2006): 735–44.

Cushing, M.L., et al. "Parkinson's disease: implications for nutritional care." *Canadian Journal of Dietetic Practice and Research* 63, no. 2 (Summer 2002): 81–87.

DiGiacomo, R.A., et al. "Fish-oil dietary supplementation in patients with Raynaud's phenomenon: a double-blind, controlled, prospective study." *American Journal of Medicine* 86, no. 2 (February 1989): 158–64.

Doron S., et al. "Probiotics: their role in the treatment and prevention of disease." *Expert Review of Anti-Infective Therapy* 4, no. 2 (April 2006): 261–75.

Eby, G.A., and Halcomb, W.W. "Ineffectiveness of zinc gluconate nasal spray and zinc orotate lozenges in common-cold treatment: a double-blind, placebo-controlled clinical trial." *Alternative Therapies in Health and Medicine* 12, no. 1 (January–February 2006): 34–8.

Evans, D.L., et al. "Mood disorders in the medically ill: scientific review and recommendations." *Biological Psychiatry* 58, no. 3 (2005): 175–89.

Fahey, J.W., et al. "Sulforaphane inhibits extracellular, intracellular, and antibiotic-resistant strains of Helicobacter pylori and prevents benzo[a]pyrene-induced stomach tumors." *Proceedings of the National Academy of Sciences of the United States of America* 99, no. 11 (May 28, 2002): 7610–5.

Farchi, S., et al. "Dietary factors associated with wheezing and allergic rhinitis in children." *European Respiratory Journal* 22, no. 5 (November 2003): 772–80.

Fernandez-Banares, F., et al. "Randomized clinical trial of Plantago ovata seeds (dietary fiber) as compared with mesalamine in maintaining remission in ulcerative colitis. Spanish Group for the Study of Crohn's Disease and Ulcerative Colitis (GETECCU)." *American Journal of Gastroenterology* 94, no. 2 (February 1999): 427–33.

Forastiere, F., et al. "Consumption of fresh fruit rich in vitamin C and wheezing symptoms in children. SIDRIA Collaborative Group, Italy (Italian Studies on Respiratory Disorders in Children and the Environment)." *Thorax* 55, no. 4 (April 2000): 283–8.

Foster, Tammy. "Bulimia." http://www.emedicine.com (accessed March 28, 2005).

Gassull, M.A. "Review article: the role of nutrition in the treatment of inflammatory bowel disease." *Alimentary Pharmacology and Therapeutics* 20, Suppl no. 4 (October 2004): 79–83.

Genever, R.W., et al. "Fracture rates in Parkinson's disease compared with age- and gender-matched controls: a retrospective cohort study." *Age and Ageing* 34, no. 1 (2005): 21–24.

Godfrey, H.R., et al. "A randomized clinical trial on the treatment of oral herpes with topical zinc oxide/glycine." *Alternative Therapies in Health and Medicine* 7, no. 3 (May–June 2001): 49–56.

Gordon, Andrea E., and Shaughnessy, Allen F. "Saw palmetto and prostate disorders." *American Family Physician* 67, no. 6 (March 15, 2003).

Grant, J.E., et al. "Analysis of dietary intake and selected nutrient concentrations in patients with chronic fatigue syndrome." *Journal of the American Dietetic Association* 96, no. 4 (April 1996): 383–6.

Grant, W.B. "Epidemiology of disease risks in relation to vitamin D insufficiency." *Progress in Biophysics and Molecular Biology* 92, no. 1 (September 2006): 65–79.

Hamilton-Miller, J.M. "Probiotics and prebiotics in the elderly." *Postgraduate Medical Journal* 80, no. 946 (August 2004): 447–51.

"Health risks and benefits of alcohol consumption." *Alcohol Research and Health* 24, no. 1 (2000).

Heliovaara, M., et al. "Serum antioxidants and risk of rheumatoid arthritis." *Annals of the Rheumatic Disease* 53, no. 1 (January 1994): 51–3.

Henneman, Alice, and Boeckner, Linda. "Nutrition and osteoporosis." *Food Reflections.* May/June 2001. Online newsletter. http://lancaster.unl.edu/food/ftm-j01.htm

Hill, D.J., et al. "Effect of a low-allergen maternal diet on colic among breastfed infants: a randomized, controlled trial." *Pediatrics* 116, no. 5 (November 2005): 709–15.

Jakobsson, I., et al. "Cow's milk proteins cause infantile colic in breast-fed infants: a double-blind crossover study." *Pediatrics* 71, no. 2 (February 1, 1983): 268–71.

Kendall, S.N. "Remission of rosacea induced by reduction of gut transit time." *Clinical and Experimental Dermatology* 29, no. 3 (May 2004): 297–9.

Kerr, Martha. "Probiotics significantly reduce symptoms of IBS, ulcerative colitis." *Medscape Medical News.* www.medscape.com/viewarticle/455964 (accessed May 21, 2003).

Kim, L.S., et al. "Efficacy of methylsulfonylmethane (MSM) in osteoarthritis pain of the knee: a pilot clinical trial." *Osteoarthritis and Cartilage* 14, no. 3 (March 2006): 286–94.

Kontiokari, T., et al. "Dietary factors protecting women from urinary tract infection." *American Journal of Clinical Nutrition* 77, no. 3 (March 2003): 600–4.

Kose, K., et al. "Plasma selenium levels in rheumatoid arthritis." *Biological Trace Element Research* 53, no. 1–3 (Summer 1996): 51–6.

Kotimaa, A.J., et al. "Maternal smoking and hyperactivity in 8-year-old children." *Journal of the American Academy of Child and Adolescent Psychiatry* 42, no. 7 (July 2003): 826–33.

Laitinen, K., et al. "Breast milk fatty acids may link innate and adaptive immune regulation: Analysis of soluble CD14, prostaglandin E2, and fatty acids." *Pediatric Research* 59, no. 5 (May 2006): 723–7.

Leitzmann, C. "Vegetarian diets: what are the advantages?" *Forum of Nutrition*, no. 57 (2005): 147–56.

Levri, K.M., et al. "Do probiotics reduce adult lactose intolerance? A systematic review." *The Journal of Family Practice* 54, no. 7 (July 2005): 613–20.

Lucassen, P.L., et al. "Infantile colic: crying time reduction with a whey hydrolysate: a double-blind, randomized, placebo-controlled trial." *Pediatrics* 106, no. 6 (December 2000): 1349–54.

Massey, L. "Magnesium therapy for nephrolithiasis." *Magnesium Research* 18, no. 2 (June 2005): 123–6.

McElroy, B.H., et al. "An open-label, single-center, phase IV clinical study of the effectiveness of zinc gluconate glycine lozenges (Cold-Eeze) in reducing the duration and symptoms of the common cold in school-aged subjects." *American Journal of Therapeutics* 10, no. 5 (September–October 2003): 324–9.

McHughes, M., and Lipman, A.G. "Managing osteoarthritis pain when your patient fails simple analgesics and NSAIDs and is not a candidate for surgery." *Current Rheumatology Reports* 8, no. 1 (February 2006): 22–9.

Mickleborough, T.D., et al. "Protective effect of fish oil supplementation on exercise-induced bronchoconstriction in asthma." *Chest* 129, no. 1 (January 2006): 39–49.

Nandurkar, S., et al. "Relationship between body mass index, diet, exercise and gastrooesophageal reflux symptoms in a community." *Alimentary Pharmacology and Therapeutics* 20, no 5 (September 1, 2004): 497–505.

Nishida, M., et al. "Calcium and the risk for periodontal disease." *Journal of Periodontology* 71, no. 7 (July 2000): 1057–166.

Nishida, M., et al. "Dietary vitamin C and the risk for periodontal disease." *Journal of Periodontology* 71, no. 8 (August 2000): 1215–23.

Nordmark, G., et al. "Effects of dehydroepiandrosterone supplement on health-related quality of life in glucocorticoid treated female patients with systemic lupus erythematosus." *Autoimmunity* 38, no. 7 (November 2005): 531–40.

Obermuller-Jevic, U.C. "Lycopene inhibits the growth of normal human prostate epithelial cells in vitro." *Journal of Nutrition* 133, no. 11 (November 2003): 3356–60.

Oken B.S., et al. "Randomized controlled trial of yoga and exercise in multiple sclerosis." *Neurology* 62, no. 11 (June 8, 2004): 2058–64.

O'Mahony, R., et al. "Bactericidal and anti-adhesive properties of culinary and medicinal plants against Helicobacter pylori." *World Journal of Gastroenterology* 11, no. 47 (December 21, 2005): 7499–507.

Ozgocmen, S., et al. "Vitamin D deficiency and reduced bone mineral density in multiple sclerosis: effect of ambulatory status and functional capacity." *Journal of Bone and Mineral Metabolism* 23, no. 4 (July 2005): 309–13.

Pattison, D.J., et al. "Does diet have a role in the aetiology of rheumatoid arthritis?" *Proceedings of the Nutrition Society* 63, no. 1 (February 2004): 137–43.

Pixley, F. and Mann, J. "Dietary factors in the aetiology of gall stones: a case control study." *Gut* 29, no. 11 (November 1988): 1511–5.

Pixley F., et al. "Effect of vegetarianism on development of gallstones in women." *British Medical Journal* (Clinical Research Ed) 6, no. 291(6487) (July 1985): 11–2.

Prager, N., et al. "A randomized, double-blind, placebo-controlled trial to determine the effectiveness of botanically derived inhibitors of 5-alpha-reductase in the treatment of androgenetic alopecia." *Journal of Alternative and Complementary Medicine* 8, no. 2 (April 2002): 143–52.

Rabkin, J.G., et al. "Placebo-controlled trial of dehydroepiandrosterone (DHEA) for treatment of nonmajor depression in patients with HIV/AIDS." *American Journal of Psychiatry* 163, no. 1 (January 2006): 59–66.

Rall, L.C., and Roubenoff, Ronenn. "Nutrition and connective tissue disease." *Nutrition Today* 35, no. 4 (July/August 2000): 142–9.

Rannem, T., et al. "Selenium status in patients with Crohn's disease." *American Journal of Clinical Nutrition* 56, no. 5 (November 1992): 933–7.

Reilly, A., and Snyder, B. "Raynaud phenomenon." *American Journal of Nursing* 105, no. 8 (August 2005): 56–65.

Rennard, B.O., et al. "Chicken soup inhibits neutrophil chemotaxis in vitro." *Chest* 118, no. 4 (October 2000): 1150–7.

Rhee, D.J., et al. "Complementary and alternative medicine for glaucoma." *Survey of Ophthalmology* 46, no. 1 (July/August 2001): 43–55.

Rindone, J.P., and Murphy, T.W. "Warfarin-cranberry juice interaction resulting in profound hypoprothrombinemia and bleeding." *American Journal of Therapeutics* 13, no. 3 (May/June 2006): 283–4.

Ritch, R. "Complementary therapy for the treatment of glaucoma: a perspective." *Ophthalmology Clinics of North America* 18, no. 4 (December 2005): 597–609.

Ricciardi, Nikki. "Boric acid effective treatment for chronic yeast infections." College Pharmacy press release. www.collegepharmacy.com.

Rogers, M.A., et al. "Consumption of nitrate, nitrite, and nitrosodimethylamine and the risk of upper aerodigestive tract cancer." *Cancer Epidemiology, Biomarkers and Prevention* 4, no. 1 (January/February 1995): 29–36.

Romano, L., et al. "In vitro activity of bergamot natural essence and furocoumarin-free and distilled extracts, and their associations with boric acid, against clinical yeast isolates. *Journal of Antimicrobial Chemotherapy* 55, no. 1 (January 2005): 110–4.

Romieu, I., et al. "Fruit and vegetable intakes and asthma in the E3N study." *Thorax* 61, no. 3 (2006): 209–15.

Scott, M., et al. "Gastroesophageal reflux disease: diagnosis and management." *American Family Physician* 59, no. 5. www.aafp.org (accessed November 21, 2006).

Segasothy, M., et al. "Vegetarian diet: panacea for modern lifestyle diseases?" *QJM* 92, no. 9 (September 1999): 531–44.

Seidner, D.L., et al. "An oral supplement enriched with fish oil, soluble fiber, and antioxidants for corticosteroid sparing in ulcerative colitis: a randomized, controlled trial." *Clinical Gastroenterology and Hepatology* 3, no. 4 (April 2005): 358–69.

Simon, J.A., et al. "Serum ascorbic acid and gallbladder disease prevalence among U.S. adults." *Archives of Internal Medicine* 160, no. 7 (April 10, 2000): 931–6.

Sivam, G.P., et al. "Protection against Helicobacter pylori and Other Bacterial Infections by Garlic." *Journal of Nutrition* 31, no. 3S (March 2001, supplement): 1106S–1108S.

Staudte, H., et al. "Grapefruit consumption improves vitamin C status in periodontitis patients." *British Dental Journal* 199, no. 4 (August 27, 2005): 213–7.

Stommel, M., et al. "Depression and functional status as predictors of death among cancer patients." *Cancer* 94, no. 10 (May 15, 2002): 2719–27.

Stone, J., et al. "Inadequate calcium, folic acid, vitamin E, zinc, and selenium intake in rheumatoid arthritis patients: results of a dietary survey." *Seminars in Arthritis and Rheumatism* 27, no. 3 (December 1997): 180–5.

Suvarna, R., et al. "Possible interaction between warfarin and cranberry juice." *British Medical Journal* 327, no. 7429 (December 20, 2003): 1454.

Taylor, E.N., et al. "Obesity, weight gain, and the risk of kidney stones." *Journal of the American Medical Association* 293, no. 4 (January 26, 2005): 455–62.

Taylor, E.N., et al. "Dietary factors and the risk of incident kidney stones in men: new insights after 14 years of follow-up." *Journal of the American Society of Nephrology* 15, no. 12 (December 2004): 3225–32.

Thys-Jacobs, S. "Micronutrients and the premenstrual syndrome: the case for calcium." *Journal of the American College of Nutrition* 19, no. 2 (April 2000): 220–7.

Trost, L.B., et al. "The diagnosis and treatment of iron deficiency and its potential relationship to hair loss." *Journal of the American Academy of Dermatology* 54, no. 5 (May 2006): 903–6.

Tsai, C.J., et al. "Long-term intake of trans-fatty acids and risk of gallstone disease in men." *Archives of Internal Medicine* 165, no. 9 (May 9, 2005): 1011–5.

Walker, A.F., et al. "Magnesium supplementation alleviates premenstrual symptoms of fluid retention." *Journal of Women's Health* 7, no. 9 (November 1998): 1157–65.

Williams, A.L., et al. "Do essential fatty acids have a role in the treatment of depression?" *Journal of Affective Disorders* 93, no. 1–3 (July 2006): 117–23.

Wilt, T., et al. "Pygeum africanum for benign prostatic hyperplasia." *Cochrane Database Systematic Review*, no. 1 (2002): CD001044.

Wong, K.W. "Clinical efficacy of n-3 fatty acid supplementation in patients with asthma." *Journal of the American Dietetic Association* 105, no. 1 (January 2005): 98–105.

Yusuf, S., et al. "Obesity and the risk of myocardial infarction in 27,000 participants from 52 countries: a case control study." *The Lancet* 366, no. 9497 (November 5, 2005): 1640–9.

# Web Sites

**AIDSINFO**
www.aidsinfo.nih.gov

**AMERICAN ACADEMY OF ALLERGY ASTHMA AND IMMUNOLOGY**
www.aaaai.org

**AMERICAN ACADEMY OF DERMATOLOGY**
www.aad.org

**AMERICAN ACADEMY OF FAMILY PHYSICIANS**
www.familydoctor.org

**AMERICAN ACADEMY OF PERIODONTOLOGY**
www.perio.org

**AMERICAN CANCER SOCIETY**
www.cancer.org

**AMERICAN COUNCIL FOR HEADACHE EDUCATION**
www.achenet.org

**AMERICAN DENTAL ASSOCIATION**
www.ada.org

**AMERICAN DIABETES ASSOCIATION**
www.diabetes.org

**AMERICAN DIETETIC ASSOCIATION**
www.eatright.org

**AMERICAN HEART ASSOCIATION**
www.americanheart.org

**AMERICAN LUNG ASSOCIATION**
www.lungusa.org

**AMERICAN SOCIETY OF COLON AND RECTAL SURGEONS**
www.fascrs.org

**ARTHRITIS FOUNDATION**
www.arthritis.org

**ASTHMA AND ALLERGY FOUNDATION OF AMERICA**
www.aafa.org

**BREAKING THE VICIOUS CYCLE**
www.breakingtheviciouscycle.org

**CENTERS FOR DISEASE CONTROL AND PREVENTION**
www.cdc.gov

**CLEVELAND CLINIC HEALTH INFORMATION CENTER**
www.clevelandclinic.org

**CROHN'S AND COLITIS FOUNDATION OF AMERICA**
www.ccfa.org

**EMEDICINE**
www.emedicine.com

**ELSON HAAS, M.D.**
www.elsonhaas.com

**EPILEPSY.COM**
www.epilepsy.com

**FEINGOLD DIET**
www.feingold.org

**FOURFOLD PATH TO HEALING**
www.fourfoldhealing.com

**EPILEPSY FOUNDATION**
www.epilepsyfoundation.org

**GLAUCOMA RESEARCH FOUNDATION**
www.glaucoma.org

**HEALTHY PLACE**
www.healthyplace.com

**THE HELICOBACTER FOUNDATION**
www.helio.org

**HEPATITIS FOUNDATION INTERNATIONAL**
www.hepfi.org

**IRRITABLE BOWEL SYNDROME SELF-HELP AND SUPPORT GROUP**
www.ibsgroup.org

**KID'S HEALTH**
www.kidshealth.org

**KUSHI INSTITUTE**
www.kushiinstitute.org

**LUPUS FOUNDATION OF AMERICA**
www.lupus.org

**MAYO CLINIC**
www.mayoclinic.com

**MEDLINE PLUS**
www.nlm.nih.gov/medlineplus

**MERCK MANUAL**
www.merck.com

**NATIONAL CANCER INSTITUTE**
www.cancer.gov

**NATIONAL HEART, LUNG, AND BLOOD INSTITUTE**
www.nhlbi.nih.gov

**NATIONAL INSTITUTE ON ALCOHOL ABUSE AND ALCOHOLISM**
www.niaaa.nih.gov

**NATIONAL INSTITUTE OF ARTHRITIS AND MUSCULOSKETAL AND SKIN DISEASES**
www.niams.nih.gov

**NATIONAL INSTITUTE OF DIGESTIVE AND DIABETES AND KIDNEY DISORDERS**
www.niddk.nih.gov

**NATIONAL INSTITUTE OF MENTAL HEALTH**
www.nihm.nih.gov

**NATIONAL INSTITUTE OF NEUROLOGICAL DISORDERS AND STROKE**
www.ninds.nih.gov

**NATIONAL KIDNEY FOUNDATION**
www.kidney.org

**NATIONAL PARKINSON FOUNDATION**
www.parkinson.org

**NATIONAL PSORIASIS FOUNDATION**
www.psoriasis.org

**NATIONAL ROSACEA SOCIETY**
www.rosacea.org

**NATIONAL WOMEN'S HEALTH INFORMATION CENTER**
www.womenshealth.gov

**OFFICE OF DIETARY SUPPLEMENTS**
www.dietary-supplements.info.nih.gov

**NORTH AMERICAN MENOPAUSE SOCIETY**
www.menopause.org

**PDRHEALTH.COM**
www.pdrhealth.com

**PREVENT BLINDNESS AMERICA**
www.preventblindness.org

**PUBMED**
www.pubmed.com

**RAY SAHELIAN, M.D.**
www.raysahelian.com

**REBECCA WOOD ASHLAND COOKING SCHOOL**
www.rwood.com

**SPECIFIC CARBOHYDRATE DIET WEB LIBRARY**
www.scdiet.org

**SCLERODERMA FOUNDATION**
www.sclero.org

**SJOGREN'S SYNDROME FOUNDATION**
www.sjogrens.org

**THE SKIN CURE DIET**
www.skincurediet.org

**UNIVERSITY OF MARYLAND MEDICAL CENTER**
www.umm.edu

**UNIVERSITY OF PENNSYLVANIA HEALTH SYSTEM**
www.pennhealth.com

**UNIVERSITY OF PITTSBURGH MEDICAL CENTER**
www.upmc.com

**UNIVERSITY OF WASHINGTON MEDICINE**
www.uwmedicine.org

**VETERANS AFFAIRS NATIONAL HEPATITIS C PROGRAM**
www.hepatitis.va.gov

**VARICELLA-ZOSTER VIRUS (VZV) RESEARCH FOUNDATION**
www.vzvfoundation.org

**WEB MD**
www.wedmd.com

**WESTON A. PRICE FOUNDATION**
www.westonaprice.org

**WILD FERMENTION**
www.wildfermentation.com

# ACKNOWLEDGMENTS

Writing a book is never completely a solo endeavor, despite the many hours a writer toils alone. I owe my gratitude to many people, and I'd like to start by thanking my editors at Fair Winds—Wendy Gardner, Holly Schmidt, and Amanda Waddell—as well as the other staff members who have helped bring this project to fruition.

None of this would have been possible without the help of some extraordinary medical experts who gave me their time, energy, and wisdom. I'd like to thank Susan M. Calne, Lisa Dorfman, Theodore C. Friedman, Christine Gerbstadt, Lise Gloede, Kathleen Hall, Marielle Kabbouche, Michele Kearney, Andrew Larson, Ivy Larson, Elizabeth Lipski, Mary Ann LoFrumento, Susan Krantz, Thomas Lyons, Michael McNett, Mary Jane Minkin, Jeannie Moloo, Amy Neuzil, Mildred M.G. Olivier, Lola O'Rourke, Fred Pescatore, Joseph Petrosino, Richard Price, Marie Savard, Janet Scloss, Carl Stafstrom, Melvin Stjernholm, Laura Stevens, Milton Stokes, Lynn Sutton, Marilyn Tanner, and Jacob Teitelbaum. I'd also like to thank Jennifer Starkey at the American Dietetic Association.

And finally, I'd like to thank my friends and family, especially Jeff, Samantha, and Annie.

# ABOUT THE AUTHOR

Winnie Yu is a freelance writer who writes frequently on health and nutrition for national magazines, such as *Woman's Day, Weight Watchers, Redbook,* and *Fitness.* She has a B.A. in magazine journalism and psychology from Syracuse University and lives in upstate New York with her husband and two daughters.

# INDEX

## A

acetylcholinesterase, 33

acid-alkaline imbalances, 42

acidic foods, 78, 180, 286, 312, 315

*acidophilus*, 78, 143–44, 162, 194, 209, 282, 283, 309, 313, 315

acne, 12–14

acupuncture, 195, 294

additives, 29, 53

adenosylmethionine (SAM-e), 110, 143, 290

ADHD
 *See* attention deficit hyperactivity disorder (ADHD)

adrenal function, 223

advancing age, 15–18

African pygeum, 268

aging, 15–18

AHCC (active hexose correlated compound), 99, 199

AIDS/HIV infection, 19–22

alcohol

 advancing age and, 17

 AIDS/HIV infection and, 21

 anxiety and, 40

 bad breath and, 163

 bulimia and, 60

 cancer and, 69, 71

 cold sores and, 93

 depression and, 110

 diabetes and, 114–15

endometriosis and, 131

fever and, 139

fibroids and, 319

fibromyalgia and, 142

hangover and, 164–65

hepatitis and, 177

herpes and, 180

high blood pressure and, 184

hyperthyroidism and, 188

insomnia and, 201

kidney stones and, 213

Lyme disease and, 224

menopause and, 232

moderation in, 337

mononucleosis and, 234

MS and, 241

osteoporosis and, 245

pregnancy and, 261

Raynaud's phenomenon and, 275

rosacea and, 282

SAD and, 289

Sjogren's syndrome and, 296

stress and, 299

ulcers and, 312

varicose veins and, 326

 weight gain and, 55

alcoholism, 23–26

alfalfa sprouts, 220

allergies, 27–30, 40
 *See also* food allergies

Alzheimer's disease, 31–34

American diet, changes in, 8

anaphylaxis, 28

anemia, 35–37

antibiotics, 13, 51, 72, 76, 89, 123, 282, 285

antidepressants, 86, 208

antidiarrheal drugs, 119

antioxidants
 *See also* specific antioxidants

 AIDS/HIV and, 22

 Alzheimer's disease and, 32

 cancer and, 67, 69

 fibromyalgia and, 141

 foods rich in, 28

 glaucoma and, 153

 hepatitis and, 176

 macular degeneration and, 227

 MS and, 241

 psoriasis and, 272

 stress and, 298

antiretroviral drugs, 22

anti-seizure medications, 134

antiviral remedies, 94, 180–81, 332–33

anxiety, 38–40

appetite problems, 106

arginine, 93, 180, 294, 332

arnica, 64

artery-clogging foods, 33
 *See also* saturated fats; trans-fatty acids

arthritis, 41–44
    psoriatic, 271
    rheumatoid, 277–80
artificial sweeteners, 60, 109–10, 142, 289
aspartame, 60, 109–10, 142, 289
aspirin, 48, 173, 185, 235, 304, 313
asthma, 73
atherosclerosis, 45–48, 301
atrophic vaginitis, 322
attention deficit hyperactivity disorder (ADHD), 49–53
autoimmune disorders
    lupus, 218–21
    multiple sclerosis, 239–42
    rheumatoid arthritis, 277–80
    scleroderma, 284–87
    Sjogren's syndrome, 295–96
*avena sativa*, 294

# B

babies
    candidiasis and, 73
    colic in, 95–96
    transmission of herpes to, 180
back pain, 54–57
bacterial vaginosis, 322
barbecues, 71
berberine, 76, 323
beta carotene, 228, 278
betaine HCL, 196
*Bifidobacteria,* 309
bilberry, 153, 228, 327
biofeedback, 168, 306
bioflavanoids, 43, 63

biotin, 159, 160
bisphosphonates, 246
black cohosh, 232
blackheads, 12
bladder infections
    *See* urinary tract infections
blood clots, 45, 46, 301
blood glucose, 112–13, 116, 203, 204
body mass index (BMI), 172, 183
bone fractures, 249
    *See also* osteoporosis
boric acid, 324
boswellia, 224, 280
bowel management program, 251
BRAT diet, 118
breakfast, 52
breast cancer, 69
breastfeeding, 96, 124, 125, 127
breath odor, 161–63
bromelain, 64, 280, 309
bulimerexia, 59
bulimia, 58–61
bursitis, 62–64
butcher's broom, 327
B vitamins
    *See also* folic acid; thiamin
    ADHD and, 52
    advancing age and, 16
    AIDS/HIV infection and, 22
    alcoholism and, 26
    Alzheimer's disease and, 34
    anemia and, 36, 37
    anxiety and, 39, 40
    arthritis and, 43

bursitis and, 63
canker sores and, 78
CFS and, 86
Crohn's disease and, 106
depression and, 110
endometriosis and, 130, 132
fibroids and, 319, 320
fibromyalgia and, 141
hair loss and, 159
heart disease and, 173
high blood pressure and, 184
indigestion and, 196
kidney stones and, 213
PMS and, 265
rheumatoid arthritis and, 278
SAD and, 290
shingles and, 293
sources of, 78
stress and, 298, 299
stroke and, 304
TMJ and, 306

# C

caffeine
    anxiety and, 39–40
    bulimia and, 60
    cancer and, 69
    cold sores and, 93
    constipation and, 101
    depression and, 110
    diarrhea and, 118
    endometriosis and, 131
    fibromyalgia and, 142
    glaucoma and, 153

dysphagia, 250

dysthymia, 111

   *See also* depression

# E

ear infections, 123–25

eating disorders, 58–61

echinacea, 98, 198

eczema, 126–28

egg whites, 159

elderberry, 199

elderly

   *See also* aging

   osteoporosis and, 243–46

   pneumonia and, 255

elimination diet, 118, 124, 127, 142, 168, 272, 279, 309

emphysema, 88–89

endometrial cancer, 69

endometriosis, 129–32

environmental pollutants, 178

enzyme-linked immunoassay (ELISA) test, 223

epilepsy, 133–36

epinephrine, 300

Epstein-Barr virus (EBV), 233, 235

estrogen, 17, 130, 268, 318

evening primrose oil, 128, 132, 266, 320

exchange system of eating, 114

exercise

   aging and, 18

   anxiety and, 40

   arthritis and, 44

   back pain and, 56

   cancer and, 71

candidiasis and, 76

CFS and, 86

constipation and, 102

COPD and, 90

Crohn's disease and, 107

depression and, 111

diabetes and, 116

diverticulitis and, 122

endometriosis and, 132

epilepsy and, 135–36

fibromyalgia and, 144

gallstones and, 147

GERD and, 150

hair loss and, 160

headaches and, 169

heart disease and, 174

high blood pressure and, 185

hypothyroidism and, 193

indigestion and, 196

insomnia and, 202

insulin resistance and, 203, 206

lupus and, 221

macular degeneration and, 229

menopause and, 232

MS and, 242

osteoporosis and, 246

PCOS and, 259

PMS and, 266

pregnancy and, 262

Raynaud's phenomenon and, 275

rheumatoid arthritis and, 280

rosacea and, 283

SAD and, 290

scleroderma and, 286

stress and, 299

stroke and, 304

ulcerative colitis and, 310

varicose veins and, 327

exophthalmos, 187

# F

fast foods, 149, 323

fats

   *See also* saturated fats; trans-fatty acids

   ADHD and, 51

   cancer and, 71

   choosing wisely, 335

   diabetes and, 114

   diarrhea and, 118

   hepatitis and, 176

   hypothyroidism and, 191

   IBS and, 208

   insulin resistance and, 205

   lupus and, 220

   macular degeneration and, 227

   monounsaturated, 46, 172, 183, 191, 204, 258, 303

   polycystic ovarian syndrome and, 258

   polyunsaturated, 204–5, 258

febrile seizures, 138

Feingold Program, 29, 53

fermented foods, 20, 28, 101, 105, 210, 308, 337

fever, 137–39

feverfew, 144

fiber

   advancing age and, 16

   anxiety and, 39

herpes and, 180

## O

oats, 82

obesity, 8, 32
*See also* overweight

oils, 241

olive leaf extract, 94, 181, 332

olive oil, 146, 241

omega-3 fatty acids
acne and, 13
allergies and, 28, 29
Alzheimer's disease and, 32, 33
arthritis and, 42
bursitis and, 63
depression and, 109, 110
eczema and, 127
hair loss and, 159
health benefits of, 335
heart disease and, 46, 48, 172, 173
high blood pressure and, 183, 184
lupus and, 219, 220
macular degeneration and, 227
menopause and, 231
MS and, 240
pneumonia and, 254
psoriasis and, 272
rheumatoid arthritis and, 278
rosacea and, 282
SAD and, 289
Sjogren's syndrome and, 296
sources of, 51, 240
stroke and, 302, 303

supplements, 33, 48, 107, 122
TMJ and, 306

omega-6 fatty acids, 51

onions, 28, 162

oral contraceptives, 73, 216

oral hygiene, 79, 157, 162

oregano oil, 94, 181, 333

oscillococcinum, 199

osteoarthritis, 41–44

osteoporosis, 231, 243–46, 278

otitis media
*See* ear infections

outdoor allergens, 30

ovaries, 256

over-the-counter medications, 30, 99, 216

overweight
*See also* weight gain
Alzheimer's disease and, 32
arthritis and, 42, 44
back pain and, 55
cancer and, 71
diabetes and, 114
gallstones and, 147
GERD and, 150
heart disease and, 172
hepatitis and, 178
high blood pressure and, 185
insulin resistance and, 203–4
kidney stones and, 213
psoriasis and, 272
stress and, 298
stroke and, 302

oxalates, 212, 245

oxalic acid, 36, 37

## P

panic disorder, 39

Parkinson's disease, 247–52

passionflower, 202, 224

pau d'arco tea, 74, 322

peppermint, 237

peppermint oil, 144, 147, 209

peptic ulcers, 311

periodontal disease, 155–57

periodontitis, 155

personal hygiene, 93

phosphorous, 245, 278

phytates, 245

phytochemicals, 71

pickles, 71

pimples
*See* acne

plantar warts, 332

plant stanols, 46

plaque, 155, 162

pneumonia, 253–55

polycystic ovarian syndrome (PCOS), 256–59

polyunsaturated fats, 204–5, 258

portions, 337–38

post-traumatic stress disorder (PSTD), 39

posture, 56, 64, 169

potassium
COPD and, 90
Crohn's disease and, 107
fibromyalgia and, 141
kidney stones and, 212
sources of, 60, 90

hyperthyroidism, 186–89

hypothyroidism, 190–93

ticks, 225

tomatoes, 268

toothpaste, 79

trans-fatty acids

ADHD and, 51

Alzheimer's disease and, 33

atherosclerosis and, 47

dangers of, 335

diabetes and, 114

gum disease and, 156

hepatitis and, 176

high blood pressure and, 184

hypothyroidism and, 192

lupus and, 220

MS and, 241

polycystic ovarian syndrome and, 258

sources of, 55

stroke and, 303

varicose veins and, 326

transient ischemic attacks (TIAs), 301

travel, motion sickness and, 236–38

traveler's diarrhea (TD), 119

trichomoniasis, 322

tryptophan, 60, 109, 201, 265

tumors, 65, 318–20

type 2 diabetes
See diabetes

tyramine, 168, 201

# U

ulcerative colitis (UC), 307–10

ulcers, 311–13

uric acid stones, 211

urinary incontinence, 317

urinary tract infections (UTIs), 314–17

uterine fibroids, 318–20

uva ursi, 76, 316, 323

# V

vaccine

flu, 197, 199, 255

pneumonia, 255

shingles, 292–93

vaginal dryness, 232

vaginal yeast infections, 321–24

vagus nerve stimulators (VNS), 133

valerian, 144, 202, 224

varicose veins, 325–27

variety, 337

vegan diet, 85, 141

vegetable oils, 241

vegetables

acne and, 13

arthritis and, 42

bursitis and, 63

cancer and, 67, 71

Crohn's disease and, 105

fermented, 20, 28, 101, 105, 210, 308, 337

gallstones and, 146

glaucoma and, 152–53

goitrogens, 188, 192

for health, 335

heart disease and, 172

hyperthyroidism and, 188

menopause and, 231–32

psoriasis and, 272

rheumatoid arthritis and, 278

rosacea and, 282

as source of antioxidants, 28, 32

stroke and, 303

yeast infections and, 322

vegetarian diets, 146

vinegar, 74

vision, ways to boost, 229

vitamin A

acne and, 13

AIDS/HIV infection and, 22

diarrhea and, 118

fibromyalgia and, 141

glaucoma and, 153

macular degeneration and, 227, 228

pneumonia and, 254, 255

vitamin B12
See B vitamins

vitamin B6 (pyrodoxine)
See B vitamins

vitamin C

ADHD and, 52

advancing age and, 16

AIDS/HIV infection and, 22

allergies and, 29

Alzheimer's disease and, 34

anemia and, 36, 37

arthritis and, 43

bursitis and, 63

canker sores and, 78

CFS and, 86

colds and, 98

ear infections and, 125

eczema and, 127, 128

endometriosis and, 132

fever and, 138, 139

fibroids and, 320

fibromyalgia and, 141

flu and, 198

gallstones and, 147

glaucoma and, 153

gum disease and, 156, 157

hair loss and, 159, 160

hyperthyroidism and, 189

kidney stones and, 213

macular degeneration and, 227, 228

mononucleosis and, 234

pneumonia and, 254, 255

pregnancy and, 261

psoriasis and, 272

rheumatoid arthritis and, 278

rosacea and, 283

stress and, 298, 299

ulcerative colitis and, 309

UTIs and, 316

vitamin D

advancing age and, 17–18

Crohn's disease and, 106

gum disease and, 156–57

high blood pressure and, 184

hyperthyroidism and, 188

lactose intolerance and, 215, 217

lupus and, 220

menopause and, 231, 232

MS and, 241

osteoporosis and, 243, 244, 246

Parkinson's disease and, 249

PMS and, 265

rheumatoid arthritis and, 278

vitamin E

AIDS/HIV infection and, 22

Alzheimer's disease and, 34

CFS and, 86

glaucoma and, 153

macular degeneration and, 227, 228

PMS and, 266

pneumonia and, 254, 255

warts and, 333

vomiting, 328–30

# W

waist circumference, 183, 204

warfarin (Coumadin), 17, 33, 315

warts, 331–33

water

*See also* fluid intake

acne and, 13

advancing age and, 17

allergies and, 28

bad breath and, 162

bulimia and, 59

fiber and, 55

gallstones and, 146

GERD and, 149

hangover and, 164

headaches and, 167

motion sickness and, 237

MS and, 240

pneumonia and, 254

scleroderma and, 285

stress and, 298

ulcers and, 312

urinary tract infections and, 315

water retention, 90

weight gain

*See also* overweight

arthritis and, 42, 44

back pain and, 55

diabetes and, 113

hypothyroidism and, 191

insulin resistance and, 203

during pregnancy, 261–62

rheumatoid arthritis and, 279

ways to limit, 33

weight loss

AIDS/HIV infection and, 21

fiber and, 183, 191–92

heart disease and, 172

Parkinson's disease and, 248, 250

polycystic ovarian syndrome and, 258

strategies for, 115, 259

stroke and, 304

wheat, 82

whey protein, 20

whiteheads, 12

whole grains, 69, 74, 176, 298, 322

wild lettuce, 224

willow bark, 224

wine, 47, 78

# Y

yeast, 13, 51, 74, 323

yeast infections, 72–76, 321–24

yoga, 306

yogurt, 74, 78, 162, 194, 215, 282, 315, 322

# Z

zeaxanthin, 153, 228

zinc

    acne and, 13

    ADHD and, 52

    alcoholism and, 24, 25

    bulimia and, 60

    colds and, 98

    cold sores and, 93

    ear infections and, 125

    flu and, 198

    glaucoma and, 153

    herpes and, 180

    macular degeneration and, 227, 228

    mononucleosis and, 234

    pneumonia and, 254, 255

    pregnancy and, 261

    prostate enlargement and, 268

    psoriasis and, 273

    sources of, 60

    warts and, 332

Zostavax, 292–93

# Also from Fair Winds

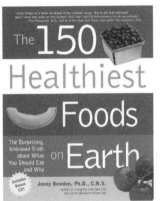

The 150 Healthiest Foods on Earth
By Jonny Bowden, Ph.D., C.N.S.
ISBN-10: 1-59233-228-5
ISBN-13: 978-1-59233-228-1
$24.99/£15.99/$32.50 CAN
Paperback; 360 pages
Available wherever books are sold.

**The sure-to-be controversial guide to what's really healthy and what's not**

In this totally unique nutrition reference guide, acclaimed nutritionist Jonny Bowden debunks old-school food myths, saves the reputations of foods long suffering from bad PR, and provides you with just the facts—what you need to know to make good, health-conscious decisions about which foods you and your family should eat.

You'll also learn the latest research findings and recommendations from around the world—amazing discoveries—about the health benefits of nutrient-packed foods you've loved since you were a kid, and some you've never tried!

• BLUEBERRIES actually help neurons in your brain communicate with one another more effectively, slowing memory loss and making them the ultimate memory food!
• PEANUTS are surprisingly high in antioxidants, ranking them in the same class as powerhouses like strawberries and blueberries!
• Recent studies have revealed that in addition relieving muscle and joint stiffness and menstrual discomfort, CINNAMON may reduce blood sugar and "bad" cholesterol!
• A handful of GOJI BERRIES . . . Hey, what are Goji berries? And why did they make it into this book?

No food provides everything. But real food—whole food with minimal processing—contains a virtual pharmacy of nutrients, phytochemicals, enzymes, vitamins, minerals, antioxidants, anti-inflammatories, and healthful fats, and can keep you alive and thriving into your tenth decade.

Learn how easy it is to find "real" food and discover what a dozen nutrition experts say are their "top 10" best foods on earth.

It's all the best nutrition advice you could possibly find—and it's all right here!

**About the Author**

JONNY BOWDEN, Ph.D., C.N.S., is a nationally known expert on weight loss and nutrition and is a and the author of the best-selling *Living The Low Carb Life: Choosing the Diet That's Right for You from Atkins to Zone*. The host of a popular call-in health show heard nationwide on the Health Radio Network, he frequently appears on television as a health expert and is a popular speaker at media events and seminars. He lives in Sherman Oakes, California. Visit www.jonnybowden.com.